# THE 30 DAY
# ketogenic cleanse

*Reset Your Metabolism with*
160 TASTY WHOLE-FOOD
RECIPES *& a Guided Meal Plan*

## Maria Emmerich

VICTORY BELT PUBLISHING INC.

Las Vegas

First Published in 2016 by Victory Belt Publishing Inc.

ISBN-13: 978-1-628601-16-9

The author is not a licensed practitioner, physician, or medical professional and offers no medical diagnoses, treatments, suggestions, or counseling. The information presented herein has not been evaluated by the U.S. Food and Drug Administration, and it is not intended to diagnose, treat, cure, or prevent any disease. Full medical clearance from a licensed physician should be obtained before beginning or modifying any diet, exercise, or lifestyle program, and physicians should be informed of all nutritional changes.

The author/owner claims no responsibility to any person or entity for any liability, loss, or damage caused or alleged to be caused directly or indirectly as a result of the use, application, or interpretation of the information presented herein.

Front and Back Cover Photography by Hayley Mason and Bill Staley

Interior Design by Yordan Terziev and Boryana Yordanova

Meal Plan by Craig Emmerich

Printed in Canada

TC 0417

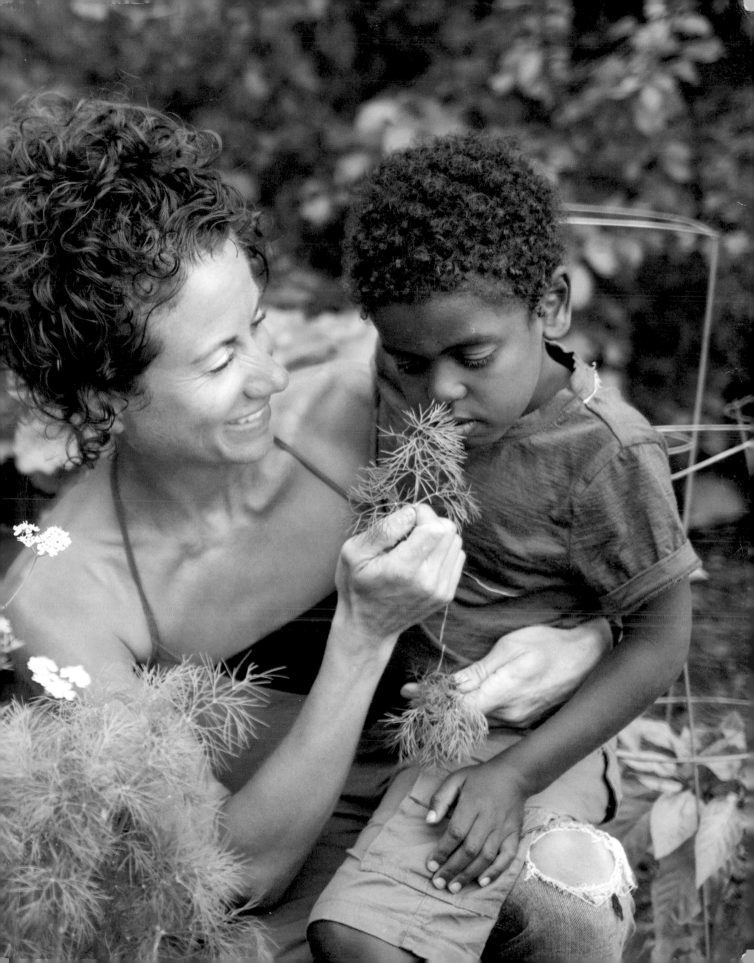

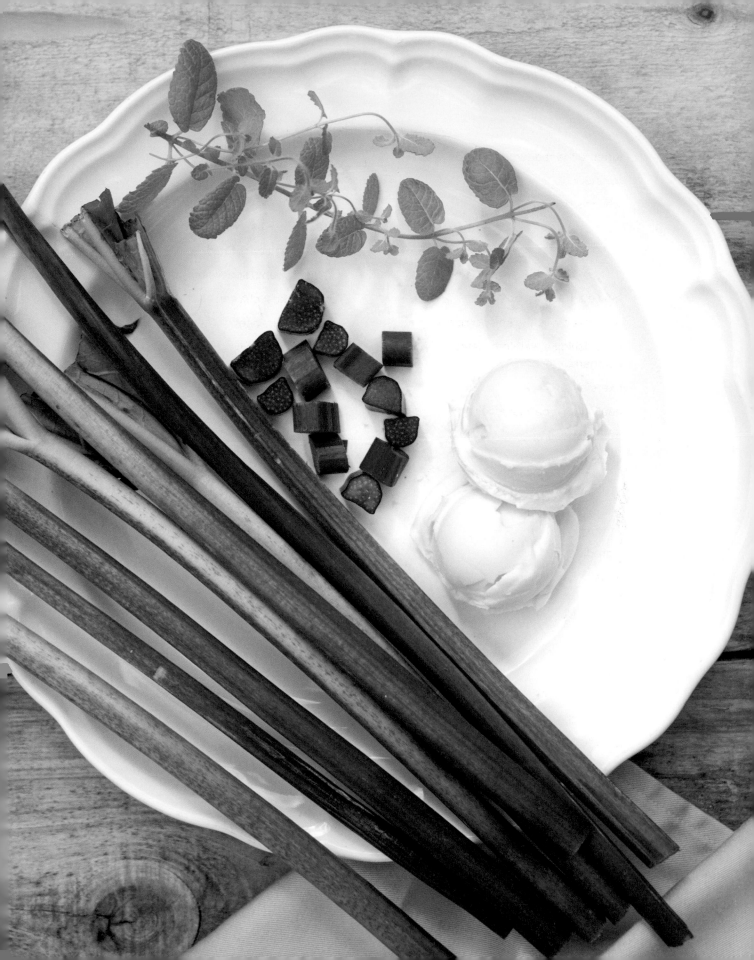

# contents

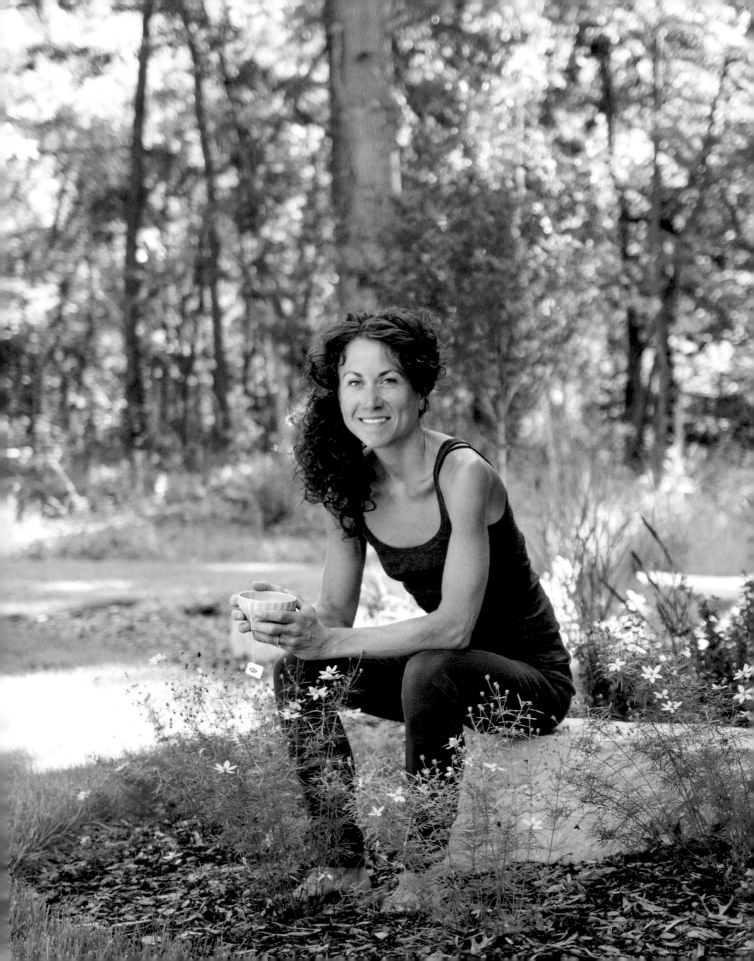

# letter to the reader

You wouldn't put diesel fuel in a gasoline engine and expect it to run, but that's what many of us are guilty of doing to our bodies on a daily basis. We fuel our bodies with processed, packaged foods that evolutionary science has proven make our bodies run much less efficiently. Before I discovered the ketogenic diet, I was guilty of this habit myself.

I struggled with food and my weight throughout adolescence and into adulthood. I was a "fat restrictor" and exercised constantly. Still fat and frustrated after graduating from college, I decided to add a nutritional component to my exercise regimen and put into practice all the information I was about to preach to the world. After decades of being told by marketing geniuses that going fat-free was the way to lose weight, eating real fat was scary for me. But in the first week that I added fat to my diet, I slept deeper and felt calmer and better than I ever had.

Now, years later, I understand the biochemical reasons why restricting fat is not the answer. All my life I'd been taught that good-tasting foods make you fat. After years of antifat brainwashing, it's almost too much to imagine that we can feel totally sated *and* lose weight by eating a low-carb diet that emphasizes fatty foods like avocados, meats, and even sugar-free desserts. But it has been over ten years since I made fat the major component of my diet, and I feel amazing. I traded a lifetime of overexercising and restricting fat for a nutrient-dense, fat-filled diet, *and I lost weight in the process.*

Once I found the secrets to healing my mitochondria—the fat-burning powerhouses of the body's cells—with the right type and amount of food, hydration, sleep, and exercise and overhauled my bathroom cabinet to rid it of unhealthy products, losing weight became an easy goal to achieve. By transitioning to a very-low-carb, high-fat, moderate-protein diet, I resensitized my biochemistry to the hormone insulin and the lesser-known hormone leptin, which turn off severe food cravings.

Best of all, unlike my previous low-fat diets, my new high-fat diet did not leave me feeling deprived, even while I was losing weight! The nutrient-rich, relatively high-fat cooking style that I have developed is what finally helped me achieve peace with food, something I never imagined possible. Even more weight came off than I was originally aiming for.

By beginning to follow the ketogenic lifestyle, you too will learn how to eat to balance your hormones, sleep better, feel better, and lose weight! The tasty keto recipes in this book will keep you satisfied and enhance your physique. You will even get to enjoy desserts; after all, we need to enjoy the sweetness of life.

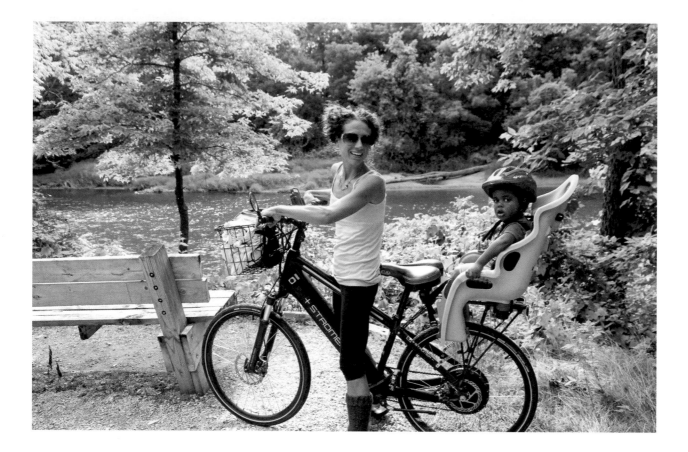

# my story

I am passionate about helping people heal their bodies through food because the medical profession has failed me and my family numerous times.

When I was a young teen, I suffered from severe acne. My mom took me to the doctor, and without even asking about my diet, he put me on a strong dose of antibiotics. I can now pinpoint that event as having a huge negative impact not just on my physical health but on my mental health as well. Sure, I was thrilled that the acne was gone, but my moods started to spiral downward. I'd been a really happy kid, but at about that time I began to experience feelings of sadness.

"Just because of an antibiotic?" you might ask. Yes, those powerful drugs that teens are still being prescribed for acne wreak havoc on the gut, where serotonin (a "feel-good" chemical) is produced. Gut health directly correlates to mood. Sadly, I was on antibiotics for years without realizing the damage they were doing. This long-lasting deterioration of my gut health caused intense sugar cravings, which led to weight gain. The added weight further dampened my happy-go-lucky spirit. If only my doctor had asked me what I was eating and had known that the cereal and skim milk I consumed every morning were the cause of my acne, I wouldn't have experienced all those issues. But, of course, they brought me to where I am today!

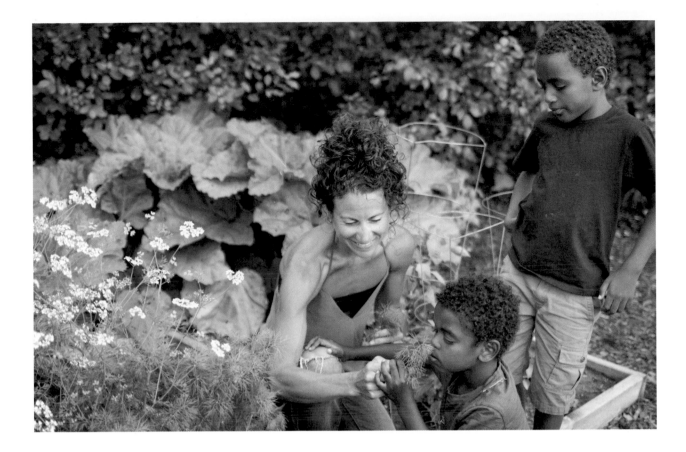

In addition to my own story, there are sadder and more serious stories in my family's medical history that led me to become a passionate advocate of healing through food.

I was a lucky little girl who had two fantastic grandpas. My dad's father, Grandpa Vince, was a kind man who I believe gave me the work ethic that I have today. He owned a plumbing and heating business. He also loved taking me fishing and teaching me how to garden. Grandpa Vince survived his first heart attack at age thirty-two, but with the low-fat diet that his doctors recommended, it is no wonder that his heart never healed. He eventually required heart surgery at age forty-five, and then again at age fifty-two. At that point, the doctors gave him five years to live; he made it nine more years and died at age sixty-one on Thanksgiving morning. My dad was the one who tried to revive him, and he believes his father might still be alive if he hadn't received such bad nutrition advice from his doctors, such as never to eat eggs, butter, or saturated fat. Vince was living off butter substitutes and popcorn.

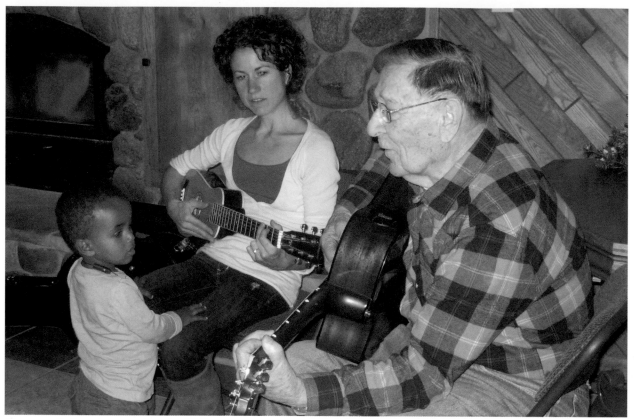
*My grandfather Jerry and me in 2010.*

My mom's father, Grandpa Jerry, was a totally different kind of man. He was a musician, and he always made me laugh. I am honored that I was able to play the guitar alongside him at every holiday get-together until the day he died from type 2 diabetes.

In the spring of 2016, I spoke at a large conference in my hometown, and the dietitian from the local hospital spoke right before me. I had to bite my tongue so I wouldn't say anything offensive in front of the crowd, because she kept saying to cut out all dietary cholesterol and saturated fat. She also said that vegetable oils and canola oil are better replacements.

I realized that my presentation would contradict everything she had just told the audience. When it was my turn to speak, I started by saying, "Did you know that breast milk is made up mainly of cholesterol and saturated fat? Yep! I don't think that this marvel was put in place to harm babies. It was put in place to help babies grow and form healthy hormones. Cholesterol is needed to make hormones, build a healthy immune system, and develop healthy brains!" The audience was very receptive to what I had to say after that. They adored the fact that man-made foods such as canola oil, not natural foods that are high in cholesterol (such as eggs), are the primary cause of inflammation.

The saddest part of this story is that this woman was also the dietitian at the nursing home where my Grandpa Jerry stayed before he passed away. I can only wonder how much her ill-informed nutrition advice must have exacerbated his diabetes.

Through my writing and teaching, I try to reach as many people as I can in the hope that the ketogenic lifestyle will keep others and their families from suffering needlessly like my grandpas and I did.

# why this book?

I used to love Fridays because the arrival of the end of the week meant eating whatever I wanted. During the week I ate "healthy," or what I thought was healthy, but on weekends, I "cheated." I wasn't a terrible cheater—I'd have a few french fries here, a glass of wine there—but I wasn't comfortable in my skin. What I know now is that my "healthy" weekday diet was filled with foods that were turning into sugar in my blood, keeping me constantly craving sugar.

Cheating on a keto diet isn't like cheating on other diets. One of the most common complaints I hear from my clients is that when they slip and consume junk, they feel almost hungover the next day. That sick feeling doesn't happen when you cheat on a low-fat diet filled with whole grains. Sure, you may feel depressed because the number on the scale goes up after a donut bender, but you don't feel physically ill. But the ketogenic diet is so powerful at healing that if you go on a bender after getting your blood sugar within a healthy range, you will totally feel the effects. Conversely, when your diet focuses on calorie restriction for weight loss, your blood sugar is all over the place, so you aren't going to suffer because of the cheating.

This is why keto eating is so powerful! If you go all-in, you'll see amazing results. Only after you go all-in will you start to realize how low your energy level was. I say "all-in" because you can't do an 80/20, or even a 90/10, keto diet. It doesn't work that way. You can't do keto 80 percent and expect 80 percent results; it needs to be 100 percent. But most of my clients don't find that to be a challenge because keto foods naturally leave you feeling satisfied, so you no longer feel the urge to cheat!

Keto isn't a diet for me; it's a lifestyle. I love food and I will always love food, but even more, I love the way I feel when I eat like this! That's why I've spent so much time creating new, delicious recipes for you. I want you to be able to commit 100 percent.

*The 30-Day Ketogenic Cleanse* is not only for those of you who want to try a ketogenic diet for the first time and be assured of success right off the bat, but also for those of you who have tried a ketogenic diet on your own and didn't see the results you were looking for. In this book, you will find recipes designed to have the perfect ketogenic ratios of fat, protein, and carbs to take you into ketosis while keeping your body satisfied. At the end of the thirty days, you'll notice that you no longer want to nap in the afternoon, you have shed belly fat, your skin looks amazing, joint pain is no longer an issue, and you are no longer hungry or thinking about food all day. Sure, it may take you more time to plan and prepare meals, but we all have to prioritize our time. When you feel and look great, you won't regret the time you put into it!

Giving keto a try for thirty days may be your goal. But *my* goal is for you to do the 30-Day Ketogenic Cleanse and feel so fantastic that you no longer want to eat any other way!

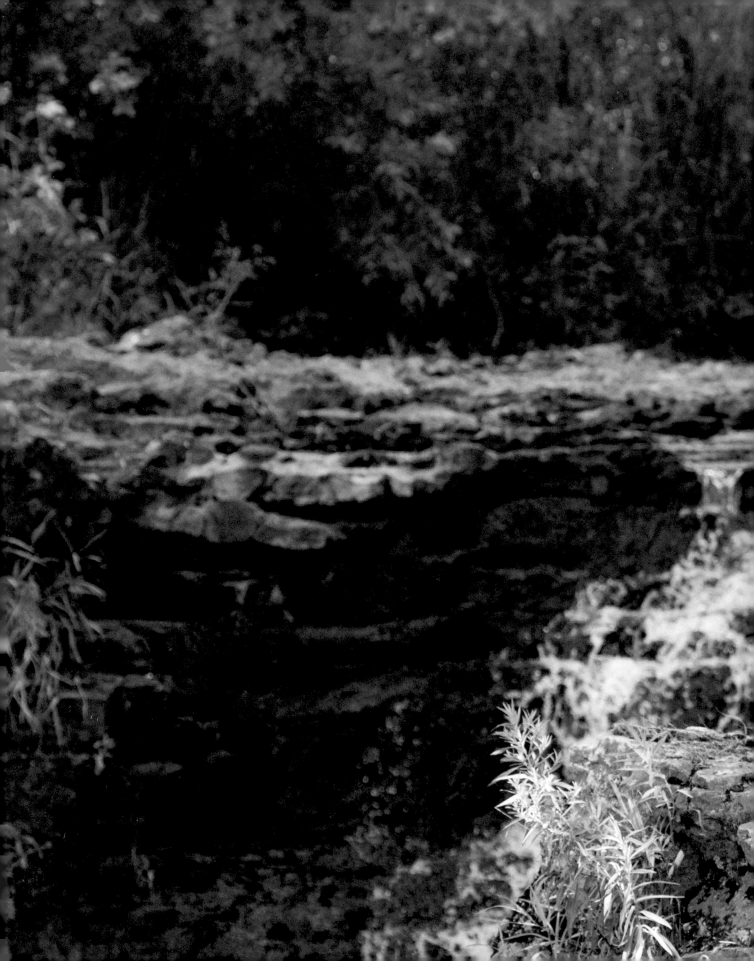

PART 1:

# heal your
# body

# how our bodies work

Before I give you the nuts and bolts of what a well-formulated ketogenic diet is and how to implement it so that you can begin to reap the benefits, I want to explain how our bodies work and why the modern diet has produced such disastrous results. I'll give you an overview first, followed by a more in-depth discussion of the major players in our overall health: cholesterol, carbohydrates, fat, sugar, and insulin. I will take you through how fat is stored, but more importantly, I want to demonstrate how we become at risk for diabetes, heart disease, and other serious maladies.

Let's begin with the causes of weight gain and inflammation.

After you eat carbohydrates and/or protein, your blood sugar (glucose) rises. When you eat too much carbohydrate and/or protein, your body cells quickly become full of glucose, so excess glucose stays in your bloodstream. This glucose acts like tar, clogging arteries, binding with proteins to form damaging AGEs (advanced glycation end products), and causing inflammation. It also causes triglycerides (a type of fat in your blood) to go up, increasing your risk for coronary artery disease.

Almost all carbohydrates, including both starch and sugar, are stored as fat. (Starch is just glucose molecules hooked together in a long chain, which the digestive tract breaks down into glucose—so a sugary diet and a starchy diet are essentially the same thing, despite what you may have heard about "healthy" whole grains.) Any carbohydrates not immediately used by the body are stored in the liver and muscles in the form of glycogen. Once the liver and muscle reach storage capacity for glycogen, glucose has to be converted to fat and stored in the fat cells, which have an unlimited capacity.

Insulin is the hormone that moves glucose into cells. Excess carbohydrates cause an increase of insulin into the bloodstream, and this is not good. Insulin is toxic at high levels, causing cellular damage, cancer, and plaque buildup in the arteries (which is why diabetics are more likely to have heart disease), as well as many other inflammatory issues, such as nerve damage and pain in the extremities. Starch and sugar also destroy nerve tissue, causing tingling and retinopathy, which in turn cause glaucoma and loss of eyesight. Even worse, eventually, consistently high insulin levels cause cells to stop responding to insulin at all, like a kid tuning out her mother's shouts. This is insulin resistance, and it can lead to type 2 diabetes and is associated with heart disease, cancer, Alzheimer's, and more.

I have still more bad news: cells become so damaged after a lifetime of cereal and skim milk for breakfast that not only does insulin resistance block glucose from entering cells, but AGEs form a crust over cells that blocks amino acids from entering. Amino acids are the building blocks of protein, and therefore create muscle. So now you can't even maintain your muscles! Plus, your muscles become cannibals. Because insulin resistance makes the body thinks there is not enough stored glucose in the cells, it sends signals to start consuming valuable muscle to make more glucose. The results: you lose muscle and get fatter. Instead of feeling energetic after you eat, you feel tired and crave more carbohydrates. Since you now have less muscle, exercise becomes too darn difficult, and the sad cycle continues.

Now comes even more bad news: because of everything your body has been through, thyroid disorders can occur. When the liver becomes insulin resistant, it can't convert the thyroid hormone T4 into T3, so you may get those unexplained thyroid problems that lower energy and slow metabolism.

If you don't want any of this to happen to you, there is good news! Combining a well-formulated ketogenic diet (see pages 25 to 35) with the right amount and type of exercise (described on pages 36 to 45) can break this vicious cycle and get you on your way to better health.

# on cholesterol

Contrary to popular belief, cholesterol is not a bad guy; in fact, it is vital to every cell in the human body. You cannot live without it! Cholesterol is one of the body's repair substances, and it is essential for hormone function, particularly during stressful times. Its elevated presence in your system tells you that your body is trying to heal something, such as inflammation.

I like to refer to cholesterol as the firefighter in the body: like a firefighter putting out a fire, cholesterol goes to work putting out inflammation. When you eliminate the firefighter (cholesterol), does the fire (inflammation) stop burning? No, it doesn't. Using statin drugs to reduce cholesterol instead of focusing on eliminating the foods causing the inflammation, such as sugars and carbs, is the wrong answer; it only causes muscles to deteriorate, which slows your metabolism.

Cholesterol is so important to the human body that nature has devised a backup plan in the event that your diet falls short of delivering sufficient cholesterol: your liver makes cholesterol. In its natural, unstressed state, the liver makes 75 percent of the cholesterol that the body needs. The rest you have to eat in the form of meat, shellfish, and eggs—my favorite food groups!

However, if you deprive your body of dietary cholesterol, your liver overproduces cholesterol to make up the difference and stock up. This overdrive state doesn't shut off until you start eating cholesterol again. So a low-fat, high-carbohydrate diet can actually lead to heart disease!

Here's why: Coronary artery disease occurs when an LDL cholesterol particle, which is small and dense, gets lodged in a lesion in an artery wall. (Lesions are caused by inflammation—which in turn is caused by sugar and carbs) The particle then releases its cholesterol into the artery wall, which triggers the formation of plaque. So if you have very low inflammation and therefore no arterial lesions for the LDL particle to get stuck in, your cholesterol numbers aren't really relevant.

If you want to know your risk for heart disease, get a calcium score (CAC test). It tells you how much calcium (or plaque) buildup is in the arteries around your heart. It is quick and cheap, and a score above 100 means the risk of heart disease is 800 percent greater than a score of 0. Scores over 1,000 have a 1,600 percent increased risk. In fact, CAC score is highly correlated to all causes of mortality. So it is really a great test to assess your health.

# on carbohydrates

One common question or complaint I hear from clients is "Why can't I eat 'normal'?" Sure, there are people who can eat potatoes, rice, and pasta and not be overweight, but this doesn't mean they are healthy. I've had a handful of female clients who weighed around 115 pounds but had very high blood sugar and had to be put on insulin. It's not just diabetics and people who want to lose weight who should limit their intake of carbohydrates; everyone should. We are all, in an evolutionary sense, predisposed to becoming diabetic as a result of ingesting too many carbohydrates. After you eat excess carbohydrates, your blood sugar increases and stays elevated because it can't get into the cells fast enough. This harmful level of blood sugar ends up clogging arteries and causing inflammation.

But diabetes isn't the only risk from eating too many carbohydrates: heart disease and obesity are additional likely outcomes. We're relentlessly told that carbs are nutritional good guys, so we should eat large amounts of them. Following these words of "wisdom," Americans are gobbling cereal, bread, and pasta, trying desperately to make carbohydrates 75 to 85 percent of total calories, as advocated by the medical establishment. However, overeating carb-laden foods inhibits the body's ability to utilize fat for energy (which is why I find it interesting that someone going to the gym to "burn fat" will consume a fruity yogurt or granola bar before working out). It is a terrible paradox: people are eating less fat and getting fatter!

Sadly, many people don't really know what a carbohydrate is. Most people will say that carbohydrates are sweets and pasta. They often think of vegetables and fruits as foods that they can eat in unlimited amounts without gaining weight. This may come as a surprise, but sweets, pasta, vegetables, and fruits are all carbohydrates. Carbohydrates are merely simple sugars linked together in long chains. Any carbohydrates not immediately used by the body are stored in the form of glycogen. The body has two storage sites for glycogen: the muscles and the liver. Glycogen stored in the muscles is inaccessible to the brain. Only the glycogen stored in the liver can be sent back to the bloodstream to maintain adequate blood sugar levels for proper brain function. The liver's capacity to store glycogen is very limited and can easily be depleted within ten to twelve hours. So the liver's glycogen reserves must be continually maintained.

What happens when you eat too many carbohydrates? The body's total storage capacity for glycogen is quite limited. The average person can store 300 to 400 grams in the muscles and only 60 to 90 grams in the liver.

Once the storage space for glycogen is filled, excess carbohydrates have to be converted to fat and stored. So even though carbs are fat-free, excess carbohydrates end up as body fat! But that's not the worst part. Any meal or snack that is high in carbs will trigger a rapid rise in blood glucose. In response, the pancreas secretes the hormone

## type 3 diabetes–aka alzheimer's!

*Do you know anyone suffering from Alzheimer's or dementia? Sadly, I do. My Grandma Rosemary has severe Alzheimer's, and as I write this book, she doesn't know who I am (or who anyone is, really). I tried to tell my parents that Alzheimer's is sometimes referred to as type 3 diabetes, but that is a hard concept for them and many others to wrap their heads around.*

*The brain prefers to use ketones, created from burning fat, for energy, rather than glucose. In Alzheimer's patients, the brain can no longer convert glucose for energy. Ketosis is very healthy for these patients because ketones are a source of energy that their brains can utilize!*

## overconsumption of carbohydrates leads to:

 **Brain fog:** Are you sending your kids off to school on a bowl of cereal with skim milk? Not a good idea. If you want your kids to focus well in class, the ketogenic diet is great for mental abilities.

 **Low blood sugar:** What goes up must come down. If you feel "hangry" or dizzy or crave sweets, those are key signs of low blood sugar.

 **Lack of energy:** Instead of feeling energetic after you eat, you are tired and you crave more carbohydrates, and since you have less muscle, exercise is getting too darn difficult . . . and the sad cycle continues.

 **Gut damage:** Carbohydrates cause inflammation of the gut. A scary fact is that only 8 percent of celiacs truly heal because they consume gluten-free grains, which are often higher in carbs than gluten-containing grains.

 **Increased levels of A1c:** A1c (or HbA1c or glycated hemoglobin) is a test that provides information about a person's average blood glucose levels over the last three months. Red blood cells are constantly forming and dying, but on average, they live for about three months. So this test gives a good average of how glycated your red blood cells are over their lifetime (three-month average). It is a great test for determining many factors of health and has strong correlation to many health problems (higher equals more heart disease, cancer, Alzheimer's, etc.). You want your A1c to be 5.4 or less (ideally 5.0 or less).

 **Increased blood pressure:** Doctors now recognize that most people with hypertension have too much insulin and are insulin resistant. There is often a direct relationship between the level of insulin and blood pressure: as insulin levels increase, so does blood pressure.

 **Depression:** Carbohydrates are a natural downer; it is not uncommon to see depressed persons with insulin resistance. Carbs change brain chemistry. They produce a depressed or tired feeling. On the flip side, protein is a brain stimulant that picks you up mentally.

 **Alcoholism:** Insulin resistance is also prevalent in people addicted to alcohol, caffeine, cigarettes, or other drugs. Often, alcohol is the secondary problem, with insulin resistance being the primary one. Alcohol becomes sugar in our bodies. This is why recovering alcoholics often overeat sweets, which causes a relapse. They never kicked the true addiction: sugar!

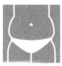 **Increased fat storage and weight gain.**

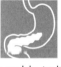 **Diabetes:** Over time, after years of high-carbohydrate meals, your body becomes unable to handle the amount of sugar produced in the blood and your cells become resistant to the effects of insulin.

 **Alzheimer's disease:** In patients with Alzheimer's (aka type 3 diabetes), the brain has become insulin resistant and can't process glucose for energy.

insulin into the bloodstream. Insulin then lowers the level of blood glucose. The problem is that insulin is mainly a storage hormone; it works to put aside excess carbohydrate calories in the form of fat in case of a future food shortage. The insulin that's stimulated by too many carbs assertively promotes the accumulation of body fat.

To recap, when you eat too much carbohydrate, insulin sends a message to your body that states, "Store this as fat." It also tells your body not to release any stored fat, since there's plenty of glucose available for fuel. When this happens, you can't use your own body fat for energy. So the excess carbs in your diet not only make you fat, they also make sure you stay fat.

After you eat carbohydrates, your pancreas releases insulin and your blood sugar increases. Insulin makes sure that your cells receive some blood sugar, which is necessary for life, and increases glycogen storage. But it also tells your body to use more carbohydrate and less fat for fuel. Insulin also converts almost half of your carb intake to fat for storage in case of an energy emergency. If you want to burn fat for energy, the insulin response must be decreased. Eating refined sugars releases a lot of insulin, allowing less stored fat to be burned.

A very-low-carbohydrate diet stimulates the burning of fat for fuel, which is why people lose weight on a keto diet. Cutting out carbs and keeping protein moderate also reduces insulin levels. A normal blood glucose level is the equivalent of 1 teaspoon of sugar. Many Americans consume over 63 teaspoons a day! If you can conquer abnormal blood sugar, you will reduce the problems associated with high insulin levels, such as insulin resistance, high blood pressure, metabolic syndrome, weight gain, and sleeplessness.

# on fat

In the fat-free propaganda of the 1980s, all dietary fats became linked to elevated cholesterol levels, cardiovascular problems, and obesity. Evidence recently came out that the sugar industry deliberately funded studies that looked for a link between fat and heart disease in order to take the focus off of sugar.

We reacted by radically changing our eating habits and removing as much fat from our diets as possible. With everyone cutting the fat, you'd think we'd all be skinny-minnies by now, but the opposite has happened! Limiting our intake of fat increases our desire for sugary processed foods; when fat is removed from foods, it is usually replaced with sugar.

Even the most health-conscious foodies went overboard with fat-free carbohydrates, and many became overweight in the process. The problem was that refined carbs, such as bagels, as well as complex carbs, such as whole-grain bread, were viewed as "free" foods. These foods produce a quick spike in blood sugar levels, which raises insulin, our fat-storing hormone. In fact, corn has a higher glycemic index than most candy bars! Too much insulin blocks the body's ability to burn stored fat for energy and creates a rapid fall in blood sugar, resulting in more hunger, and then we grab more unfulfilling calories. Here's something to think about: conventionally raised cows, which consume only corn, fatten up in just six months, compared to the two years required for grass-fed cows. Here's another interesting fact: sumo wrestlers eat fat-free diets centered around rice and sugar!

The food industry is responsible for a detrimental lie—that processed and imitation food is just as good as real food. Just because a food takes away our hunger pangs doesn't mean that it nourishes our bodies properly. Billions of dollars are made from the sale of that "food." But to make that money, companies have to spin things so that people don't know enough to question their behavior. Advertising geniuses know that if you keep on repeating a lie, a lot of people end up believing it.

The bottom line is that fat does not make you fat. Your body's response to excess carbohydrates is what makes you gain weight. The body has a limited capacity to store excess carbs, but it can easily convert those excess carbs into excess body fat.

# on sugar

Sugar is so gratifying. That first bite of a heavenly sweet can calm us down and give us energy at the same time. It's like magic, with the power to flip our mood 180 degrees. That's the upside. The downside is that the more you eat sweets, the more you want them. Excess sugar causes a hormonal imbalance that leads to carbohydrate cravings and weight gain, literally turning your body into a fat-making, fat-storing machine. However, I've got good news: you are in charge, and you can get off the fast track to diabetes, naturally. Overconsumption of fat-free foods and a sedentary life can lead to insulin resistance, which is a physical imbalance that makes the body respond abnormally to carbohydrate-rich foods and causes weight gain.

Sugars are the simplest forms of carbohydrate. They can be natural, such as lactose (milk sugar) and fructose (fruit sugar), or refined, such as sucrose (table sugar). When digested, they are immediately absorbed into the bloodstream, causing an increase in the hormone insulin. Insulin clears sugar and fat from the blood to be stored in the tissues for future use. This causes weight gain.

No matter where the carbohydrate comes from, 4 grams of carbohydrate equals 1 teaspoon of sugar in the body. Let me say that again: 4 grams of carbohydrate equals 1 teaspoon of sugar. So a small Blizzard has 530 calories and 83 grams of carbohydrate, which equals 21 teaspoons of sugar. A 9-ounce bag of potato chips equals 32 teaspoons of sugar. Add a soda, and that's another 16 teaspoons of sugar.

In 1890, the average person consumed 2 teaspoons of sugar per day. Today, the average person consumes 56 teaspoons, mostly in the form of refined white sugar. Wow! This added sugar is high in calories and devoid of nutrients. Extra sugar is added to prepackaged foods. A piece of bread now contains refined sugar. Chocolate cake and other sweet delights can contain as much as 25 teaspoons of refined sugar, and that doesn't include the refined flour turning into sugar in the bloodstream! It's not just white sugar that needs to be consumed in moderation; brown sugar, powdered sugar, honey, and maple syrup are all sources of refined sugar. Eating too much sugar is part of an addictive cycle. When you eat sugar, it's digested and burned quickly, and it causes peaks and valleys in your energy level that leave you craving more.

## hospital food nightmare

*My father-in-law had a mild stroke and had to stay in the hospital for 24 hours. He is fine now, and we are thankful for that. My brother-in-law was there with him, and he sent me a photo of the breakfast they offered: cereal, skim milk, juice, and toast.*

*I replied, "What are they trying to do, induce a heart attack!?" It drives me crazy that hospitals feed patients food that makes them sicker. It's even worse when they feed diabetic patients lots of low-fat, high-sugar, and high-carb foods and then have to give them huge doses of insulin as a result.*

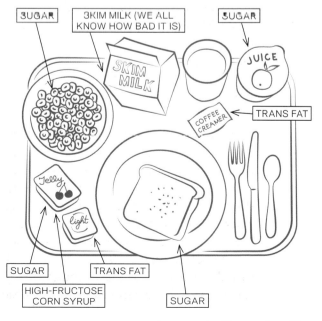

It is a dangerous situation when uninformed medical professionals recommend a high-complex-carbohydrate, low-saturated-fat diet. A high-complex-carbohydrate diet is nothing more than a high-sugar diet.

The body's primary way of getting rid of sugar, because high levels are toxic, is to burn it with exercise. The sugar your body can't burn is stored as glycogen. But we can hold only so much glycogen, so when our reserves are full, sugar is stored as fat. Insulin also prevents you from burning fat for fuel. If you eat sugar, your body will burn that sugar first instead of burning fat.

The more sugar you eat, the more you crave it. If you start your day with cereal and skim milk, you aren't going to be able to walk by the candy jar at 2 p.m. without grabbing a piece! Check out this breakfast comparison:

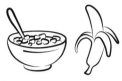 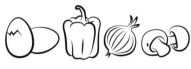 

**Option 1**

1 cup Smart Start cereal,
1 cup skim milk, and a banana

| calories | carbs | fiber |
| --- | --- | --- |
| 472 | 105g | 4g |

= 26¼ teaspoons of
sugar in blood

**Option 2**

2 eggs with 2 cups of mushrooms,
bell peppers, and onions

| calories | carbs | fiber |
| --- | --- | --- |
| 190 | 9g | 3g |

= 2¼ teaspoons of
sugar in blood

**Option 3**

Homemade donut made
with coconut flour

| calories | carbs | fiber |
| --- | --- | --- |
| 217 | 7.4g | 4.6g |

< 2 teaspoons of
sugar in blood

# on insulin

Insulin has a very important job in the body: it responds to elevated blood sugar. First it uses sugar for energy. Then it sends what's left over to be stored in the muscles and liver as glycogen.

The problem is that most people have room to store only about 500 grams of glycogen at any given time. After these storage areas fill up, insulin pushes the leftover glycogen into fat cells.

Insulin works hard at helping your body preserve energy from food, and it does so in three ways:

1. It tells your body to eat, particularly sugar or carbohydrates. If you follow those cravings, it rewards you with a feeling of extreme gratification.

2. It escorts the energy from these foods, which is now blood sugar, to wherever in the body it is needed, and tells the liver to turn any extra into triglycerides (blood fat) to be stored in the fat cells.

3. It orders your body to keep food energy locked inside the fat cells, not burn it for energy, in case of famine.

Under ideal conditions, this regulation mechanism works perfectly. When you're a kid and you eat candy, your blood sugar increases and your pancreas releases a little insulin, which drives your blood sugar back down rapidly. The pancreas releases only a small amount of insulin, because a child's cells are very sensitive to this hormone. We may think that it's fine for kids to enjoy the simple pleasures of junk food, but over time they can, just like adults, lose their sensitivity to insulin, a condition known as insulin resistance.

This begins a cruel cycle of needing more insulin to keep the system going. As the body releases more insulin in an attempt to push through the resistance and force the precious blood sugar to the muscles and liver, the extra insulin leads to carbohydrate cravings. In an attempt to calm our desire for carb-filled foods, even more insulin is released, and to protect itself from too much insulin, the body becomes even more insulin resistant. Eventually, the fat cells will shut down while the insulin gets stuck in the bloodstream, which leads to type 2 diabetes. As we overconsume refined carbs and sugar over the years, our bodies require higher levels of insulin to metabolize food appropriately and keep our blood sugar in the normal range.

High insulin levels also suppress two important hormones: growth hormone and glucagon. Growth hormone is used for developing muscle and building new muscle mass. Glucagon promotes the burning of fat and sugar. Eating a high-carbohydrate meal also stimulates hunger. As blood sugar increases, insulin rises, causing an immediate drop in blood sugar. This results in hunger, often only a couple of hours after the meal. Cravings, usually for sweets, are frequently part of this cycle, leading you to snack on more carbohydrates. Not eating makes you feel ravenous, shaky, moody, and ready to crash. This cycle causes you to hang onto that extra stored fat and decreases your energy.

Most people do not know that the thyroid hormone T4 is converted into activated T3 in the liver, not in the thyroid. So when the liver gets tired and toxified from all the excess carbohydrates, unexplained thyroid issues can start to crop up, further causing lethargy, a sluggish metabolism, and low moods.

Does this sound like you? My best suggestion for utilizing more fat is to moderate the insulin response by limiting your intake of refined sugars and focus on carbohydrates coming from nonstarchy vegetables, leafy greens, and herbs. I have eliminated all grains from my diet—that means no pasta, rice, oatmeal, cereal, or any of those government-recommended "healthy whole grains"—and have never felt better.

Insulin responses are different in everybody, but decreasing carbohydrates and increasing fats will help bring your body back into balance. By moderating your carb intake, you can burn more fat, which is an optimal fuel source.

# what exactly is the ketogenic diet?

For hundreds of thousands of years, people ate mostly meat and vegetables—the so-called caveman diet. With the onset of modern civilization and the development of agriculture, the human body was asked to digest and metabolize larger amounts of starches and refined sugars. But our bodies are unable to utilize a large amount of carbohydrates. Therefore, symptoms develop. The good news is that the ketogenic diet offers a solution—a practical and healthy method for reversing the modern plague of poor health and obesity.

## a quick overview

The ketogenic diet is a high-fat, moderate-protein, low-carb style of eating that has powerful health benefits. Originally developed in the early 1920s to treat epileptic seizures, the diet fell out of favor in the medical establishment once antiseizure medications became available. More than seventy years later, it was rediscovered as an effective alternative to pharmaceuticals. Since then, it has grown in popularity and has received increasing media attention for the variety of maladies that it treats.

The ketogenic diet is too often viewed as simply a sugar-elimination diet. But really, it is a low-carb diet, and that is an important distinction. The keto diet eliminates or drastically reduces all the foods that turn into sugar in the body, which include carbohydrates and even protein, as well as refined and natural sugars. After all, complex carbohydrates (including "healthy" whole grains and root vegetables) are just glucose molecules hooked together in a long chain. The digestive tract breaks it down into glucose . . . also known as sugar!

So often people focus on calorie reduction for weight loss because they are told that metabolism comes down to calories in, calories out. But our bodies are much more complex than that. It's hard to lose weight simply by restricting calories. Eating less and losing excess body fat do not necessarily go hand in hand. A low-calorie, high-carbohydrate diet sets off a series of biochemical signals in your body that take you out of balance, making it more difficult to access stored body fat for energy. As a result, you reach a weight-loss plateau beyond which you simply can't lose any more weight. Furthermore, diets based on limiting calories usually fail because people on these restrictive diets get tired of feeling hungry and deprived. Unsatisfied, they go off their diets, put the weight back on, and then feel like failures for not having enough willpower or discipline to stay on the diet.

In reality, though, successful weight loss has little to do with discipline. It's more about focusing on what to eat than how much. On a ketogenic diet, you can eat enough food to feel satisfied and still lose body fat, without obsessively counting calories or fat grams.

# how the ketogenic diet works in the body

There are two available sources of fuel for the human body: sugar (glucose) and fat. Ketones are produced when the body burns fat, and these are what fuel cells. The goal of the ketogenic diet is to get the body to metabolize fat rather than sugar. Being a fat burner is called being keto-adapted, and it is the preferred metabolic state of the human body. It usually takes two to four weeks on a ketogenic diet for a person to reach this state.

Too many people remain slaves to the belief that glucose is the only source of fuel. As a result, they live in fear of running low on glucose. But fat is the ideal energy source and has been for most of human evolution. That's why we have fat on our bodies! We actually need only minimal glucose, most or all of which the liver can supply as needed on a daily basis.

The sad fact that carbohydrates and sugar are so cheap and readily available doesn't mean that we should depend on them as a primary fuel source. It is this blind allegiance to the "carb paradigm" that has driven so many people to experience the vast array of metabolic problems that threaten to overwhelm our health-care system.

## health benefits of the ketogenic diet

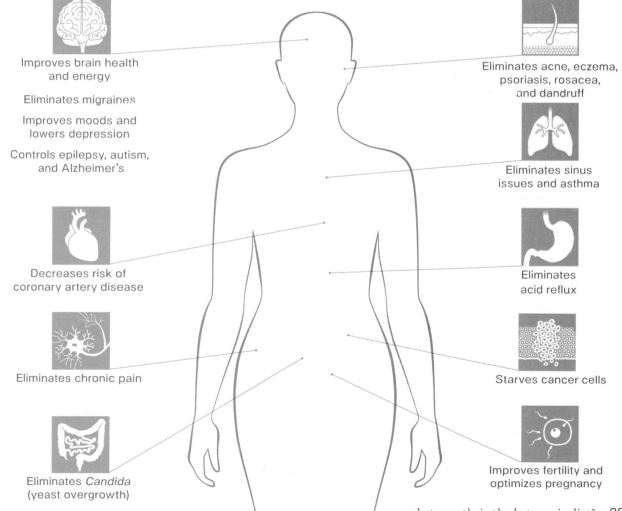

Improves brain health and energy

Eliminates migraines

Improves moods and lowers depression

Controls epilepsy, autism, and Alzheimer's

Decreases risk of coronary artery disease

Eliminates chronic pain

Eliminates *Candida* (yeast overgrowth)

Eliminates acne, eczema, psoriasis, rosacea, and dandruff

Eliminates sinus issues and asthma

Eliminates acid reflux

Starves cancer cells

Improves fertility and optimizes pregnancy

# what it means to be a sugar burner

In order to understand what it means to be keto-adapted, it is useful to examine what it means to be a sugar burner.

A sugar burner can't easily access stored fat for energy. That means a sugar burner's muscles can't oxidize (or break down) fat. I know, the runner's magazine you are reading says that your body burns glucose for energy, which is why marathoners eat a huge pasta dinner the night before a race and then have oatmeal for breakfast. I did that for years and ran some pretty good marathons, but I was overweight and had a lot of joint pain. I essentially wanted to be hooked up to a glucose IV drip because I was always hungry or "hangry" (hungry + angry). When I went two, three, or four hours without food, or even—dare I say it—skipped a meal, the people around me needed to watch out! I was the definition of a suffering sugar burner.

The human body evolved to depend on the oxidation of fat for the majority of its energy needs. In a keto-adapted body, fat tissue releases a bunch of fatty acids four to six hours after eating and during fasting, because the muscles are able to use them for fuel. But because I kept eating bananas, granola bars, and other carbs, my cells were burning sugar, not fat. Once my blood sugar was used up, hunger would set in again, and I would reach for yet another banana.

If you are a sugar burner, you cannot process the fat you eat for energy. The detrimental side effect is that more fat—from carbs, remember, not dietary fat—is stored than burned. Unfortunately, sugar burners end up gaining a lot of body fat. A low ratio of fat-to-carbohydrate oxidation is a solid predictor of future weight gain.

A sugar burner relies on a short-lived source of fuel for energy. You can store only about 50 to 90 grams of glycogen, the storage form of glucose, in your liver for energy conversion, which really isn't a lot. You can also store glycogen in your muscles, a process that varies quite a bit from person to person (athletes usually have larger storage sites if they train with carbohydrates). You can't store very much glycogen, however, unless you count the grams of sugar in the snacks in your pockets. For example, a very lean man with 12 percent body fat who weighs 160 pounds has over 19 pounds of fat to burn for oxidation, but the glycogen in his muscles and liver is limited to about 500 grams. Would you rather have 19 pounds (8,618 grams) of energy or 500 grams of energy? I choose the longer-lasting energy source.

Another major issue with the limited storage room for glycogen in our bodies is that while you're asleep, you can't eat to replenish this glycogen. So when sugar burners sleep, their bodies runs out of glucose and starts breaking down protein—muscle and bone—to make more glucose. Over time, this causes less lean mass and contributes to issues like osteoporosis.

# establishing a well-formulated ketogenic diet

Fat, protein, and carbohydrate are the three macronutrients that human beings need for growth and health. A well-formulated ketogenic diet can be thought of as a distribution of these three macronutrients in that order, from high to low. Here is a good breakdown for most people to follow:

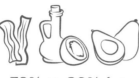 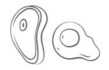 

70% to 80% fat          10% to 20% protein          5% carbs

These percentages are approximate because each person is different. Exactly how much of each macronutrient you can consume and become (or remain) keto-adapted is best pinpointed through testing; see pages 28 to 29.

Broadly speaking, though, a well-formulated ketogenic diet focuses on three steps:

 1. Eliminate sugar and high-carbohydrate foods.

2. Moderate consumption of protein; focus on fatty rather than lean protein.

 3. Include plenty of healthy fats.

For a discussion of maintaining a healthy balance of micronutrients (vitamins and minerals) while eating a keto diet, see pages 30 to 32.

## step 1: eliminate sugar and high-carbohydrate foods

By now you understand that sugar causes inflammation, and even complex carbohydrates are just glucose molecules hooked together in a long chain that your digestive system breaks down into glucose—sugar. So step 1 of your ketogenic cleanse is to cut out sugar and carbohydrates.

To get your body to start burning fat, focus on making carbs only 5 percent of your total food intake. For diabetics, this level may need to be lowered even further to counteract insulin resistance (see page 21). A good carb intake is about 30 grams per day or less; for a type 1 diabetic, it should be lower still, about 20 grams per day or less.

Even the carbohydrates in vegetables are broken down into sugar in your body, so if you want to enter ketosis, limiting starchy vegetables—along with refined sugars and grains, of course—is essential.

## step 2: limit consumption of protein and focus on fatty rather than lean protein

Our Paleolithic-era ancestors got about 80 percent of their calories from fat and only about 20 percent from protein. During prolonged periods of starvation or extended physical exertion, the body burns fat to produce ketones, the preferred energy source for highly active tissues, like those found in the heart and muscles.

Clients ask me all the time, "How much protein is too much?" Well, everyone has a different tolerance, just like with carbohydrates. Testing for ketones (see pages 28 to 29) will help you determine your own levels. The typical range is 50 to 75 grams per day, but I work with some extreme diabetics who can't eat more than 60 grams of protein a day (about 20 grams at each meal) or they will be kicked out of ketosis.

Don't eat lean protein! Choose chicken thighs instead of breasts, pork belly instead of pork chops. Our bodies do not tolerate it well. Eating only lean protein causes an excess intake of nitrogen, which can lead to hyperammonemia, a buildup of ammonia in the bloodstream that is toxic to the brain. A diet that is high in healthy fats, however, is sustainable for a lifetime. Many traditional societies survived on a diet made up solely of animal products, which are naturally high in fat.

### how much protein do we need?

*To answer this question, I think it's important to consider breast-fed babies. I think we all would agree that breast milk is the best food for a growing baby. Since breast milk is 60 percent fat, babies are in a ketogenic state. I think we also would agree that because they are growing so rapidly, babies have the highest protein requirement per kilogram of body weight. So how much protein does a baby get from breast milk? It comes out to about 1 gram of protein per kilogram of body weight per day. This is nature's protein intake at its highest time of need. Fully grown adults need even less.*

*A ketogenic diet is great for preserving muscle mass. So this is one of those situations in which the traditional thinking based on the Standard American Diet doesn't apply. You require less protein when in nutritional ketosis.*

## step 3: eat plenty of healthy fats

If you cut out sugar and carbohydrates and limit protein, what's left? The f-word—yep, fat. It's key macronutrient that has been wrongfully demonized for decades. When you are keto-adapted, healthy fat, and lots of it, is your fuel source. Fat is also what keeps you feeling full and satisfied and keeps cravings at bay. Once you become keto-adapted, you'll feel full with fewer calories; don't force extra fat into your diet to try to raise ketone levels—you will burn your own fat to make ketones and you'll lose weight faster.

In order to become keto-adapted, you need to turn up your healthy fat intake to push yourself over the adaptation divide as quickly as possible. The amount of fat you need to eat will depend on your caloric needs. To lose weight, you want to consume fewer calories than you burn. Most clients I work with find that 1,000 to 1,400 calories is a good target range once they're keto-adapted. The following is a good equation to determine the amount of fat in grams you need to consume per day:

(calories x 0.8) / 9 = grams of fat per day

So if you are shooting for 1,400 calories a day with 80 percent of those calories coming from fat, then you get:

$$(1400 \times 0.8) / 9 = 124 \text{ g of fat per day}$$

If you are shooting for 70 percent of calories from fat, then adjust the equation accordingly:

$$(calories \times 0.7) / 9 = \text{grams of fat per day}$$

When it comes to which fats and oils to consume, the higher the amount of saturated fatty acids (SFAs) they contain, the better. Saturated fats like MCT oil, coconut oil, tallow, and lard are your best choices: they are stable, anti-inflammatory, and less prone to oxidation, which can cause inflammation. Grass-fed and organic sources are best if you can get them.

MCT stands for "medium-chain triglycerides," which are chains of fatty acids. Consuming fats with an abundance of MCTs is particularly beneficial because, unlike long-chain triglycerides, MCTs are used quickly by the body and not stored in the fat cells. A bonus: any MCTs not immediately utilized are converted to ketones, which can be helpful when becoming keto-adapted. Until the body is efficient at generating ketones from body fat, ketones from MCT oil can help feed the brain, which only uses ketones or glucose. MCTs are found naturally in coconut oil and palm oil, as well as butter and ghee. MCT oil is extracted from coconut oil or palm oil and contains a higher amount of MCTs. Unlike coconut oil, MCT oil stays liquid even when refrigerated.

Avoid polyunsaturated fatty acids (PUFAs), which are unstable. PUFAs are found in products like margarine, vegetable oil, and vegetable shortening—all products that you should steer clear of at all times!

Trans fats also should be avoided. They come from adding hydrogen to unsaturated fats (partially hydrogenating them). The food industry uses trans fats because they are less expensive and extend the shelf life of foods. But trans fats are very detrimental to health.

In a study that focused on heart health and fats, scientists studied two groups: one consumed trans fats and the other saturated fats. Not only did saturated fats not cause heart disease, but the trans-fat group gained three times more weight, even though they ate the same number of calories! And that extra weight was visceral fat, the estrogen-dominant fat stored in the abdominal area that puts people at high risk for cancer and cardiovascular disease.

Not all fats are equal. You need to be a detective when it comes to feeding your family! If you buy prepared foods, check the labels for trans fats or partially hydrogenated oils, which are a source of trans fats. But the best way to avoid trans fats and other unhealthy fats is to eat meals that you've made yourself. I encourage my clients to create the foods they crave at home; I've even made chili cheese fries! If you make the dish at home, you are less likely to put on weight, even if it has the same number of calories as a commercially prepared version.

## trans fats and aging

*We all want to stay youthful, which is why there is a multibillion-dollar industry focused on making people look younger. Food is something we often ignore when it comes to looking youthful, but in many ways, trans fats are a huge age accelerator, from the inside out.*

*One way that trans fats age cells is by inhibiting neurons' ability to communicate. Neurons, or nerve cells, are coated in a fatty substance called myelin, which allows them to send impulses throughout the body. Trans fats become incorporated into myelin and affect neurons' ability to send those impulses.*

*Trans fats are also very inflammatory, which leads to aging. We often focus on cutting out sugar and starch in a ketogenic diet in an effort to reduce inflammation, but if you are eating foods filled with trans fats, they too are causing long-lasting inflammation!*

# fine-tuning your ratio of macronutrients

Often my clients think that they didn't quite get to 70 to 80 percent fat, so they start adding in bulletproof coffee (a blended mixture of coffee, butter, and MCT oil) or eating an extra tablespoon of coconut oil just to correct the ratio. I do not recommend this practice if you are eating keto for weight loss. Your body is a marvel and can create ketones from the stored fat in your body.

As long as your carb intake is right (30 grams or less per day, ideally 20 grams or less) and your protein intake is moderate (50 to 75 grams a day for most people), then you will achieve ketosis, a state in which your body can use dietary fat and body fat equally well. If there isn't enough dietary fat, your body will use stored fat for fuel—exactly what you want for weight loss.

So eat fat just until you are full or until you reach your calorie limit for the day, whichever comes first. I say "calorie limit" because early on, if you have leptin resistance, you can overeat fat and hold yourself back. If you have leptin resistance, you never feel full, even after a large meal: the hormones that signal you are full are not working as they should. A ketogenic diet will start to heal your body and hormones will start to fire as they should. After leptin resistance is healed, it is hard to overeat fat when your carb and protein amounts are correct, because you will feel full and satisfied.

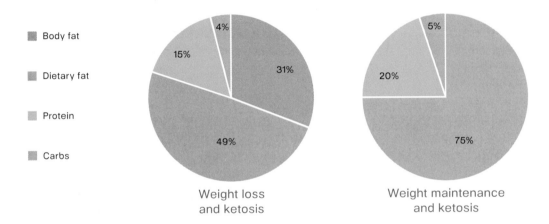

Body fat

Dietary fat

Protein

Carbs

Weight loss
and ketosis

Weight maintenance
and ketosis

# testing for ketones

After two to four weeks of following a well-formulated ketogenic diet, you should achieve nutritional ketosis, a state in which your body is burning fat rather than sugar. To determine whether you have become keto-adapted, you can test yourself for ketones, which should be at a certain level if you're in ketosis. There are a few ways to do it.

## three types of ketone bodies

To understand the methods of testing, you need to know a little bit about ketone bodies. Functionally, there are three types of ketone bodies: acetone, acetoacetate, and beta-hydroxybutyrate (BHB).

The liver converts long- and medium-chain fatty acids into BHB and acetoacetate, which live in reversible equilibrium (they can transform back and forth). Acetoacetate can also be turned into acetone, but after being converted to acetone, it cannot be converted back. Acetone is typically excreted through the urine or breath.

Each kind of test for ketones looks for one of these three ketone bodies. Acetone is tested in the breath, acetoacetate in the urine, and BHB in the blood.

## three methods for testing ketones

There are three methods for testing ketones. Each has its advantages and disadvantages.

### urine test strips (ketostix)

Our bodies excrete excess ketones in two ways: through the urine and through the breath. When you test your urine for ketones, you will typically see higher levels in the early stages of following a ketogenic diet because your body isn't using ketones for fuel yet. After you are fully keto-adapted, you will see fewer and fewer ketones in your urine because your body is using the ketones for fuel instead of excreting them.

Urine test strips are also susceptible to changes in your state of hydration. The more hydrated you are (and we should all be drinking more water in a ketogenic lifestyle), the lower the ketone level on the urine test strip will be.

### breath ketone testing (ketonix breath analyzer)

Breath testers test your breath for acetone. Your breath acetone level gives you a good idea of how much your body is turning fat into fuel, but it doesn't directly correlate to the BHB in your blood.

### blood ketone testing

Blood ketone testing (I like the Precision Xtra model best) is the best indicator of your true state of ketosis. At a BHB range of 0.5 to about 5.0 mmol, the body is in ketosis and using ketones as its primary fuel source.

Remember that more is not better when it comes to ketones. Many studies have shown that above a BHB level of 4 to 5 mmol, there is no added metabolic benefit. And if you are metabolically damaged (or insulin resistant; see page 21), you won't be able to utilize ketones for fuel as efficiently, which can result in higher ketone levels. Your focus should be on moderating protein and getting total carbs to 20 grams or less. If you do those two things correctly, your body will get into ketosis regardless of your blood ketone measurements.

### ketosis in athletes

*Blood ketone levels are simply the difference between ketones produced and ketones used. So if you work out a lot, you might have lower levels, as your body uses more of the ketones in your blood for fuel. Some athletes and bodybuilders can be in ketosis but have blood ketone levels of 0.3 because they are using all the fuel (ketones) that their bodies generate. That's why the absolute level of blood ketones isn't that relevant to weight loss and healing. Some people do great at 0.3 or 0.6, and others do well at 2.0 or higher.*

# maintaining a healthy balance of micronutrients

While macronutrients are the focus on a ketogenic diet, it's also important to ensure that you're getting adequate amounts of certain micronutrients, the vitamins, minerals, and electrolytes that the body needs. Maintaining a healthy balance of these micronutrients can mean the difference between feeling great during your 30-day cleanse and feeling so awful that you want to give up.

## sodium and electrolytes

When people adopt a ketogenic lifestyle, one of the first effects they experience is a rapid improvement in sensitivity to insulin. Low-carb eating causes insulin levels to fall quickly, and the body starts to recover from insulin resistance. As insulin levels fall, the kidneys begin to release fluid promptly. A common complaint I hear from clients who are just getting started is that they have to urinate more often than usual in the middle of the night. This effect will go away eventually.

The good news is that when your kidneys release excess fluid, it becomes easier for your body to oxidize fat. The bad news is that as the extra water goes, essential sodium and electrolytes go, too. When sodium falls below a certain level, which can happen quickly, undesirable side effects can occur, such as headaches, dizziness, cramping, and low energy.

Soon after you start your 30-day cleanse, you might notice that if you stand up quickly, you feel faint. This is because you are dehydrated! Just drinking water isn't going to work, though. You need more sodium, too. Salt is not the evil that your doctor may have warned you about; you've got to start thinking differently. Just as it's important to know that eating more fat lowers your risk of heart disease, it's also important to understand that a well-formulated keto diet requires a lot more sodium.

Even if you don't experience any obvious side effects, you will need extra water and sodium. Eliminating all packaged foods removes a lot of sodium from your diet, and the recommended keto foods don't contain a lot of liquid, so you will want to drink at least half your body weight in ounces of water each day. If you get the fierce headaches that some people get when starting out, add sodium. Try to get about 6 grams of sodium a day.

My favorite way to get more sodium (as well as electrolytes and a ton of minerals) is to consume homemade bone broth—see page 108 for a recipe. (Store-bought broth will not convey these benefits.) It is so easy to make—you can even do it in a slow cooker! It takes at least a day to cook, and up to three days for ultra-rich broth, but I often make a huge batch in the pot that Craig used to use for home brewing (yes, we have come a long way in our journey!). I freeze it in small containers, and it keeps for a long time.

If you really don't want to make your own bone broth, you can use store-bought bouillon: it has a lot of sodium, tastes good as a hot drink, and can eliminate carbohydrate cravings. But please watch out for MSG and gluten. Not all brands are healthy.

In addition to drinking broth, I suggest that you replace your typical table salt with liberal amounts of real salt, such as a quality sea salt or rock salt. Real salt is essential for electrolyte balance and will boost your energy. Celtic sea salt and Himalayan rock salt are good options. These salts are either harvested from ancient sea beds or made by evaporating seawater with a high mineral content, and they contain about 70 percent of the sodium of regular table salt (which has been refined, bleached, and processed until it is pretty much pure sodium chloride, often with anticaking agents added). The other 30 percent consists of minerals and micronutrients (including iodine) found in mineral-rich seas. I greatly prefer the taste of these salts to regular salt; they are well worth the extra bucks. Do not make the mistake of using a brand of sea salt that adds dextrose (a form of sugar) as an anticaking agent and is devoid of iodine and other nutrients.

## potassium

If you don't want to lose lean muscle, pay attention here! Since you excrete a lot of sodium through the diuretic effect of a keto diet (even a well-formulated one), you will eventually lose a lot of potassium as well. Keeping your potassium level up safeguards your lean muscle mass as you lose weight. Just like sodium, adequate potassium also prevents cramping and fatigue. A deficiency in potassium causes low energy, heavy legs, salt cravings, and dizziness, and you may cry easily.

I often teach nutrition classes, and at the end of each class, I answer participants' questions. One question I frequently hear is, "How do you recommend getting potassium if you don't recommend eating bananas or potatoes, especially if someone has high blood pressure?"

I think it's interesting that doctors often recommend bananas and potatoes to their patients who have high blood pressure. Sure, those things taste great, and people love them. But in reality, those two foods are causing the problem, not fixing it! And there are foods that are much higher in potassium than the insulin-increasing banana and potato. Dried herbs, for example, contain a lot more potassium without any of the sugar or starch.

To ensure that you are getting adequate potassium, start adding potassium-rich foods like these to your diet:

Dried herbs: basil, chervil, dill, oregano, parsley, saffron, tarragon, turmeric

Avocados

Paprika, red chili powder

Cocoa powder, unsweetened baking chocolate

Fish: halibut, pompano, salmon, tuna

You can also take 99 milligrams of potassium supplements twice a day. Keeping your sodium as well as your magnesium intake up will help preserve your potassium level, too.

## magnesium

A main source of magnesium for many people is fortified whole grains ("fortified" just means that a magnesium supplement has been added). So if you remove grains from your diet, you are eliminating a major source of magnesium. Taking calcium supplements also increases your chance of a magnesium deficiency, as calcium competes with magnesium for uptake. That being said, a well-formulated ketogenic diet does not cause a massive depletion of magnesium, as a high-carb diet does. Your body uses 54 milligrams of magnesium to process just 1 gram of sugar or starch! That creates a high demand for magnesium. No wonder it is one of the most common deficiencies that I see in clients. About 70 percent of people don't get even the minimum recommended dietary allowance of magnesium, which isn't that high. Most people who have metabolic syndrome or high blood pressure and/or are overweight, insulin resistant, or diabetic are deficient in magnesium. As your insulin level increases, so does your blood pressure. Insulin stores magnesium, but if your insulin receptors are blunted and your cells grow resistant to insulin, you can't store magnesium; therefore, it passes out of your body through urination. Magnesium in your cells relaxes your muscles. If your magnesium level is too low, your blood vessels will constrict rather than relax, which raises your blood pressure and decreases your energy level.

It is not entirely necessary to get a blood test to see if you are deficient; the fact is, most people don't get enough. I will always take a magnesium supplement. It helps repair muscles, naturally relaxes blood vessels and tight muscles, and is a miracle cure for migraines and many other ailments. Good magnesium levels help regulate potassium levels. I suggest supplementing children with it as well, since it helps with sleep issues. There are topical magnesium gels and lotions that are readily absorbed.

You may be wondering why we need to supplement with minerals if our ancestors never did. Well, most of the magnesium they ingested was found in the water they drank from streams and wells. Today, most people drink treated, softened, or bottled water, which is devoid of magnesium. Magnesium salts in water leave deposits in water pipes and make it difficult to get a decent lather with soap. These problems were solved with the development of water softeners, but the softening process created a new problem in that it gets rid of the magnesium that our bodies need.

Since our water is now depleted of magnesium and adequate amounts are not found in foods, I suggest taking at least 400 milligrams of a quality chelated magnesium supplement per day. Most people find magnesium relaxing, so taking it at bedtime helps them get quality sleep. But on rare occasions, magnesium is energizing, so if you find yourself unable to sleep after taking it, I suggest taking 400 milligrams at breakfast and, if needed, another dose at lunch. Everyone has a different tolerance.

When purchasing supplements, note that chelated magnesium is combined with an amino acid agent for absorption. So if the dosage is 1,000 milligrams of magnesium citrate, the amount of magnesium isn't 1,000 milligrams. The chelated amino acid is heavier than magnesium; about 15 percent of the weight is magnesium and the rest is the agent. The only way to really know how much magnesium you're getting is to look at the Recommended Daily Intake (RDI). The RDI for magnesium is 400 milligrams, so if you see that a dose of the supplement contains 50 percent of the RDI, then you know that each dose contains 200 milligrams of magnesium.

The only problematic side effect to magnesium is loose stool. This is more likely to occur if you purchase magnesium oxide, which is a nonabsorbable form. Look for magnesium glycinate, which I have only been able to find online. If you are taking a small dose and still have issues with loose stool, I suggest that you use a topical magnesium or Epsom salts in a bath.

# intermittent fasting

When I first heard about intermittent fasting, I thought, "No, no, no—this is not good for anyone who wants to maintain muscle." But after diving into what happens when you fast while on a well-formulated ketogenic diet, I realized that you not only maintain muscle but also reap other amazing benefits. As I put intermittent fasting into practice, I experienced physical benefits, and the mental benefits were outstanding!

## Why fast? Here are some of the benefits:

 It heightens brain function.
Neuroscientist Mark Mattson found that intermittent fasting increases levels of a protein called brain-derived neurotrophic factor, or BDNF. This, in turn, stimulates new brain cells in the hippocampus, the region of the brain that is responsible for memory. (Shrinking of the hippocampus has been linked to dementia and Alzheimer's disease.)

 It reduces blood pressure.
As insulin increases, so does blood pressure. Insulin stores magnesium, but if your insulin receptors are blunted and your cells grow resistant to insulin, you can't store magnesium; it ends up passing out of your body through urination. Magnesium in your cells relaxes muscles. If your magnesium level is too low, your blood vessels will constrict rather than relax, raising your blood pressure and decreasing your energy level.

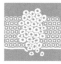 It inhibits cancer growth.
Fasting cleans out damaged mitochondria. It turns on certain genes that repair tissues that would not be repaired in times of surplus. Studies have shown that intermittent fasting can reduce spontaneous cancers in animals due to a decrease in oxidative damage or an increase in immune response.

 It improves mood. BDNF also suppresses anxiety and elevates mood. When Mattson injected BDNF into rats' brains, it had an antidepressant effect.

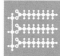 It increases the effectiveness of insulin, the hormone that affects our ability to process sugar and break down fat.

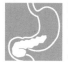 It reduces triglycerides.
Insulin up-regulates lipoprotein lipase (LPL) on fat tissue and inhibits activation on muscle cells. On the other hand, glucagon up-regulates LPL on muscle and cardiac tissue while inhibiting the activation of fat.

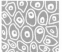 It extends life.
Fasting allows certain cells to live longer (as repaired cells) during famine since repairing a cell is energetically less expensive than dividing and creating a new one. Fasting reduces the amount of IGF-1, an insulin-like growth hormone, that the body produces, according to Valter Longo at the University of Southern California. Lower IGF-1 has been shown to reduce the risk of many age-related diseases. You need adequate IGF-1 and other growth factors when you are young and growing, but high levels later in life appear to lead to accelerated aging and cancer.

Fasting is not a diet; it is a pattern of eating. It runs counter to the way we tend to live today, but it really isn't as drastic as it sounds. While you sleep, you are starting to fast a little. The point of intermittent fasting is to stretch that window of not eating. During the first eight hours after eating, you are digesting and absorbing nutrients. Only after not eating for eight hours do you get into a fasted state. So if you limit your window of eating to eight hours a day—meaning you fast for sixteen hours—then you can maintain a fasted state, in which you can burn fat more efficiently.

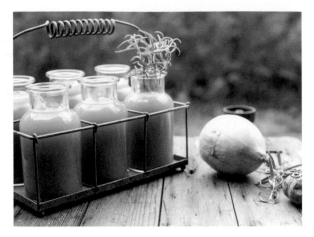

### water fast only!

*Bone broth contains high levels of glutamine, which are easily turned into sugar in the blood. One cup of broth can have 1,000 milligrams of glutamine. Many clients experience a large increase in ketones and a decrease in blood sugar when they follow my instructions and stop fasting with broth. If you have intestinal damage and want to consume broth for health reasons, that is fine and healthy, but I would stick to 1 cup a day.*

Fasting also affects our hormones, which are what ultimately determine weight loss or gain. Hormones go up and down throughout the day like ocean waves. Insulin and human growth hormone are antagonists, and since insulin is the more powerful of the two, it always wins. So when you eat carbohydrates, insulin rises and shunts the rise of human growth hormone. The largest natural surge of human growth hormone occurs thirty to seventy minutes after you fall asleep, but eating a bowl of ice cream or some toast with peanut butter and honey just before bed (which I always did as a kid) stops that precious fat-burning hormone from helping you burn fat while you slumber. When you wake up in the morning, you still have glycogen in your liver and you haven't burned any fat.

What I find interesting is that with most diets, the mental part is easy but the physical part is hard. But with fasting, it is the mental part that blocks many of my clients from even trying it. I thought it seemed impossible, too. When I was a sugar burner, I always wanted to eat. Now that I'm keto-adapted, I save so much time by not being plagued by thoughts of food all day.

There are a lot of ways to incorporate fasting into your life. I suggest skipping dinner once or twice a week, maybe on a day you will get home late and would be eating too close to bedtime. I like this option because it keeps you from bingeing later in the day and causes human growth hormone (the fat-burning hormone) to be at a high level when you fall asleep. During the evening fast, you can have plain water, chamomile tea without additives, or water from a soda streamer sweetened with stevia.

You can also fast in the morning—an especially good option for people who like to do cardio in the morning. If you skip eating before your workout, your body will burn fat instead, as your fat-burning human growth hormone level will remain high. Do not feel that you need to eat right after your workout. If you aren't hungry, do not force food, especially not a protein shake if you are trying to lose weight. You can take branched-chain amino acids to build muscle without calories if you like. During the morning fast, you are allowed organic decaf caffè Americano, tea, or water. (Regular decaf coffee is often made with a chlorinated filtration process, and chlorine inhibits thyroid function. Caffè Americano is made with espresso, which uses a water filtration process and has less caffeine than coffee.) I also recommend taking certain amino acids, such as L-carnitine, when you wake up. This will help shuttle triglycerides to the mitochondria, where you burn fat.

Or you can do a combination fast. For example, have dinner no later than 3 p.m., then go to bed at around 10 p.m. and wake up at 6 a.m. After you wake up, consume only calorie-free liquids, such as water, green tea, or decaf caffè Americano; I also take L-carnitine at this time. I then recommend exercising. You might eat at around 9:30 or 10 a.m. This is a total of over eighteen hours between meals.

I like to fast in the morning. I wake up at 5 a.m., take my amino acids, and then work. I run on an empty stomach from 8 a.m. to 9 a.m., and then I eat breakfast. Craig and I practice intermittent fasting daily, and in most cases, our fast lasts close to twenty hours. For some people, however, this is too extreme or doesn't fit their work schedule. So trying to fit in intermittent fasting a few days a week is a great goal.

## willpower is a muscle!

*If you're having a hard time with cravings, don't blame yourself. Willpower is a muscle in the brain that can get overworked. You need to limit temptations. You have only a finite amount of willpower, so try to save it for emergencies. Work and family obligations may require all your willpower, and you end up giving in to food temptations. I notice that if I stay up too late to work, my mind starts to wander to food, and those thoughts eventually become overwhelming. If I had a pantry filled with junk, it would be too tempting. But since I live way out in the country and I'm not going to turn on the oven to bake, I take L-glutamine to help calm the cravings and then go to bed. I suggest that you do the same.*

*Here are some more tips to help you stay the course:*

*• Clean out your pantry before beginning your 30-day cleanse. Nobody needs that stuff!*

*• Don't put temptations near you. Just putting food where you can see it depletes your willpower.*

*• Supplements like bifidobacteria, magnesium, and zinc can help with those nasty cravings.*

*• Cravings, frustration, and desire can all become overwhelming. After your 30-day cleanse, you can make "healthified" brownies and ice cream. I keep these in my freezer at all times, especially in the summer, when I feel the desire to eat sugar- and wheat-filled treats!*

*In the short term, self-control is a limited resource. But over the long haul, you can develop it like you would a muscle. Practice, practice, practice! It will get easier every day.*

# exercise

Sometimes when we want to lose weight, we focus on the number on the scale and forget about the importance of losing body fat. The majority of body fat (over 80 percent) is stored in fat cells. To get rid of it, you need to use it for energy.

This is one of the great things about ketosis: when your body is accustomed to burning fat for fuel, it can use body fat as well as dietary fat. And when you increase the amount of energy your body needs by exercising, all that extra energy comes from burning more fat! But if you are a sugar burner and fuel your body with carbs, you just burn sugar instead, making it much harder to lose body fat.

Ketosis is great for athletic performance, too. Our bodies can store over 40,000 calories of fat but only 2,000 calories of carbs, so when we're burning fat instead of sugar, there's a lot more fuel available at any given time. This is why carb-burning marathoners "hit the wall" during a race and need gel packs and Gatorade—they've used up the glucose they had available for fuel. They are low in performance at the end of the race, too, due to the depletion of carbs in their muscles and liver. Here's something to think about: migratory birds and whales rely on stored fat to fuel their long journeys.

Developing your fat engine will increase the amount of energy you can generate and reduce the amount of carbs you use. Added together, you have a more stable and enduring energy supply, better endurance, and faster finish times.

In this section, I'll look at some of the most effective kinds of exercise and offer my tips for getting the best results from exercise.

# cardio

Awesome things happen to your body when you work out at an intense rate. Not only does cardiovascular exercise improve the efficiency of your heart and lungs, it also increases the rate at which your body burns fuel. Over time, burning more fuel means that you will lose weight.

I know that those of you who are fans of Gary Taubes, who wrote *Why We Get Fat*, will think I am wrong. He believes exercise has nothing to do with weight loss, and I understand his points, but I have seen the benefits of exercise and cardio, especially when it comes to losing body fat. Studies show that a number of metabolic changes occur with cardiovascular exercise that uniquely enhance fat metabolism, including the following:

1. A major boost in the number and size of mitochondria. These parts of a cell are the only places where fat is burned and oxidized. They are the cell's fat-burning furnaces.

2. An increase in the oxidative enzymes that speed up the transport of fatty acid molecules to be used for energy during cardiovascular exercise (in other words, fat gets to the mitochondria faster, so the body can use it for fuel during exercise)

3. Increased oxygen delivery through blood flow, which helps cells oxidize and burn fat more proficiently

4. Amplified sensitivity of muscles and fat cells to epinephrine, which helps increase the release of triglycerides into the blood and muscles to clear them from the body. Since triglycerides—a kind of fat found in the blood—are linked to increased risk of heart disease, this is great news for your heart.

## pumping iron

*Iron is needed to carry oxygen to the mitochondria of your cells, where fat is burned during oxidation. (As you might guess from the name, oxidation requires oxygen.) If you have an iron deficiency, therefore, it is hard for your body to burn fat. Worse, when you push yourself too hard, you end up depleting this mineral even more. Women, take note: if you are feeling tired, losing your hair, and not losing weight with exercise, you are likely low in iron. About 90 percent of women who are low in iron can attribute the deficiency to three causes: menstruation (loss of blood equals loss of iron); a diet filled with gluten, which inhibits the body's ability to absorb iron; and/or excess cardio.*

5. An increase in the rates at which specialized protein transporters move fatty acids into the muscle cells, making fat more readily available for energy

6. A boost in the amount of fatty acids allowed into the muscle, which also makes fat more readily available for energy

All this data shows that with consistent, progressive cardiovascular exercise, we can truly expand our bodies to be awesome fat-burners. When our bodies are tired and we want to stop exercising, it's gratifying to know that when we push through the pain, we are creating more fat-burning furnaces (mitochondria)!

# strength training

Most women use their valuable time for cardiovascular or aerobic exercise, and I used to be one of them. I would run twelve miles a day and compete in marathons, but the scale didn't budge. I finally started taking a fitness class called BodyPump, which uses light to moderate weights, and the pounds began to melt off. I stopped running so much and started strength training.

I found that there are other benefits to strength training, too, in addition to weight loss:

• **It helps lift your mood.** Studies prove that watching yourself lift heavier and heavier weights builds confidence and reduces depression, even if you aren't losing weight.

• **It builds healthy bones.**

• **It helps you develop a strong and healthy body for daily movement throughout life.**

The most beneficial movements are multi-joint exercises, which use more than one muscle in a single movement—one example is a bench press, which uses both the shoulder and elbow joints as well as several muscle groups. Your metabolism and heart rate are directly related to the total volume of muscle mass being used, so multi-joint movements burn more calories by stimulating more muscles.

Some people are concerned that a low-carb diet, like the ketogenic diet, will prevent them from building muscle with strength training. However, in a well-designed low-carb, high-fat diet, there is less protein oxidation and double the fat oxidation, which means muscle is preserved while you burn fat!

### are you gaining weight with strength training?

*One reason women say their pants fit tighter after lifting heavier weights is that they are overconsuming carbohydrates or protein. Don't grab oatmeal and skim milk—or worse, a brownie—after all your hard work. Did you know a pound of fat is 3,500 calories and running a whole marathon burns only about 2,500 calories? So don't think that just because you performed a kick-butt workout, you can have a bag of Twizzlers. Learn the proper ways to fuel your body—it's essential for your health and outward appearance. And treat yourself in other ways! A one-hour massage is a great way to reward your muscles for their hard work.*

There are a lot of myths floating around about strength training. Let's take the top myths down one by one.

### Myth 1: For weight loss, I should do only cardio exercise.

While cardio is important, it isn't the only type of exercise that can help you lose fat. Strength training increases muscle mass, and the more muscle you have, the more calories you'll burn all day long.

Muscle is denser than fat and takes up less space. That means when you lose fat and gain muscle, you'll be slimmer and trimmer.

### Myth 2: To tone my muscles, I should use lighter weights and do more reps.

In order to create strong muscles, you must lift enough weight to break down the muscles, so they can be repaired to be even stronger. Muscles break down as you lift, and they repair and grow as you rest. If you plan on doing fifteen triceps extensions, choose a weight that allows you to only do fifteen reps. You want your body to feel the difficulty of lifting the weight in order for the muscle to become defined. That lean, defined look comes from losing body fat, which means heavy weights equals more fat-burning!

### Myth 3: Strength training makes women bulk up.

This popular myth continues regardless of the fact that women don't have the amount of testosterone required to build huge muscles. In fact, even men struggle to gain muscle and spend hours lifting to create a muscular physique.

Lifting heavy weights can benefit both men and women. In fact, challenging your body with heavy weights is the only way you'll really see results and get stronger. I've been lifting heavy weights for years, and I have never even come close to looking like a bodybuilder; most women who lift weights regularly would agree. Remember, muscle takes up less space than fat. Adding muscle (along with doing cardio and eating a healthy diet, of course) helps you lose fat, which means that you'll be leaner and more defined.

# interval training

Interval training is my favorite way to burn the most calories possible. Not only do you burn a ton of calories while you're doing it, it also stimulates your metabolism to a far greater degree than lower-intensity training. This is referred to as the afterburn effect. Interval training causes your muscles to go crazy with activity; I call it a metabolic disturbance. This crazy metabolism boost causes lots of calorie-burning after exercise to get your body back to normal. The result is that you end up burning more fat and calories in the post-exercise period as your body tries to get things under control.

Interval training is basically what it sounds like, alternating intervals of high-intensity and low-intensity exercise. It's based on a simple concept: go fast, go slow, repeat. It sounds simple, but this formula has an incredible number of potential variations and strategies.

Here are the basics of interval training:

1. **To begin, start your workout at an easy pace and slowly increase your heart rate for at least five minutes.** You can use a heart rate monitor or just use a "rate of perceived exertion" test to judge how hard your workout is on a scale of one to ten; one is resting, ten is working as hard as possible.

2. **When you're warmed up, you're ready for an explosion of high-intensity work.** Break into a jog or sprint, depending on what "high-intensity" means to you; your rate of perceived exertion should be around eight, and you shouldn't be able to carry on a conversation. Your body's ability to swap oxygen and carbon dioxide will be reduced, and you should feel the "burn" as your body eliminates lactic acid and your muscles start to lose their ability to contract. You should be working so hard that you aren't physically able to continue this level of intensity for long.

3. **After a few minutes, reduce the intensity level to something you can maintain for a longer period**, but don't slow down so much that your pulse dips too low, because you will lose the aerobic effect completely. This is called the active recovery period. Your body increases the exchange of oxygen and carbon dioxide to deliver nutrients to your muscles. The lactic acid burn should diminish, and your rate of breathing should slow a bit. After you complete this period for a few minutes, you have accomplished one cycle.

4. **Repeat this process of feeling the burn and recovering for at least thirty minutes.** The high-intensity periods should be shorter than the active-recovery periods, particularly when you first start. For example, when you begin to introduce your body to interval training, walk for five minutes, then run for one minute. As you become more proficient, increase the time you spend in high-intensity periods.

Here's why high-intensity interval training is awesome:

• **It saves time.** If you normally spend an hour and a half in the gym following the "fat-burning zone" philosophy, know that you'll work yourself just as hard in forty-five minutes with interval training.

• **Higher intensities stimulate your metabolism far more after the workouts than lower-intensity training.** This means you continue to burn calories and fat for long periods after you're done training—an extra 150 to 250 calories burned without any extra work!

• **It combats boredom.** It's fun, and time flies during each session because you're working in cycles of high and low intensity instead of spending a long time at any one activity. I like to make a playlist of songs to match the intensity of the workout: a warm-up song, a fast-paced song, a recovery-paced song, and repeat!

• **It challenges your aerobic and anaerobic systems at the same time, so you're improving your body's capacity to burn calories at a higher rate.**

• **It helps you add new muscle, which speeds up your metabolism of fat even at rest.**

• **It's an aerobic workout that burns lots of calories.**

• **It's effective for pushing beyond a weight-loss plateau.**

Many studies have proven the value of interval training. One followed a group of overweight women and assigned them to one of two groups. The first group worked out using high-intensity intervals, which involved two minutes of maximum effort followed by three minutes at a lower intensity. The second group worked out at a constant pace the whole time. The lengths of the workouts were varied so that both groups burned 300 calories. At the conclusion of the study, fitness levels in the interval group had improved by 13 percent, while no improvements were found in the steady-state group. The first group also continued to burn calories after the workout was finished.

---

### human growth hormone

*Human growth hormone is necessary for building muscle (which, in turn, increases metabolism), but it's also the fat-burning hormone. The combination of the two means that more growth hormone is great for losing weight.*

*Growth hormone is inversely related to insulin: if one is high, the other is low. So if you eat something (especially carbohydrates) before a workout, you will be spiking your insulin level and your growth hormone level will be low. This is one reason it's helpful to exercise on an empty stomach (see page 43 for other reasons). Short, high-intensity workouts are also awesome for stimulating growth hormone, and when lifting weights, that burn that you feel at the end means an increase in growth hormone.*

---

# circuit training: strength + cardio

Circuit training is a combination of strength training and cardiovascular exercise. If you're looking for a workout that provides allover fitness benefits, from revving up your metabolism to extending your endurance, look no further than circuit training.

A circuit-training workout combines cardio activity like jogging with a resistance workout, with little to no rest between exercises. The absence of long rest periods makes circuit training as effective as a cardio-based high-intensity interval workout (see page 39), which raises your heart rate and boosts metabolism by building muscles. Like interval training, circuit training burns a ton of calories, not just during the workout but for hours afterward—the afterburn effect. Minimizing rest time between exercises is as important as the exercises themselves. The more downtime between movements, the more your heart rate and metabolic rate decrease.

I love a circuit-training class at my local gym called Bootcamp. We rotate stations that include one strength-training activity and one cardiovascular activity, and two people share each station. For example, one station might be biceps curls for one person and explosive step-ups over an elevated step for the second person; you switch every minute or two. Once you are done with a station, you quickly do fifteen push-ups, sit-ups, or squats and then move on to the next heart-pumping station.

Here is one circuit-training workout that's an efficient way to burn fat:

1. **Warm up for 5 minutes, then jog for 5 minutes.**

   **First set:** Do 10 push-ups, then 10 sit-ups

   **Second set:** 9 push-ups, 9 sit-ups

   **Third set:** 8 push-ups, 8 sit-ups

   **Following sets:** 7, 6, 5 . . . all the way down to 1 each

2. **Jog for another 5 minutes.**

   **First set:** Do 10 triceps dips, then 10 biceps curls

   **Second set:** 9 triceps dips, 9 biceps curls

   **Following sets:** 8, 7, 6 . . . all the way down to 1 each

3. **Jog for another 5 minutes.**

   **First set:** Do 10 squats, 10 jumping jacks

   **Second set:** 9 squats, 9 jumping jacks

   **Following sets:** 8, 7, 6 . . . all the way down to 1 each

For a more advanced workout, repeat the whole cycle. Then walk to cool down and stretch!

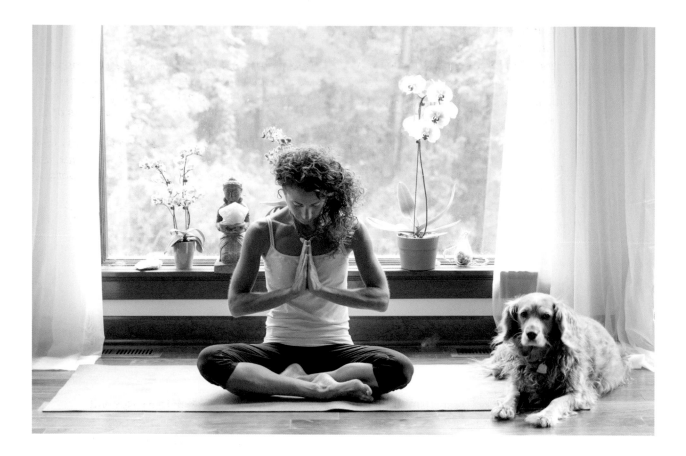

# yoga

About eight years ago, I taught yoga at the Andersen Windows corporate office over the lunch hour. Just about everyone in the class was brand-new to yoga. They mostly wanted a break from their desks and a time to relax. But after the first class, they all were surprised at how much they sweated and "felt the burn" while de-stressing at the same time. They were hooked. I loved hearing after each class that yoga had changed their lives in some way—they had less back pain, were making better food choices, felt happier and calmer, and more.

Yoga is one of the most helpful workouts for fighting stubborn fat stores. Research has found that yoga decreases levels of stress hormones and increases insulin sensitivity, which helps the body burn rather than store energy. In addition, stress, bad food habits, lack of energy, and thyroid problems can all be sources of weight gain, and practicing yoga can help with all of these.

That said, most types of yoga don't have the calorie-burning abilities of aerobic exercise. A 150-pound person will burn 150 calories in an hour of yoga, compared to 311 calories in an hour of walking at 3 miles per hour. Yoga's best benefit when it comes to weight loss is that it puts you in touch with your body in a way nothing else can.

Yoga isn't just exercise; it is a mind-body connection. It helps us become more in touch with our bodies and how we feel. It creates a sense of mindfulness, which is the ability to monitor what is happening internally. It helps change the relationship between the mind and body, and in time, that translates into a change in eating habits. The strong mind-body connection forged in yoga makes you more aware of what you eat and how it feels to be full, and the conscious awareness of your body translates to better appetite control. You become more aware of which foods nourish you and which make you feel lethargic.

So if you think you want to change your routine or the way you approach food, or get over harmful eating patterns, yoga can help you make those changes.

## exercise helps break bad habits

*Habits are hard to break. Instead of just stopping a bad habit, I like to help people form new healthy habits in its place—it makes stopping the bad habit much easier, and of course it offers benefits of its own. Exercise can be an effective tool as one of those helpful good habits. Here's an example from my own life: I grew up eating a bedtime snack, and it was the hardest habit for me to break. Practicing a bedtime yoga routine, which calms the mind and body, helped me replace that unhealthy snack with a habit that's actually good for me.*

# exercise tips for burning more fat

There are some tricks to exercising that can increase fat-burning. Granted, these tips will not work for everyone since we need to fit in exercise whenever we can, and some people may want to enhance performance rather than burn fat. But if fat loss is your goal, check this out!

• **Exercise in the morning on an empty stomach.** If your goal is to burn fat, it's best to exercise first thing in the morning on an empty stomach. (To prevent dehydration, drink a large glass of ice water mixed with a touch of quality salt first.) This will burn 300 percent more body fat than exercising any other time of the day because there is no glycogen (stored carbohydrates) in your liver to burn, so your body has to go directly into the fat stores to get the energy necessary to complete the activity. However, if you are diabetic or have other medical issues, this is not healthy. This suggestion is only for people who have no medical conditions and are not training to win races.

• **Do cardio exercise right after weight training.** It takes twenty to thirty minutes of exercise to exhaust the glucose immediately available for fuel (unless you're working out first thing in the morning on an empty stomach—see above). It's only then that you'll start to burn body fat. By performing weight training exercises before cardio, you'll deplete your available glucose faster, so you start burning fat sooner. Lifting weights first also means you have lots of energy to focus on correct posture, decreasing the chance of injury.

• **Change the exercise.** When you do one exercise consistently, your muscles get used to it. Workouts get easier and those muscles don't have to work as hard, so you burn fewer calories. Frequently changing your exercise makes your muscles work harder and causes an increase in heart rate, which means an increase in calories burned.

• **Change the duration of exercise.** This is important because you want to prevent your body from adjusting to a constant amount of activity. As soon as the body adapts to a kind of exercise, it's easier for the muscles to perform. This is good for performance, but it becomes tougher to reach the fat-burning zone. Extending the length of your workout can compensate.

# the exercise of daily activities

There are two kinds of physical activity: planned activity, such as running on a treadmill, and the unconscious movements that we perform daily, such as tapping a foot in a meeting or simply moving to get from one place to another. Both kinds of activities require fuel and affect our metabolism, which determines how our bodies burn fuel. Overall, activity level makes up 15 to 30 percent of our metabolism.

But we often overestimate how much fuel we really burn during planned exercise. To put it in perspective, a runner burns about 2,500 calories during a marathon, and it takes 3,500 calories to burn 1 pound of fat! Plus, it can be difficult to make time for exercise; we're all so busy, it can be hard to get in three one-hour workouts a week. Here's the good news: the calories burned during unplanned activity can add up fast. Going to the grocery store and cooking dinner can burn as many calories as a boring forty-minute run on a treadmill.

So instead of going to the gym after work, stressing out on the way home because you don't have anything planned for dinner, and stopping at a restaurant for takeout, go to the grocery store, power shop, and go home and make your family a healthy meal! You'll have burned the same amount of calories, and you'll be giving your body the healthy fuel it needs to thrive.

This is not to say that exercise is unimportant. It definitely is! It strengthens your heart, lungs, and muscles, which is important for overall health. Recent studies have found that exercise is more helpful in treating depression than antidepressant medications. But when it comes to weight loss, it's not everything. Do I exercise? Yes, I run, bike, walk, lift weights, practice yoga—I love to move. But I did all this when I was fat, too. Nutrition was the missing key to successful weight loss.

I see exercise as a tool to help you live a healthy lifestyle. Do not push yourself by living at the gym or on a treadmill in order to lose more weight. It is more about what you put into your mouth than how many miles your legs can run.

### fitness tip: wear a pedometer!

*Every car has an odometer that records the miles it has traveled. Similarly, a pedometer measures steps. Walking 10,000 steps a day burns 300 to 400 calories. Wearing a pedometer can enhance your motivation to increase your number of daily steps. Focus on one day at a time. Over time, you will find yourself going for an extra walk, taking extra steps from the parking lot, and expending a few more calories here and there. These small changes add up over time and lead to stable, lifelong results.*

# the dangers of too much exercise

I love to exercise for so many reasons. I love my morning run in the country: the silence, the feeling of gratitude, seeing deer. But it took me years to enjoy running. When I first started, I was aiming for a half mile, and even that was tough for me. Now I run every morning without hardship, and I do it not for weight loss but because I enjoy it.

I did, however, sign up for a marathon for weight loss six years ago, and guess what happened while I was running twice a day? I *gained* weight, even though I was eating the same low-carb diet. What was going on?! I was overtraining. My high-intensity exercise routine had pushed my body's stress response too far, which led to a cascade of biochemical responses that damaged my health.

Most people do cardiovascular exercise to lose weight. Unfortunately, too much cardio stimulates cortisol, a stress hormone that tells your body to hang on to fat stores. Cortisol is released when the body is under all kinds of stress—work, family life, lack of sleep, poor eating habits, and, yes, excess exercise (such as marathon training) can all stimulate cortisol.

Chronically high levels of cortisol aren't just a problem for weight loss. They also increase your risk for a variety of health issues, such as depression, sleep disturbances, and digestive issues. Also, cortisol and testosterone seem to conflict; the more aerobic work you do, the more cortisol is released and the less testosterone is available to build muscle (plus, for men, lower testosterone has all kinds of effects on libido and erectile function).

Aside from cutting back on excessive intense exercise, there's a simple way to lower cortisol: get more sleep! (This is why people tend to gain weight in the summer: with the longer days, they're not getting enough sleep.)

Stress, whether from excess cardio or other life stressors, also affects neurotransmitters such as serotonin, GABA, and dopamine. These are our feel-good, antianxiety brain chemicals, and burning them out with stress and too much intense exercise can lead to depression, chronic fatigue, and sleep disorders. A shortage of these neurotransmitters also can cause serious thyroid conditions, such as hypothyroidism, which is known to cause weight gain, depression, and digestive dysfunction. Plus, low serotonin levels are associated with cravings for carbohydrates and binge eating.

If you are already living a life filled with stress from work, school, or family, know that exercise is another stressor. True, exercise is known to be more of a "healthy stress," but your adrenal glands don't know the difference. If you have adrenal fatigue, you may want to read the section on yoga, which is a great low-impact exercise that can also help you de-stress (see page 42).

# healing on a cellular level

This section may have some of the most incredible information you will ever read about the future of healthy living. It starts where the ketogenic diet leaves off, going to the next level of understanding about how to heal our bodies on a cellular level—especially our mitochondria, the fat-burning furnaces of our cells. Yes, this may venture kind of far beyond the idea of a 30-day cleanse, but this information is so important to our overall health that I feel it would be wrong to leave this information out.

It all starts with water, a critical element to life. The human body is 80 percent water, but over 99 percent of the molecules in our bodies are water molecules. That is pretty astounding!

Water is pretty straightforward, right? $H_2O$ is a simple molecule that has three states: gas, liquid, and solid. That's what we're taught in school, and most scientists haven't bothered to investigate it much further. Recently, though, a few scientists, led by University of Washington professor of bioengineering Gerald Pollack, decided to take a closer look. This decision kicked off a series of experiments that will forever change the way we look at water.

Even before Dr. Pollack and his team began their experiments, there were a lot of unexplained mysteries about water. For example, why do the molecules clump up and accumulate into clouds? And why do water droplets remain intact for up to ten seconds when dropped onto the surface of water? There were no good explanations for these mysteries, so the scientists started to investigate.

They found that when water comes in contact with any hydrophilic surface (a surface on which water likes to spread out), a barrier of negatively charged water develops. This exclusion zone (EZ) of negatively charged water accumulates and pushes out everything else. The next thing they found was that when they shined light, especially infrared light, onto the water, the exclusion zone increased in size.

This EZ water is the fourth state of water (it is actually $H_3O_2$). As it turns out, this is the phase that water goes through when it freezes and thaws. It is an ordered state of water. Some scientists have called this discovery the most influential of our generation.

Dr. Pollack's team also observed that when a small tube is placed in water, the water flows through the tube, without any obvious mechanism. They then applied light and found that the rate of the water's flow increased, especially under infrared light. Light was adding energy (electrons) to this EZ water. This, in combination with the way light causes the exclusion zone to increase in size, shows that light actually gives energy to the water.

You might be asking yourself, "What does this have to do with health?" Let's look at blood flow as one example. It's been observed that some of the capillaries that supply our cells with blood are as small as 3 micrometers in diameter. But red blood cells are at least twice that size—6 to 8 micrometers. So how do red blood cells get through these tiny capillaries? They have to bend. It was first thought that the heart's pumping action forces them through. But a Russian scientist did the calculations and found that forcing red blood cells through capillaries would take one million times the pressure that the human heart can exert.

Everything in the body, like cell walls, is hydrophilic. Much, if not all, of the water in the body, then, is EZ water. Infrared light, which is part of sunlight, can penetrate into the body and adds energy to this water, which creates a series of benefits, including giving it the energy to pump red blood cells through the smallest capillaries. The water is essentially like a battery, and the energy light adds enables red blood cells to flow through the smallest capillaries.

In fact, the body is like one huge battery, fueled by sunlight and magnetism. The more sunlight (especially morning light) and magnetism (from the earth's negative charge) we're exposed to, the more negative charge the body accumulates, as EZ water stores this energy. A negative charge makes the body slightly alkaline, which is what you want—it's associated with a lower risk of cancer and reduced systemic inflammation.

# a four-part action plan

This new information about how light and water interact in the cells in our body has real implications for health.

I want you to understand how to use this information to hack your lifestyle and improve your health, sleep, and vitality. So I'm going to break it all down into a four-part action plan that you can use to leverage this quantum biology in your body.

## part 1: getting sunlight and blocking blue light at night

Plants need sunlight to grow, but what about humans? Interestingly, the human body can use light of a certain wavelength (670 nm) to make adenosine triphosphate (ATP), a carrier of energy.

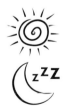

Getting exposure to morning sunlight and blocking blue light at night are two of the most important things you can do to enhance your environment and improve your health and sleep.

The first, and maybe the most important, thing is increasing exposure to morning sunlight and UV light. Both can be very helpful in healing, sleep, and longevity.

I preach over and over how important good sleep is. Getting at least eight hours of sleep can be the key to health, weight loss, mental clarity, and so much more. One of the best ways to ensure a restful night of sleep is to get your circadian clock in rhythm so that your body naturally produces melatonin at the right times.

The human eye has a receptor that responds to the presence of light—specifically blue light—and signals the activation of the suprachiasmatic nucleus (SCN) in the brain. The activation of the SCN, due to the presence of blue light in the eye, prevents the pineal gland from producing melatonin, the hormone that signals sleep. A lack of blue light in the eye signals to the pineal gland to produce melatonin, inducing drowsiness.

So it's critical to support this process to enable good sleep cycles. There are two parts to keeping your circadian clock in rhythm:

**Get direct sunlight for twenty minutes within two hours of waking.** Ideally, you want direct sunlight in your eyes to stimulate the SCN and energize you for the day. Go outside and face the sun; if you wear glasses or contacts, take them off. By removing some clothing and exposing skin to UV light, you will also energize your body, get vitamin D, and generate cholesterol sulfates, which improve mood and the health of your cells.

The UV and infrared light that you get from sunlight help with many health processes. We all know how important vitamin D is for mood and strong bones. You might be getting 5,000 IU of D3 from a supplement, but in a bright, sunny location, you can make 1,000 IU per minute of skin sun exposure. As with many things, the current thinking about UV light is wrong. Third-degree sunburns are harmful, yes, but UV light in itself is not harmful.

Infrared light energizes our cells and the EZ water in those cells to create a "mammalian battery." This gives you energy and makes your mitochondria more efficient. It can even enable your body to produce ATP from sunlight (just like plants!).

**Limit blue light in the evening.** Our modern environments are very bad in this regard and contribute to poor sleep cycles. Interior lighting, smartphones, computers, and TVs all emit blue light that inhibits the pineal gland from producing melatonin in a natural cycle. If you plan to use devices or watch TV in the evening, get a pair of blue-blocking glasses. They block all blue light so you can watch TV and use your devices while still allowing your brain and pineal gland to produce melatonin at the right time to enable sleep. Start wearing them three to four hours before bed.

The pitfalls of blue light exposure are becoming well known. Even iOS devices like the iPhone and iPad now have a setting to limit blue light. Just go to Settings, click on Display & Brightness, and turn on Night Shift. Set it to the warmest setting. I have mine set to turn on at about 6:30 p.m.

# part 2: staying hydrated

I always discuss the importance of getting enough water: half of your body weight in ounces a day at a minimum. I shoot for a gallon a day. The best source for cellular health is spring water. There are quite a few sources out there. Just make sure to avoid water that contains fluoride and chlorine.

The second component to hydration is to energize this water by getting good circadian light, as discussed in Part 1. You can also energize your body by grounding (below).

# part 3: getting grounded

The earth has a negative charge. We have long known that there are many benefits to having a slightly alkaline body, such as a lower risk of cancer, better sleep, and reduced inflammation. Making our bodies more negatively charged makes them more alkaline.

When we connect to the earth through an electrical ground, we are negatively charging our bodies (making them more alkaline). But we almost never accomplish this feat today. We wear rubber-soled shoes at home and at work, and in our cars we are electrically isolated from the earth.

So how do you hack this? First, you can wear grounding shoes, which have a section that conducts electricity, so they ground you to the earth as you walk. There are many styles out there. You can also just go barefoot outdoors. To hack the environment in your home or office, you can use a grounding (or "earthing") mat that plugs into an electrical outlet that has an earth ground (the round hole at the bottom). You can use a grounding mat at your computer, in bed, or anywhere else you spend a lot of time.

## part 4: chilling out

 Cold therapy has been used for some time to speed recovery in athletes, but being cold is important for everyone's cellular health. Cooling your body shrinks your mitochondria, and smaller mitochondria are more efficient at burning fat.

If this section was a bit too much like a biology class for you, here is a quick overview of how to hack your environment, improve the health of your cells and your body, and heal your mitochondria:

• **Eat keto.** Sugar causes inflammation in the cells; a keto diet reduces that inflammation.

• **Fast daily.** When you fast, your body can stop focusing on digesting and using food and focus instead on breaking down failing mitochondria and creating new and healthy ones. I refer to this as the body's mechanism for reversing aging and curing a damaged metabolism. (See page 33 for more.)

• **Sleep eight to ten hours a night.** Sleep is not just about putting your head down; it is a vital time when the brain cycles through frequencies in the tissues of the body, matching them briefly through a process called magnetic resonance. One sweep through all the tissues in the body creates one sleep cycle, which partially restores the charge on your fatigued cells from the day's activities. After the sleep cycle is completed, you are ready for the day. A magnetic sleeping pad can help promote this process.

• **Wake up early and turn a UV light on, especially in the winter, when there is less sunlight.** I love this time of year for taking pictures—the clouds make a beautiful shade—but my body craves the light. Getting more light helps you sleep well!

• **Lift heavy weights every other day.** Exercise also helps with mitochondrial health.

• **Drink ice-cold water in the morning.** There was a time when I loved coffee. Heck, I worked at a coffee shop in high school and at another one in college! But with time, I came to understand the connections among caffeine, the adrenal glands, hormones, and insulin. So I switched to decaf caffè Americano, chocolate safari tea, green tea, and ice-cold water. I also chew on ice.

• **Run in the cold.** Being cold is important for cellular health.

• **Walk barefoot on the earth whenever you can,** and consider wearing grounding shoes (which help with plantar fasciitis, too!).

• **Be very particular about what you put on your skin.** No chemicals. This is quite freeing for me: I no longer need to shop at stores for toothpaste, lotions, and other toxic products that change the health of my cells. (See page 408 for more.)

• **Practice cold therapy about an hour before bed.** I start by placing my feet in a large bucket. I fill it slowly with ice-cold water from the hose outside, which gradually gets me used to the cold temperature. I used to take an ice-cold shower, but I find that starting with my feet is easier. Once my feet and legs are submerged in the ice water, I spray my arms, head, and then back. This cools my body down for a nice long sleep!

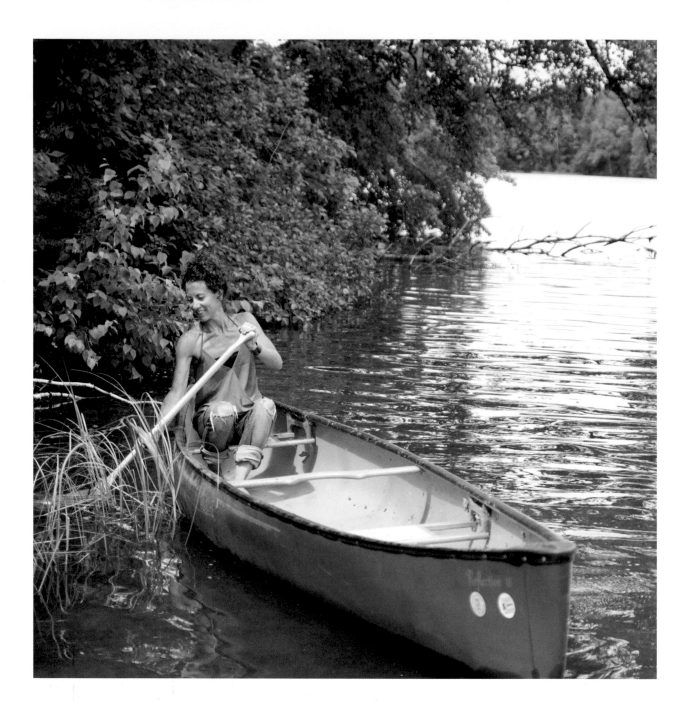

By utilizing the quantum properties of our bodies and the water that makes up our bodies, we can see great improvements in overall health—better sleep, moods, energy, and focus. But it also improves the health of our mitochondria, the fat-burning furnaces in our cells. Mitochondria can be damaged and become less efficient because of many things in our environment: dark cubicles, artificial light all day and night, no connection to the earth, and toxins from food. The great thing is, though, that just some simple lifestyle changes can help heal your mitochondria and energize your body.

# how to heal your mitochondria

## MORNING:

 Wake up with the sun, and get outside and expose as much skin to the sunlight as possible for 20 minutes within two hours of waking. This starts your circadian clock.

 Work out outside. Get sunlight! Even in below-zero weather in January, I run outdoors. Those runs have many benefits: I get outside with nature, sunlight, and cold therapy.

 Drink ice-cold water instead of hot coffee; it shrinks your mitochondria, and smaller mitochondria are more efficient. Plus, good water (containing no chlorine or fluoride) is essential for cellular health.

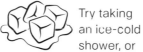 Try taking an ice-cold shower, or make the water as cold as you can handle for the last few minutes of your shower.

Work out if possible: exercise builds healthy mitochondria! The best time to burn fat is first thing in the morning, on an empty stomach, after drinking a large glass of water or green tea to avoid dehydration. You burn 300 percent more body fat in the morning on an empty stomach than at any other time of the day because your body does not have much glucose readily available to burn, so it has to go directly into the fat stores to get the energy necessary to complete the activity. You also increase your level of human growth hormone, which is the fat-burning hormone. Human growth hormone and insulin counteract each other. If one is high, the other is low, like a seesaw. So if you eat something, especially carbohydrates, before a workout, you will spike your insulin level, meaning that your human growth hormone level will be low. (See page 40 for more.)

## MIDDAY:

 Break-your-fast with a ketogenic meal.

Wear grounding shoes or walk barefoot; use a grounding mat under your desk to make your cells more alkaline (negatively charged).

Drink lots of water. Our cells are 99 percent water molecules.

Get outside in the sun. Sunlight is important to health, and water in the body can get a charge (become more alkaline) from infrared light.

## EVENING:

 Limit blue light: set electronics to lower blue light (use the Night Shift setting on iOS devices) and wear blue-blocking glasses when watching TV or working on a computer.

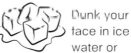 Dunk your face in ice water or jump into ice-cold water (I swim in a spring-fed river before bed).

Have a keto snow cone to lower your body temperature.

Limit vigorous exercise in the evening; stick to gentle walking or yoga.

## BEDTIME:

 Do not eat within three hours of bedtime.

68°F Lower the temperature in your bedroom. Keep it below 68 degrees; lower is better. I have a cooling mattress pad, too!

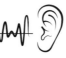 Use light-blocking blinds to keep the bedroom dark.

 Use a sound machine in the bedroom to help with sleep.

 Use an essential oil diffuser to emit lavender.

 Sleep eight to ten hours every night!

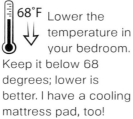

# troubleshooting

A well-formulated ketogenic diet has the proper macronutrient ratios and includes keto-enhancing foods, as well as extra electrolytes and salt. Many of my new clients claim that they eat ketogenically, but it later comes out that they'd been consuming foods that were keeping them from ketosis and weight loss. Some people are so metabolically damaged that even adding a slice of lemon to their water can take them out of ketosis!

If you find yourself hitting some roadblocks during your 30-day cleanse, this section is here to help you troubleshoot.

## common keto mistakes

Here are some common pitfalls that can keep you from achieving and maintaining ketosis.

### ☒ adding fruit and high-carb veggies to "feel better"

Some people experience ill effects when they first go low-carb, such as hair loss, tiredness, depression, and heavy legs—this is the so-called low-carb flu. A common mistake is to start adding fruit and higher-carb veggies like spaghetti squash to your diet because the extra carbohydrates make you feel better. But the problem isn't that you need to eat more carbs; it's that your keto diet isn't well formulated. It is too low in sodium and electrolytes. You need to supplement properly to feel better and more energized; see page 30 for more information.

### ☒ counting net carbs, not total carbs

Subtracting fiber from vegetable carbohydrates in order to calculate net carbs is another common mistake that low-carb dieters make. I have many clients who are kicked out of ketosis with too much fiber. My meal plan (beginning on page 94) contains only the highest-nutrient veggies without high total carb counts.

## ☒ consuming too many nuts, nut flours, seeds, and psyllium husk

Too much fiber is a common problem when people first try a ketogenic diet and overconsume nuts, nut flours, seeds, and psyllium husk. Ketosis isn't just for weight loss; you may be trying to gain weight, put on muscle, or just maintain good health. But if you are undertaking this keto cleanse with the goal of losing weight, cut out all nuts, nut flours, seeds, and psyllium husk for at least the first two weeks. Weigh yourself the first day, then weigh yourself again two weeks later. After two weeks, try adding ¼ to ½ cup per day of the nuts that are lowest in total carbs (walnuts and macadamia nuts are good options; refer to the following chart) and see how you feel.

| NUT | TOTAL CARBS PER OUNCE |
|---|---|
| Macadamia nuts | 3 g |
| Walnuts | 3.8 g |
| Almonds | 6 g |
| Hazelnuts | 5 g |
| Brazil nuts (high in selenium for thyroid health) | 3.5 g |
| Pistachios | 7.6 g |
| Cashews | 7.8 g |

## ☒ consuming dairy

Cut out all dairy, even "low-carb," high-fat dairy, during your 30-day cleanse. Skip the butter, cream, whey protein, cheese, yogurt, cream cheese, and whey protein powder. The recipes in this book can all be made without dairy.

I find that eliminating dairy helps so many people reach their goal weight. For 50 percent of my clients, dairy is insulin-spiking and holds them back from losing any weight. Other problems can occur with dairy as well: When your gut is damaged and inflamed, a phenomenon called "atrophy of the villi" occurs. Dairy is digested at the ends of the villi, which are little fingerlike pieces that line the intestinal wall. If your villi are damaged, dairy may not be well absorbed, leading to symptoms of acid reflux, indigestion, gas, and/ or bloating. Once you heal the intestinal wall with an anti-inflammatory keto diet, you can reincorporate dairy foods (in smaller amounts at first). I usually recommend taking healing supplements, such as Zinlori and aloe vera, to repair the intestinal wall faster.

To reintroduce dairy, start with goat cheese to see if your weight loss stalls or your weight creeps up. If it doesn't, try ghee next. Then progress to butter and cheese made from cow's milk if your body tolerates them.

## ☒ drinking your calories

Drinking your calories does not signal the proper hormones, such as leptin and ghrelin, that give you a sense of satisfaction and signal that you are full. Chewing is a powerful tool. Use it!

Keep in mind that if you drink bulletproof coffee in an effort to "fast" until noon, you are no longer fasting. Consuming more than 40 to 50 calories takes you out of intermittent fasting, which is a powerful tool for ketogenic dieting (see page 33 for details). And butter is dairy, which you should cut out during your 30-day cleanse.

## ☒ eating when you're not hungry

Adhering to the belief that you need to eat breakfast within an hour of waking is not helping your waistline. If you are constantly fueling your body and increasing insulin, you will burn sugar rather than ketones, and you will not get into fat-burning mode. Do not eat every two hours; wait until you are truly hungry. Breakfast isn't the most important meal of the day—"breaking your fast" is!

## ☒ drinking alcohol

I once had a client tell me that he *had* to have a few glasses of wine in the evening so he would blow ketones in the morning using his Ketonix breath analyzer. (See page 28 for more on testing for ketones.) He said that if he didn't drink alcohol, ketones were not present. Um, what? Yep, he was right. A breath ketone tester is a lot like a Breathalyzer that police officers use. Which makes me wonder: if someone in ketosis got pulled over and was asked to blow into a Breathalyzer, would he be in trouble just for being in ketosis?

But the truth is, alcohol does not help you get into ketosis; if anything, alcohol will hold you back from being your best self, physically and mentally.

### testosterone and alcohol

*Drinking alcohol is the most efficient way to slash your testosterone level. Women, we don't want this to happen any more than men do! A single event of significant drinking raises the level of the muscle-wasting stress hormone cortisol and decreases testosterone for up to 24 hours. If you are working out to build strong fat-burning muscles yet are consuming alcohol, the result is actually a further breakdown of muscle and a slower metabolism. If you have the proper hormone levels, you break down muscle as you lift weights and repair them as you rest. If not, your body is never able to repair your muscles properly!*

When people go on a diet, they often switch to the "light" versions of their favorite alcoholic beverages in order to save a few calories. However, calories are only a small piece of the puzzle. Fat metabolism is reduced by as much as 73 percent after only two alcoholic beverages. When you drink alcohol, you're not just consuming more calories, you're impairing your body's ability to use fat for energy.

Alcohol in the body is converted into a substance called acetate. When blood acetate levels increase, the body uses acetate instead of fat for energy. To make matters worse, the more you drink, the more you tend to eat, and because your liver must work to convert the alcohol into acetate, the foods you consume will be converted into extra body fat.

If that doesn't sound bad enough, consider this: Alcohol stimulates appetite and increases estrogen by 300 percent. The infamous "beer belly" is really just an "estrogen belly." Biochemically, the higher your estrogen level, the more readily you absorb alcohol, but the slower you break it down.

Also, we all know that alcohol dehydrates us. For fat to be metabolized, it must first be released from the fat cells and then be transported in the bloodstream, where it is pushed to the liver to be used for fuel. If you are dehydrated, the liver has to come to the aid of the kidneys and can't focus on its role of releasing fat.

Alcohol affects every organ of the body, but its most dramatic impact is on the liver. The liver cells normally prefer fatty acids as fuel and package excess fatty acids as triglycerides, which they then route to other tissues. However, when alcohol is present, the liver cells are forced to metabolize the alcohol first, letting the fatty acids accumulate. Alcohol metabolism permanently changes liver cell structure, which impairs the liver's ability to metabolize fats and can lead to fatty liver disease.

## ☒ not getting enough sleep

Sleep is extremely underrated when it comes to the weight-loss puzzle! I used to I ask my clients, "How well do you sleep?" And they would respond, "Great! I sleep six hours like a baby!" So now I ask, "*How long* do you sleep?" You must get eight to ten hours daily.

If you often find yourself unable to fall asleep, I suggest taking a cortisol test in the morning and at night to determine if your cortisol level isn't falling like it should throughout the day. I also suggest a ferritin test to determine whether iron is getting into your cells properly. Low iron causes extreme lethargy throughout the day, even though you might feel so anxious that you can't sleep. Waking too early (say, you're wide awake at 3:00 a.m.) is a sign of low progesterone.

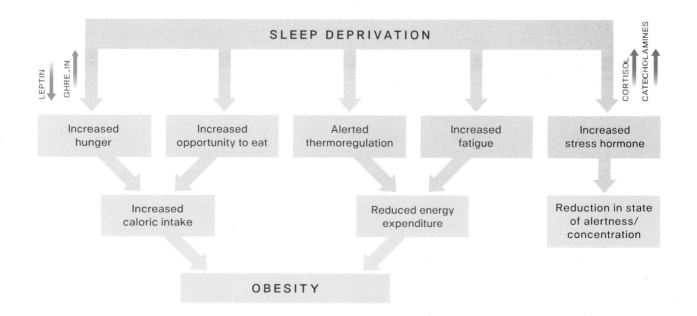

If you need help with sleep, start by working to heal your circadian rhythm, as described on page 47. Certain supplements can help, too. If you have trouble falling asleep, try taking the following supplements one hour before bed:

• **400 to 800 milligrams of magnesium glycinate** (not magnesium oxide, which is not absorbed well and will cause diarrhea). Magnesium is a natural muscle relaxant and will help you calm down (though in rare instances it can be energizing).

• **One capsule of bifidobacteria probiotic.** Bifido increases serotonin, which in turn increases melatonin production.

• **750 milligrams of GABA (gamma-aminobutyric acid).** GABA is a nonessential amino acid found mainly in the brain and eyes. It is considered an inhibitory neurotransmitter, which means that it regulates brain and nerve cell activity by inhibiting the number of neurons firing in the brain. By inhibiting overstimulation of the brain, GABA promotes relaxation, eases nervous tension, and increases quality sleep; it is the brain's natural calming agent.

• **200 milligrams of 5-hydroxytryptophan (5-HTP) or 1,000 milligrams of L-tryptophan.** These amino acids increase serotonin, which in turn increases melatonin output. Note: Do not take if on an antidepressant.

Melatonin also can help with sleep, but many people claim that melatonin supplements don't work for them, which is likely due to an absorption issue or leaky gut. I recommend melatonin patches instead. Start with 1 milligram and increase as needed.

If you have a hard time *staying* asleep, the cause is likely low progesterone (unopposed estrogen) leading to estrogen dominance. I suggest that you add a pure progesterone cream to an area of thin skin on certain days of your cycle. I prefer Pro-Gest cream, made by Emerita. Many of my women clients report feeling an immediate sense of calm when I apply this cream to their wrists.

# ☒ eating too much protein

Do not confuse the keto diet with popular high-protein diets. Too much protein becomes sugar in the blood. Do not eat too much protein at one time; split it up throughout the day. Your body cannot store excess protein.

# ☒ eating before bed and/or exercising at the wrong time of day

Weight loss is all about hormone manipulation. Adjusting your pattern of eating gives you a lot of control over not only insulin but also human growth hormone and cortisol. Your natural surge of human growth hormone occurs 30 to 70 minutes after you fall asleep, but its antagonist is insulin. If you eat before bed, insulin rises, and human growth hormone—your fat-burning hormone—will not increase because insulin is more powerful.

Cortisol is naturally high in the morning and should fall throughout the day. This is why morning exercise is awesome! If you wait until after work to exercise, you get another surge of cortisol, which messes with the natural decrease and can cause your body to store belly fat.

# ☒ suffering from adrenal fatigue

The adrenal glands are one of the most important organs in the body, yet they are often overlooked by medical professionals. Your adrenals are your main stress adaptation glands. During stressful events, they secrete hormones that help your body respond. They produce cortisol (recognized as the "belly fat" hormone), estrogen, testosterone, thyroid hormone, and many others, which regulate metabolism, the immune system, the reproductive system, and excretory functions.

Your adrenal glands also regulate water and mineral balance in your cells. Without adequate, quality salt, your blood pressure drops and your adrenal hormones suffer. People with adrenal fatigue often crave salt because they have low blood pressure.

Internal and external stressors (too much exercise, lack of sleep, family or work issues, for instance) have a huge effect on the adrenals and therefore on your hormonal output. Here are some signs of adrenal fatigue:

• Insomnia (including waking up often throughout the night)

• Lack of energy

• Anxiety from even minor stressors

• Low moods

• Low blood pressure

• Poor memory

• Low libido

• Recurring infections

• Asthma or allergies

• Need for coffee or stimulants for energy

• Hot flashes or PMS

• Loss of menstrual cycle or prolonged cycle

If you think you have adrenal fatigue, do your best to decrease stress. If you hate your job, it's time to find a new one that will embrace your new lifestyle. One client of mine quit his job to become a fitness instructor. Man, he looks like a new person!

Evaluate relationships that are causing too much stress. Are some people in your life toxic and trying to demolish your health goals? It may be time to find more supportive people in your life.

Exercise can be a stressor, too. Do not plan on running a marathon in the middle of a divorce or after a death in the family. You produce only so much stress hormone each day. During a stressful time in your life, yoga (see page 42) is a much better fit.

## ☒ eating in stressful situations

Do you often have lunch meetings at work? Do you notice that you get indigestion or diarrhea after eating in a stressful situation? While you're under stress, your heart rate goes up, your blood pressure rises, and blood is forced away from your digestive system and moved to your legs, arms, and head for quick thinking. There can be as much as four times less blood flow to your digestive system, which means that your body can't burn calories as effectively. And enzymatic output in your intestines can be decreased by as much as 20,000-fold, which means that you can't absorb nutrients properly.

During stressful situations, triglycerides and cholesterol also increase, while healthy gut bacteria decrease. So you're more susceptible to indigestion, acid reflux, or heartburn.

It is also important to note that when your body is under stress, cortisol and insulin levels rise. When cortisol is consistently raised, you may have difficulty losing weight or building muscle. Belly fat is a common external sign of frequently elevated cortisol. What's scary about belly fat is that it is a prominent contributor to the development of diabetes and metabolic syndrome.

This is why I hate it when clients have business lunch meetings. It really messes with digestion. My suggestion: keep the meetings at work and enjoy a peaceful little break for lunch. Also, try not to eat after an argument; instead, try yoga for exercise—the blood flow is going to your extremities anyway!

# common things that can kick you out of ketosis

This list isn't meant to discourage you; it is to help you understand that everybody is different, and testing your personal carbohydrate tolerance is important (see page 28 for more on testing). Some people are so metabolically damaged that they need to lower their intake of carbohydrates and protein even more than others.

**An excess of "low-carb" vegetables such as cauliflower and Brussels sprouts.** Yes, these two veggies are low in carbs, but the carbs they do contain can add up fast. You cannot subtract fiber from the total carbohydrate count.

**Dairy.** For some people, dairy increases insulin and takes them out of ketosis. Dairy products, even plain full-fat yogurt, contain natural sugar. I never recommend milk because of the sugar.

**Low-sugar fruits, such as blueberries, strawberries, raspberries, and melons.** My client Sally loves berries and allows herself to enjoy them when they are in season. She knows that she can have ¼ cup, but if she pushes it to ½ cup, her blood sugar rises and she is kicked out of ketosis. But being able to have ¼ cup keeps her happy. Knowledge is power!

**Nuts and nut flours, such as almonds and almond flour**

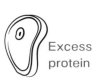
**Excess protein**

**Coconut water**

**Lemon or lime juice**

## the liver and weight loss

The liver is the main organ that governs fat loss. It processes hormones, rids cells of toxins, breaks down fats, and metabolizes carbohydrates and proteins. A liver that is constantly stressed by unhealthy food, alcohol, lack of sleep, or pollution gets tired and less capable of assisting you in your weight-loss efforts. Not only that, but low liver function causes food cravings, binge eating, and the excretion of too much cortisol, causing more liver stress. It is a vicious cycle! Antidepressants also cause more liver toxicity, which leads to more depression and further hinders your ability to lose weight.

Another important role of the liver is to ensure proper hormone balance. Estrogen dominance is a common issue. It comes from exposure to unhealthy external estrogens (found in nonorganic meat and milk, alcohol, and fructose, as well as plastics used to store food). A healthy liver detoxes estrogens. Disruptions in this process due to liver stress contribute to estrogen dominance, causing difficulty in losing belly fat. Too often we are told to calculate calories for weight loss, but I believe that it's all about hormone regulation. Insulin, estrogen, testosterone, leptin, ghrelin, glucagon, thyroid hormone, progesterone, cortisol, human growth hormone, and other hormones determine your rate of fat metabolism, cravings, energy level, sleep quality, and much more. If you fail to support your hormones, weight loss can be all but impossible, even if you run all day long and subsist on 500 calories a day.

The liver is also responsible for over half of the body's cholesterol production. Most of this cholesterol is used to produce bile, which breaks down fat. Bile salts stimulate the secretion of water into the large intestine, which helps with bowel movements. One sign of a stressed or tired liver is constipation. Here are some other signs of liver stress:

- Excess belly fat
- Fatty cysts
- Age spots
- Chronic indigestion
- Cellulite
- PMS or menopausal symptoms
- Low moods: depression/anxiety/irritability
- Muscle or joint pain
- Headaches or migraines
- Exhaustion

The good news is that the liver can heal rapidly when provided the right nutrients!

## experiencing low energy?

1. Have you increased your intake of salt and water? (See pages 30 and 48.)

2. Have you added electrolytes? (See page 30.)

3. Consider adding L-carnitine, an amino acid that increases energy, focus, and mood.

4. Are you sleeping at least 8 hours? (See pages 49 and 55.)

5. Are you low in iron? (See page 37.) Heavy periods, excessive exercise, antacids, and food allergies can all contribute to low iron levels.

6. How's your thyroid? If you have a low thyroid, you may not be able to absorb nutrients well, which can lead to low energy as well as low moods.

7. Is magnesium calming or energizing to you? Some people do better not taking it before bed. (See page 31.)

8. Are you mistakenly doing carb-ups? Or cheating on the weekends? Did you consume alcohol the night before? All three of these things cause low energy because your body doesn't know what fuel source to use, glucose or ketones. You will not benefit from the amazing energy that can come from being keto-adapted unless you commit to this lifestyle. But after 30 days of eating from this cookbook, you will feel so energized you will never want to go back!

# steps for success

Everyone is different when it comes to diet and weight loss. No two bodies are the same. I know that this book covers a lot of information, so I wanted to end this part with a checklist to help you be as successful as possible during your 30-day keto cleanse and beyond.

## ☑ get your liver as healthy as possible

The liver performs more than four hundred different jobs. It is the body's most important metabolism-enhancing organ: it clears the body of toxins, metabolizes protein, controls hormone balance, and enhances the immune system. It can even regenerate its own damaged cells! But it is not invincible. When the liver lacks essential nutrients or is overwhelmed by toxins, it no longer performs as it should.

The liver's most important function, and the one that puts it at the greatest risk for damage, is to filter the numerous toxins that attack our bodies. Working together with the lungs, kidneys, skin, and intestines, a healthy liver removes many damaging substances from the bloodstream. A tired liver may be to blame if you notice that you are on edge or easily stressed, or that you have elevated cholesterol, skin irritation, depression, sleep difficulties, indigestion, kidney damage, brain fog, hypothyroidism, chronic fatigue, weight gain, poor memory, PMS, blood sugar imbalances, or allergies.

If you have tried many ways to improve your health and energy level and nothing seems to help, it is possible that a tired liver is triggering your difficulties. Restoring liver function is one of the most essential actions you can take for your health. Here are some steps you can take to heal your liver:

• Eliminate fructose from your diet.

• Do not drink alcohol.

• **Eat cholesterol.** If you do not consume enough cholesterol, your liver will make the rest, keeping itself in overdrive.

• **Do not use topical chemicals** (see the appendix on page 408 for more information).

• **Get rid of obesogens** such as dryer sheets and scented candles.

• **Sweat! Sit in a sauna or practice hot yoga.** Just make sure to hydrate and refuel with electrolytes afterward.

## ☑ cut out all dairy, even high-fat dairy

Let me start by reminding you that I am a typical Wisconsin German girl. We love our cheese. But I also know that dairy prevents many of my clients from reaching their goals.

For the duration of your 30-day cleanse, skip the butter, cream, cheese, yogurt, and whey (including whey protein). I find that doing so helps many clients get to their goal weight. When you have an inflamed gut, a phenomenon called "atrophy of the villi" can occur, in which the villi that line the intestinal wall are damaged. Dairy is digested at the ends of the villi, so this condition damages the absorption of dairy. Once you heal the intestinal wall with an anti-inflammatory keto diet, you may be able to reincorporate dairy into your diet (in small amounts at first).

After your 30-day cleanse, conduct an experiment: weigh yourself the day before adding in some dairy and then again at the same time the next day. Try to stick to lactose-free dairy for this experiment to make sure that your weight isn't influenced by sugar (I would test with ghee or organic grass-fed butter). If the number on the scale goes up, don't panic; it's water retention. If water retention occurs, I suggest omitting all dairy for another two months and taking 3 grams of L-glutamine three times a day on an empty stomach to help heal the villi. Then try the test again.

## ☑ include overfeeding days

I'm not giving you permission to have a "cheat" day of Pizza Hut and Dairy Queen. An overfeeding day is a "healthified" high-calorie day in which you consume between 300 and 500 extra calories, mainly in the form of protein, to kick-start gluconeogenesis (the production of glucose in the body) and stimulate the thyroid. If you eat the same amount of calories every day, your thyroid may start to produce less T3, the activated thyroid hormone. You do need some sort of energy deficit, but if you have one every day for years, it may downgrade your thyroid. This is why an "overfeeding day" helps.

A lot of my clients choose Sunday for overfeeding because of the enormous amount of food served at family dinner. But I argue that you should focus on the conversation and enjoy the company. Many times we don't even remember the food we ate in large group settings. We also tend to swallow our food too soon in order to join the conversation.

I choose to overfeed when I have a slower day at work so I can chew slowly and enjoy every bite. The slower the food enters your body, the lower the insulin response will be. Walking after your meal also helps lower the insulin response.

When you overfeed, I recommend chewing your food so well that it is pretty much liquid before you swallow. I jokingly tell clients to chew thirty-two times before swallowing. I say "jokingly" because I don't really want them to count, but the number thirty-two sticks out. If you really try it, it is a lot of chewing!

## ☑ try intermittent fasting

Intermittent fasting is a pattern of eating in which you fast regularly (see page 33 for more). Craig and I limit our eating window every day; most days, our fast lasts about twenty hours, so we eat only in a four-hour window. For some people, however, this schedule is too extreme. Even a twelve-hour overnight fast, between dinner and breakfast, can be helpful. Trying to fit in daily intermittent fasting a few days a week is a great goal.

There are a lot of ways to incorporate fasting into your life. I suggest skipping dinner once or twice a week, maybe on a day you will get home late and would be eating too close to bedtime. I like this option because it stimulates human growth hormone to be at a high level when you fall asleep.

## ☑ eat fermented vegetables

I'm often asked, "How can Asians consume so much rice and noodles yet remain so thin?" The answer is that their meals often begin with kimchi and other fermented foods. Good gut bacteria help you digest food properly, can assist you with weight loss, and boost your immune system. A healthy body should have two pounds of good gut bacteria in the large intestine, but many people have none due to antibiotic use, stress, colonoscopies, or cleanses that deplete the body of this essential bacteria.

It's no wonder that I see so much depression in my office. The intestines are considered our bodies' second nervous system. You have the same amount of neurotransmitters in your gut as you do in your brain. When healthy gut bacteria are depleted, you become depleted of serotonin (the "feel-good" chemical), which causes you to be plagued with thoughts of sugar and carbohydrates. Low serotonin also causes low melatonin, which leads to poor sleep. I see this resolvable problem not only in adults, but in the majority of the children I work with, too. Cravings, depression, and sleepless nights do not have to be your fate!

Kimchi and other fermented vegetables have good gut bacteria called probiotics, which help populate and rebalance the gut flora. Studies have proven that probiotics can help heal a wide variety of ailments, such as depression, cancer, gut health, and allergies.

Yes, a lot of Asian dishes include rice or noodles, but the nutrition of those dishes must be applauded! A bowl of noodles is made with homemade beef marrow bone broth, tendons, and tripe. Asian cultures also consume large amounts of organ meats, such as beef tongue and liver.

So start your meals with fermented pickles, real sauerkraut, or kimchi to ensure proper gut balance, or take a quality probiotic that contains bifidobacteria. I assure you that the cravings will subside, your moods will be much more balanced, and your sleep will be much improved.

## ☑ cut out alcohol

Eliminating alcohol is important for sleep, mood, and metabolism. Alcohol does not help you get into ketosis; if anything, it holds you back from being your best self both physically and mentally. (See page 54 for more.)

## ☑ eliminate vegetable oils

Vegetable oils are very inflammatory and should be avoided. Most packaged foods, including marinara sauce, use canola, cottonseed, soybean, or corn oil. Even "healthy" mayonnaise, salad dressings, and roasted nuts are likely made with vegetable oils. Make your own instead using healthy fats!

## ☑ detox bad estrogens

Plastics are estrogenic. Avoid putting hot food on plastic plates or hot drinks in plastic cups. Do not microwave foods in plastic containers or drink from plastic water bottles. Eliminate nonorganic foods laced with synthetic estrogens. Eliminate obesogens such as dryer sheets and synthetic fragrances, which increase estrogen levels in women as well as men. Finally, go "number two" every day! If you don't, estrogens will be reabsorbed and locked into fat cells.

## ☑ benefit from the afterburn effect

Wait a little while to eat after a hard workout. Working out increases human growth hormone, which stimulates ketones. The afterburn effect can burn up to 400 more calories if you wait to eat. I suggest supplementing with BCAAs and L-glutamine to help repair muscles faster, then eat one hour after a hard workout.

## ☑ do not snack

If you are constantly fueling your body and increasing insulin, you cannot get into fat-burning mode. Do not eat every two hours; stick to regular meals.

## ☑ do not eat too much protein at one time

Your body cannot store protein. Any excess protein turns into sugar via gluconeogenesis. Split up your protein intake throughout the day.

## ☑ eat slowly

Eating slowly lowers the insulin response. It also helps register the hormone leptin, which gives you the signal that you are full.

## ☑ hydrate

Drinking half your body weight in ounces of water helps your kidneys and liver. When your kidneys are dehydrated, the liver stops doing its main jobs and helps out the kidneys instead. When you are well hydrated, your liver can focus on burning fat. Be nice to your liver!

## ☑ do not drink while eating

Hydration is important, but liquids dilute your digestive enzymes. Stop drinking an hour before a meal and start again an hour or two after a meal.

## ☑ avoid fluoride by drinking reverse-osmosis water and choosing organic foods

Many fruits, veggies, and other crops in the United States are sprayed with cryolite, a pesticide that contains a high amount of energy-zapping fluoride. Americans consume four times as much fluoride today as they did in 1940, when it was first added to drinking water to prevent cavities. It is found in many commercial products, like soup, soda, and black tea. Even the Centers for Disease Control (CDC) has expressed concern that over two hundred million Americans are exposed to extreme levels of fluoride. All this fluoride is wreaking havoc on our thyroids. To limit your exposure, drink reverse-osmosis water and opt for certified organic foods, which are not sprayed with pesticides.

## ☑ activate brown fat

There are two types of fat in the body. White adipose tissue (WAT) is what we normally refer to as body fat. You want to burn white fat. Brown adipose tissue (BAT) is beneficial because it helps your body burn calories and the unhealthy WAT. Cold stimulates BAT to burn excess fat and glucose for energy.

Here are some tips for activating brown fat:

• Place ice packs on your back or neck for 30 to 60 minutes while relaxing at night, when insulin levels are higher and more sensitive.

• Soak your feet in cold water at night or in the morning when you first wake up. This will stimulate heat throughout the day.

• Suck on ice cubes throughout the day.

• Have a snow cone for dessert made with flavored stevia drops, like root beer.

• Take a very cold shower upon waking.

• Lower the temperature in your house by five degrees.

## ☑ start oil pulling

I know it sounds crazy, but swishing coconut oil in your mouth for a few minutes a day—a practice known as oil pulling—is an easy, healthy, and tasty regimen. You just place a tablespoon of coconut oil in your mouth and swish it around as if it were mouthwash (if it's solid, it will melt in your mouth). My suggestion is to toss your mouthwash filled with chemicals and replace it with a jar of coconut oil.

Here are some compelling reasons to start oil pulling today:

• It removes bacteria, parasites, and toxins that live in your lymph system. Coconut oil has antimicrobial, anti-inflammatory, and enzymatic properties, which is why I suggest pulling with coconut oil over other oils. It helps kill *Streptococcus mutans,* an acid-producing bacterium that is a major cause of tooth decay. It also clears up *Candida,* which can cause thrush.

• It relieves sinus congestion and removes mucus from your throat.

• It remineralizes teeth and strengthens gums.

• It clears up skin issues like psoriasis by removing toxins, boosting the immune system.

## ☑ limit eating out

When did eating out become so common? I remember when eating at a restaurant was a rare Friday night treat. Now, if you walk into a restaurant at lunchtime, it is usually packed! Too often I hear complaints about the cost of eating healthy, when in reality eating out costs way more. My family went to brunch the other day, and we all got eggs and salmon with extra hollandaise, a side of chorizo, and a side of bacon. Craig got coffee, while the boys and I drank water. The bill was sixty-three dollars! For eggs! It is almost comical that the price of a carton of eggs had made me gasp at the store the day before.

    Control of ingredients is another reason to avoid eating out. You can never be sure which oils restaurants use for cooking, but most likely they are inflammatory vegetable oils. Inflammation-causing gluten and dairy also sneak into restaurant dishes; for example, meats are often marinated in soy sauce, which contains gluten.

## ☑ stop the negative self-talk

Tell yourself that you can do it, and surround yourself with positive people who will support you on your journey. Even an online support group can help you stay on course.

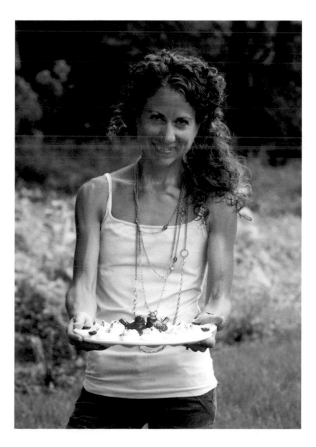

## in conclusion

With all this information in hand, I wish you luck on these first thirty days of your keto journey. I know that the ketogenic lifestyle may seem overwhelming and new, but try one new thing a week; maybe this week you will change your breakfast from cereal to eggs, and next week you'll start walking after dinner. Baby steps are what worked for me. Instead of feeling overwhelmed, feel empowered by having the tools you need for a successful trip. No more deprivation diets consisting of fat-free, man-made foods: a ketogenic diet means real food, real satisfaction, and a healthy metabolism.

If you are a visual learner like myself or want more information, I offer many Skype and online video classes at MariaMindBodyHealth.com/video-classes/

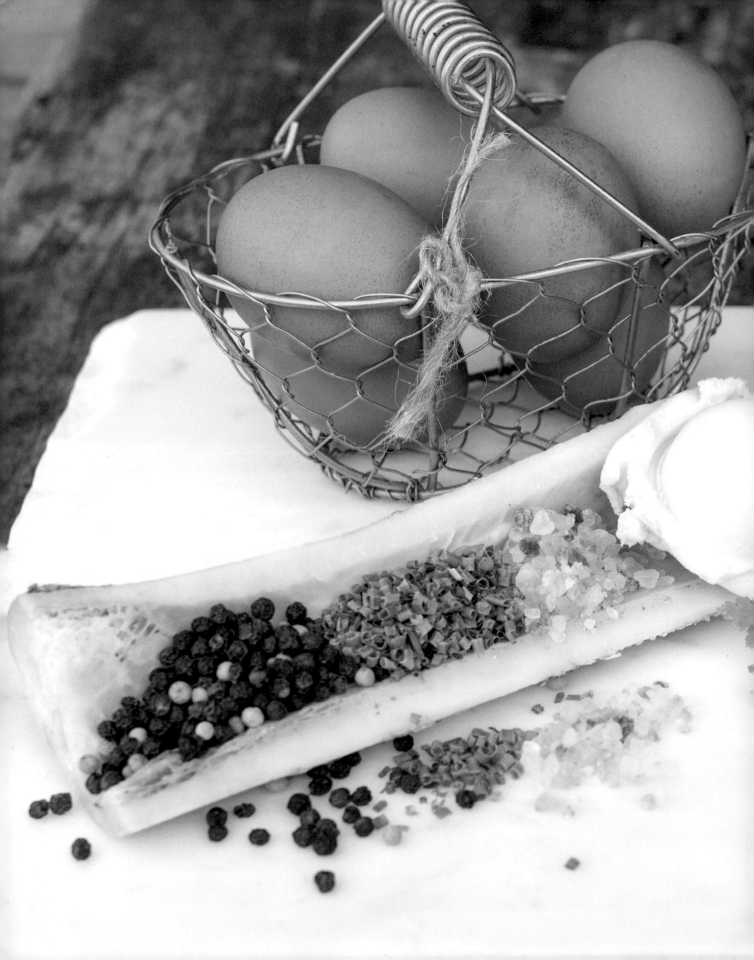

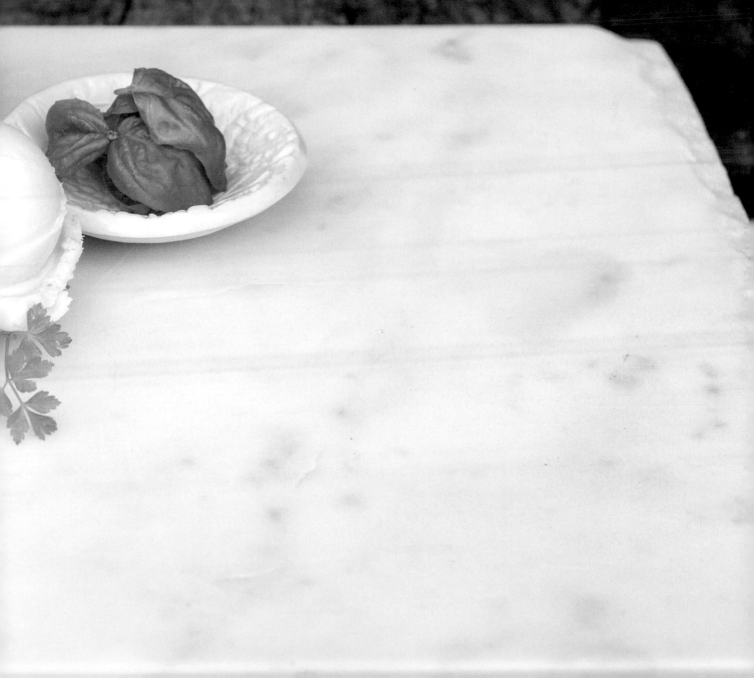

# PART 2:
# the ketogenic kitchen

# ingredients

The key to any healthy diet is eating real, whole foods. For your 30-day keto cleanse, you'll want to seek out certain ingredients and avoid others.

## fats

On a keto diet, you need lots of healthy fat to burn as fuel. But as important as it is to seek out healthy fats, it's just as important to avoid unhealthy fats.

### healthy fats

Fats with high amounts of saturated fatty acids (SFAs)—such as MCT oil, coconut oil, tallow, and lard—are best: they are stable and anti-inflammatory, protect against oxidation, and have many other important health benefits. Look for grass-fed and organic sources; these are always best. Try to avoid polyunsaturated fatty acids (PUFAs): they are prone to oxidation and are therefore less healthy. (We'll talk more about unhealthy fats on page 71.)

On the facing page is a list of the best oils and fats to use, with their SFA and PUFA content. When you see "Paleo fat" mentioned in a recipe in this book, it's fine to use any of these fats—just make sure to take into account whether you need it for a hot or a cold use.

---

### MCT oil

*MCT stands for "medium-chain triglycerides," which are chains of fatty acids. MCTs are found naturally in coconut oil, palm oil, and dairy, and they're particularly helpful on a keto diet because the body uses them quickly and any MCTs not immediately utilized by the body are converted to ketones.*

*MCT oil is extracted from coconut or palm oil and contains a higher, concentrated level of MCTs, so it's great for adding ketones to your diet. Whenever MCT oil appears in a recipe in this book, it's always my first choice, but to make the recipes as accessible as possible, I've provided alternative oil choices as well.*

| Fat | SFA | PUFA | Notes |
|---|---|---|---|
| Almond oil | 8.2% | 17% | • Has a mild, neutral flavor<br>• Works great for sweet dishes and Thai dishes<br>• Use in nonheat applications, such as salad dressings<br>• Can also be used on the skin |
| Avocado oil | 11% | 10% | • Has a mild, neutral flavor<br>• Works great for savory and sweet dishes, as well as Thai dishes<br>• Can be heated |
| Beef tallow | 49.8% | 3.1% | • Has a mild beef flavor<br>• Works great for savory dishes<br>• Can be heated |
| Cocoa butter | 60% | 3% | • Has a mild coconut flavor<br>• Works great for sweet and savory cooking<br>• Can be heated |
| Coconut oil | 92% | 1.9% | • Has a strong coconut flavor<br>• Works great for sweet dishes and Thai dishes<br>• Can be heated<br>• Can also be used on the skin |
| Duck fat | 25% | 13% | • Has a rich duck flavor<br>• Works great for frying savory foods<br>• Can be heated |
| Extra-virgin olive oil* | 14% | 9.9% | • Has a strong olive flavor<br>• Works great for Italian salad dressings<br>• Use in nonheat applications, such as salad dressings |
| Hazelnut oil | 10% | 14% | • Has a mild hazelnut flavor<br>• Works great for sweet dishes and Thai dishes<br>• Use in nonheat applications, such as salad dressings |
| High oleic sunflower oil | 8% | 9% | • Has a mild sunflower seed flavor<br>• Works great for sweet dishes and Thai dishes<br>• Use in nonheat applications, such as salad dressings |
| Lard | 41% | 12% | • Has a mild flavor<br>• Works great for frying sweet or savory foods<br>• Can be heated |
| Macadamia nut oil | 15% | 10% | • Has a mild nutty flavor<br>• Works great for salad dressings<br>• Use in nonheat applications, such as salad dressings |
| MCT oil** | 97% | less than 1% | • Has a neutral flavor<br>• Works in savory dishes and baked goods<br>• Can be heated to low or moderate heat (no higher than 320°F) |
| Palm kernel oil*** | 82% | 2% | • Has a neutral flavor<br>• Works great for baking<br>• Can be heated |

*Extra-virgin olive oil is great for cold applications, such as salad dressings, but do not use it for cooking; heat causes the oil to oxidize, which is harmful to your health.

**MCT oil can be found at most health food stores, but if you have trouble finding it, you can use avocado oil, macadamia nut oil, or extra-virgin olive oil instead, keeping in mind that avocado oil is the most neutral-flavored of the three.

***Be sure to purchase sustainably sourced and processed palm kernel oil. There are ecological concerns associated with some palm oils.

On the 30-day cleanse, I recommend avoiding all dairy—it's not included in any of the recipes in this book. Omitting dairy entirely for those thirty days gives the gut a chance to heal from any irritation or inflammation dairy may have caused.

If at the end of the cleanse you want to try adding dairy back to your diet, choose just one item and see how your body responds to it over two or three days. If you don't have any reaction, chances are you're not dairy sensitive.

If you're not dairy sensitive, the following are great healthy, keto-friendly dairy fats to add to your diet:

| Fat | SFA | PUFA |
|---|---|---|
| Butter | 50% | 3.4% |
| Ghee* | 48% | 4% |
| Heavy cream | 62% | 4% |
| Cream cheese | 56% | 4% |
| Cheese | 64% | 3% |
| Sour cream | 58% | 4% |
| Crème fraîche | 64% | 3% |

*Although I recommend avoiding ghee during your 30-day cleanse, it can be a good fat to use even if you are dairy sensitive because the milk proteins have been removed.

## purchasing keto-friendly ingredients

*You can purchase keto-friendly pantry products on my website, MariaMindBodyHealth.com/store. They're also available in most grocery stores.*

*To save money, I recommend buying ingredients in bulk—including perishables like meat and fresh veggies. They can be frozen (a chest freezer is a great investment) and thawed later.*

*Remember, choosing the best-quality organic foods is always optimal.*

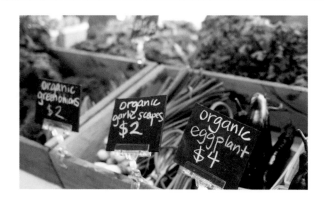

## bad fats

Two kinds of fats should be avoided on a ketogenic diet: trans fats and polyunsaturated fatty acids (PUFAs).

Trans fats are the most inflammatory fats; in fact, they are among the worst substances for our health that we can consume. Many studies have shown that eating foods containing trans fats increases the risk of heart disease and cancer.

Here is a list of trans fats to avoid at all costs:

· Hydrogenated or partially hydrogenated oils (check ingredient labels)

· Margarine

· Vegetable shortening

PUFAs should also be limited, as they are prone to oxidation. Many cooking oils are high in PUFAs. At right is a list of the most common ones.

| Fat | PUFA |
| --- | --- |
| Grapeseed oil | 70.6% |
| Sunflower oil | 68% |
| Flax oil | 66% |
| Safflower oil | 65% |
| Soybean oil | 58% |
| Corn oil | 54.6% |
| Walnut oil | 53.9% |
| Cottonseed oil | 52.4% |
| Vegetable oil | 51.4% |
| Sesame oil | 42% |
| Peanut oil | 33.4% |
| Canola oil | 19% |

# proteins

It's always best to choose grass-fed, humanely raised meat and wild-caught seafood. Not only do they offer more nutrients, but they also haven't been exposed to added hormones, antibiotics, or other potential toxins. (For help choosing sustainably sourced seafood, check out the Monterey Bay Aquarium Seafood Watch app and website, seafoodwatch.org.)

**WILD MEATS**
- Bear
- Boar
- Buffalo
- Elk
- Rabbit
- Venison

BEEF

GOAT

LAMB

PORK

**FISH**
- Ahi/mahi mahi
- Catfish
- Halibut
- Herring
- Mackerel
- Salmon
- Sardines
- Snapper
- Swordfish
- Trout
- Tuna
- Walleye
- White fish (cod, bluegill)

**SEAFOOD/ SHELLFISH**
- Clams
- Crab
- Lobster
- Mussels
- Oysters
- Prawns
- Scallops
- Shrimp
- Snails

**POULTRY**
- Chicken liver
- Duck
- Game hens
- Goose
- Ostrich
- Partridge
- Pheasant
- Quail
- Squab
- Turkey

**EGGS**
- Chicken eggs
- Duck eggs
- Goose eggs
- Ostrich eggs
- Quail eggs

NUTRITIONAL INFO (per 4 ounces)

| Pork | CALORIES | FAT | PROTEIN | CARBS | FIBER | % FAT | % PROTEIN | % CARBS |
|---|---|---|---|---|---|---|---|---|
| Chop | 241 | 12.0 | 33.0 | 0.0 | 0.0 | 45% | 55% | 0% |
| Loin | 265 | 15.5 | 30.8 | 0.0 | 0.0 | 53% | 46% | 0% |
| Pork hocks | 285 | 24.0 | 17.0 | 0.0 | 0.0 | 76% | 24% | 0% |
| Leg ham | 305 | 20.0 | 30.4 | 0.0 | 0.0 | 59% | 40% | 0% |
| Rump | 280 | 16.2 | 32.8 | 0.0 | 0.0 | 52% | 47% | 0% |
| Tenderloin | 158 | 4.0 | 30.0 | 0.0 | 0.0 | 23% | 76% | 0% |
| Middle ribs (country style) | 245 | 16.0 | 25.0 | 0.0 | 0.0 | 59% | 41% | 0% |
| Loin back ribs (baby back ribs) | 315 | 27.0 | 18.0 | 0.0 | 0.0 | 77% | 23% | 0% |
| Belly | 588 | 60.0 | 10.4 | 0.0 | 0.0 | 92% | 7% | 0% |
| Shoulder | 285 | 23.0 | 19.0 | 0.0 | 0.0 | 73% | 27% | 0% |
| Butt | 240 | 18.0 | 19.0 | 0.0 | 0.0 | 68% | 32% | 0% |
| Bacon | 600 | 47.2 | 41.8 | 0.0 | 0.0 | 71% | 28% | 0% |

NUTRITIONAL INFO (per 4 ounces)

| Beef Cuts | CALORIES | FAT | PROTEIN | CARBS | FIBER | % FAT | % PROTEIN | % CARBS |
|---|---|---|---|---|---|---|---|---|
| Rib eye | 310 | 25.0 | 20.0 | 0.0 | 0.0 | 73% | 26% | 0% |
| Rib roast | 373 | 28.0 | 27.0 | 0.0 | 0.0 | 69% | 30% | 0% |
| Beef back ribs | 310 | 26.0 | 19.0 | 0.0 | 0.0 | 75% | 25% | 0% |
| Porterhouse | 280 | 22.0 | 21.0 | 0.0 | 0.0 | 70% | 30% | 0% |
| T-bone | 170 | 12.2 | 15.8 | 0.0 | 0.0 | 64% | 36% | 0% |
| Top loin steak | 270 | 20.0 | 21.0 | 0.0 | 0.0 | 67% | 31% | 0% |
| Tenderloin roast | 180 | 8.0 | 25.0 | 0.0 | 0.0 | 40% | 56% | 0% |
| Tenderloin steak | 122 | 3.0 | 22.2 | 0.0 | 0.0 | 60% | 40% | 0% |
| Tri tip roast | 340 | 29.0 | 18.0 | 0.0 | 0.0 | 77% | 21% | 0% |
| Tri tip steak | 200 | 11.0 | 23.0 | 0.0 | 0.0 | 50% | 46% | 0% |
| Top sirloin steak | 240 | 16.0 | 22.0 | 0.0 | 0.0 | 60% | 37% | 0% |
| Top round steak | 180 | 9.0 | 25.0 | 0.0 | 0.0 | 45% | 56% | 0% |
| Bottom round roast | 220 | 14.0 | 23.0 | 0.0 | 0.0 | 57% | 42% | 0% |
| Bottom round steak | 220 | 14.0 | 23.0 | 0.0 | 0.0 | 57% | 42% | 0% |
| Eye round roast | 253 | 13.4 | 32.0 | 0.0 | 0.0 | 48% | 51% | 0% |
| Eye round steak | 182 | 9.0 | 25.0 | 0.0 | 0.0 | 45% | 55% | 0% |
| Round tip roast | 199 | 12.0 | 22.9 | 0.0 | 0.0 | 54% | 46% | 0% |
| Round tip steak | 150 | 6.0 | 23.5 | 0.0 | 0.0 | 36% | 63% | 0% |
| Sirloin tip center roast | 190 | 7.0 | 31.0 | 0.0 | 0.0 | 33% | 65% | 0% |
| Sirloin tip center steak | 190 | 7.0 | 31.0 | 0.0 | 0.0 | 33% | 65% | 0% |
| Sirloin tip side steak | 190 | 6.0 | 34.0 | 0.0 | 0.0 | 28% | 72% | 0% |
| Skirt steak | 255 | 16.5 | 27.0 | 0.0 | 0.0 | 58% | 42% | 0% |
| Flank steak | 200 | 8.0 | 32.0 | 0.0 | 0.0 | 36% | 64% | 0% |
| Shank cross cut | 215 | 6.7 | 38.7 | 0.0 | 0.0 | 28% | 72% | 0% |
| Brisket flat cut | 245 | 14.7 | 28.0 | 0.0 | 0.0 | 54% | 46% | 0% |
| Chuck 7 bone pot roast | 240 | 14.0 | 28.0 | 0.0 | 0.0 | 53% | 47% | 0% |
| Chuck boneless pot roast | 240 | 14.0 | 28.0 | 0.0 | 0.0 | 53% | 47% | 0% |
| Chuck steak boneless | 160 | 8.0 | 22.0 | 0.0 | 0.0 | 45% | 55% | 0% |
| Chuck eye steak | 250 | 18.0 | 21.0 | 0.0 | 0.0 | 65% | 34% | 0% |
| Shoulder top blade steak | 204 | 13.0 | 22.0 | 0.0 | 0.0 | 57% | 43% | 0% |
| Shoulder top blade flat iron | 204 | 13.0 | 22.0 | 0.0 | 0.0 | 57% | 43% | 0% |
| Shoulder pot roast | 185 | 7.0 | 30.7 | 0.0 | 0.0 | 34% | 66% | 0% |
| Shoulder steak | 204 | 12.0 | 24.0 | 0.0 | 0.0 | 53% | 47% | 0% |
| Shoulder center ranch steak | 152 | 8.0 | 24.0 | 0.0 | 0.0 | 40% | 60% | 0% |
| Shoulder petite tender | 150 | 7.0 | 22.0 | 0.0 | 0.0 | 42% | 59% | 0% |
| Shoulder petite tender medallions | 150 | 7.0 | 22.0 | 0.0 | 0.0 | 42% | 59% | 0% |
| Boneless short ribs | 440 | 41.0 | 16.0 | 0.0 | 0.0 | 84% | 15% | 0% |

NUTRITIONAL INFO (per 4 ounces)

| Fish | CALORIES | FAT | PROTEIN | CARBS | FIBER | % FAT | % PROTEIN | % CARBS |
|---|---|---|---|---|---|---|---|---|
| Tuna (yellowfin) | 150 | 1.5 | 34.0 | 0.0 | 0.0 | 9% | 91% | 0% |
| Tuna (canned) | 123 | 0.8 | 27.5 | 1.5 | 0.0 | 6% | 89% | 5% |
| Salmon | 206 | 9.0 | 31.0 | 0.0 | 0.0 | 39% | 60% | 0% |
| Anchovies | 256 | 15.9 | 28.0 | 0.0 | 0.0 | 56% | 44% | 0% |
| Sardines | 139 | 7.5 | 18.0 | 0.0 | 0.0 | 49% | 52% | 0% |
| Barramundi | 110 | 2.0 | 23.0 | 0.0 | 0.0 | 16% | 84% | 0% |
| Trout | 190 | 8.6 | 28.0 | 0.0 | 0.0 | 41% | 59% | 0% |
| Walleye | 156 | 7.5 | 22.0 | 0.0 | 0.0 | 43% | 56% | 0% |
| Cod | 113 | 1.0 | 26.0 | 0.0 | 0.0 | 8% | 92% | 0% |
| Sea bass | 135 | 3.0 | 27.0 | 0.0 | 0.0 | 20% | 80% | 0% |
| Halibut | 155 | 3.5 | 30.7 | 0.0 | 0.0 | 20% | 79% | 0% |
| Mackerel | 290 | 20.3 | 27.0 | 0.0 | 0.0 | 63% | 37% | 0% |
| Arctic Char | 208 | 10.0 | 29.0 | 0.0 | 0.0 | 43% | 56% | 0% |

NUTRITIONAL INFO (per 4 ounces)

| Seafood/Shellfish | CALORIES | FAT | PROTEIN | CARBS | FIBER | % FAT | % PROTEIN | % CARBS |
|---|---|---|---|---|---|---|---|---|
| Scallops | 97 | 1.0 | 19.0 | 3.0 | 0.0 | 9% | 78% | 12% |
| Mussels | 97 | 2.8 | 13.5 | 4.5 | 0.0 | 26% | 56% | 19% |
| Clams | 82 | 1.1 | 15.0 | 3.0 | 0.0 | 12% | 73% | 15% |
| Shrimp | 135 | 2.0 | 25.8 | 1.7 | 0.0 | 18% | 78% | 4% |
| Oysters | 58 | 1.9 | 6.5 | 3.1 | 0.0 | 29% | 33% | 38% |
| Crab | 107 | 2.0 | 22.0 | 0.0 | 0.0 | 17% | 82% | 0% |
| Lobster | 116 | 1.8 | 25.0 | 0.0 | 0.0 | 14% | 86% | 0% |
| Caviar | 260 | 12.0 | 31.0 | 8.0 | 0.0 | 42% | 48% | 12% |

NUTRITIONAL INFO (per 4 ounces)

| Chicken and Poultry | CALORIES | FAT | PROTEIN | CARBS | FIBER | % FAT | % PROTEIN | % CARBS |
|---|---|---|---|---|---|---|---|---|
| Chicken breast, skinless | 138 | 4.0 | 25.0 | 0.0 | 0.0 | 26% | 72% | 0% |
| Chicken breast, skin on | 200 | 8.4 | 31.0 | 0.0 | 0.0 | 38% | 62% | 0% |
| Chicken leg, skinless | 210 | 9.5 | 30.7 | 0.0 | 0.0 | 41% | 58% | 0% |
| Chicken leg, skin on | 266 | 15.2 | 29.4 | 0.0 | 0.0 | 54% | 46% | 0% |
| Chicken thigh, skinless | 165 | 10.0 | 19.0 | 0.0 | 0.0 | 55% | 46% | 0% |
| Chicken thigh, skin on | 275 | 17.6 | 28.3 | 0.0 | 0.0 | 58% | 41% | 0% |
| Chicken wings | 320 | 22.0 | 30.4 | 0.0 | 0.0 | 62% | 38% | 0% |
| Drumstick | 178 | 9.9 | 22.0 | 0.0 | 0.0 | 50% | 49% | 0% |
| Game hen | 220 | 16.0 | 19.0 | 0.0 | 0.0 | 65% | 35% | 0% |
| Pheasant | 200 | 10.5 | 25.7 | 0.0 | 0.0 | 47% | 51% | 0% |
| Turkey | 175 | 9.9 | 21.0 | 0.0 | 0.0 | 51% | 48% | 0% |
| Goose | 340 | 24.9 | 28.5 | 0.0 | 0.0 | 66% | 34% | 0% |
| Duck | 228 | 13.9 | 26.3 | 0.0 | 0.0 | 55% | 46% | 0% |

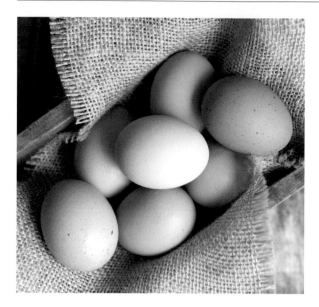

## picking the best-quality eggs

*Eggs are an amazingly nutritious food, especially the yolks, which are full of choline, healthy fats, and a ton of flavor. And high-quality eggs–those from healthy, humanely raised hens–are even more nourishing and tastier. So which eggs are the best quality?*

**Brown or White Eggs:** *There's absolutely no difference in quality here; the only thing that determines the color of an egg is the breed of the hen. Do not choose eggs based on color.*

**Egg Grades:** *Eggs can be AA, A, or B. There is little to no difference in the taste, though, and no difference in nutritional value. Grade AA eggs have the thickest, firmest whites and high, round yolks. This grade of egg is virtually free of defects and is best for frying, poaching, or methods where presentation is important. Grade A eggs are the same quality as grade AA, but the white is categorized as "reasonably" firm. Most grade B eggs are sold to restaurants, bakeries, and other food institutions and are used to make liquid, frozen, and dried egg products.*

**Vegetarian-Fed:** *The only thing this label means is that the hens are fed a diet based on corn (which is usually genetically modified). In order to ensure the hens only consume a vegetarian diet, they are kept in cages. But chickens are naturally omnivores: they evolved to eat insects, worms, and grubs as well as grass and grains. They weren't meant to be vegetarians!*

**Certified Organic:** *This label means that the hens are not in cages but in barns. They are required to have access to the sun, but that does not necessarily mean they can go outside; there may be a small window in the barn for sunlight. The hens are fed an organic, vegetarian diet that is free from antibiotics and pesticides. This label is regulated with inspections.*

**Free-Range or Cage-Free:** *This sounds like a good choice, right? Well, all this really means is that the hens are not caged. There is no requirement to let the hens outside, there are no mandatory inspections to regulate this claim, and there are no guidelines for what the birds are fed.*

**Omega-3 Enriched:** *This label indicates that the hens' feed has extra omega-3 fatty acids added to it in the form of flaxseed. But eggs already are a good source of omega-3s, so there's no need to seek out eggs with this label.*

*Since most of the labels used on egg cartons don't really help us figure out which eggs are healthiest, here are some guidelines to follow when egg shopping:*

**1.** *Be conscious of antibiotic and hormone use. While the USDA prohibits the use of hormones for egg production and the use of therapeutic antibiotics is illegal unless hens are ill, these rules aren't always enforced. The only way to ensure that the hens were antibiotic-free is to purchase organic eggs.*

**2.** *To guarantee that you eat truly free-range eggs, purchase eggs from pastured hens. Pastured hens are able to eat their natural diet of greens, seeds, worms, and bugs, and studies show that eggs from pastured hens may contain more omega-3 fatty acids, vitamins, and minerals.*

**3.** *Smaller eggs tend to have thicker shells than large eggs and are less likely to become contaminated by bacteria.*

**4.** *Be cautious of unregulated labels. Terms like "natural" and "cage-free" are often used in labeling, but these claims may not necessarily be true. Claims on eggs with the USDA shield have been verified by the Department of Agriculture, so always look for the shield when you purchase eggs from a store.*

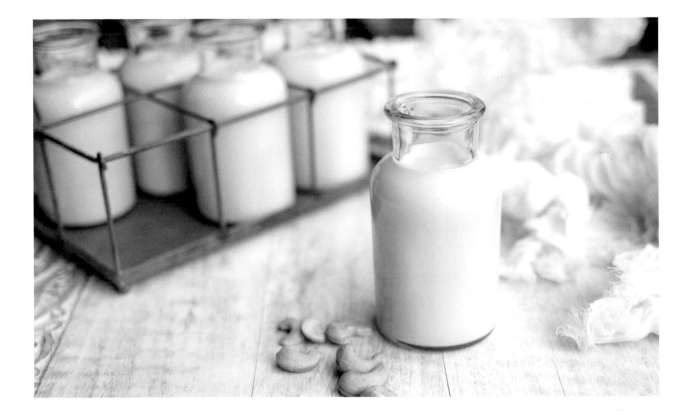

## liquids

It probably goes without saying that sodas and fruit juices should be avoided during your keto cleanse—they're full of sugars that will raise your blood sugar and kick you out of ketosis. But that doesn't mean you're limited to just water! The following are all liquids you can consume during your cleanse.

- Unsweetened almond milk
- Unsweetened cashew milk
- Unsweetened coconut milk
- Unsweetened hemp milk
- Green tea

- Organic decaf caffè Americano (espresso with water)
- Mineral water
- Water (reverse osmosis is best)

## nuts and seeds

Some nuts and seeds are fine on a keto diet, but they can take some people with metabolic syndrome out of ketosis. For that reason, I do not recommend that you consume nuts and seeds during your 30-day cleanse, and I do not use them in the recipes in this book.

# veggies

Fresh vegetables are packed with nutrients and are an important part of a keto cleanse, but to make sure you stay in ketosis, it's important to choose nonstarchy vegetables, which are lower in carbs. The following are some of the nonstarchy vegetables that I use most.

- Arugula
- Asparagus
- Bok choy
- Broccoli
- Cabbage
- Cauliflower
- Celery
- Collard greens

- Cucumber
- Endive
- Garlic
- Kale
- Kelp
- Lettuce: red leaf, Boston, romaine, radicchio
- Mushrooms

- Onions: green, yellow, white, red
- Peppers: bell peppers, jalapeños, chiles
- Seaweed
- Swiss chard
- Watercress

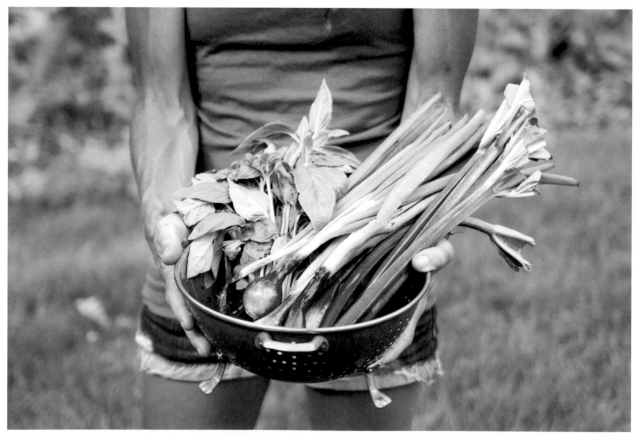

# herbs and spices

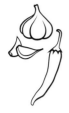

Spices and fresh herbs are the most nutritious plants you can consume. For example, everyone thinks spinach is an amazingly nutritious food, but fresh oregano has eight times its amount of antioxidants! Sure, we don't eat a cup of oregano, but it does go to show that a little bit of an herb provides a huge benefit.

- Anise
- Annatto
- Basil
- Bay leaf
- Black pepper
- Caraway
- Cardamom
- Cayenne pepper
- Celery seed
- Chervil
- Chili pepper
- Chives
- Cilantro
- Cinnamon

- Cloves
- Coriander
- Cumin
- Curry
- Dill
- Fenugreek
- Galangal
- Garlic
- Ginger
- Lemongrass
- Licorice
- Mace
- Marjoram
- Mint

- Mustard seeds
- Oregano
- Paprika
- Parsley
- Peppermint
- Rosemary
- Saffron
- Sage
- Spearmint
- Star anise
- Tarragon
- Thyme
- Turmeric
- Vanilla beans

# fruit

We tend to think of fruit as a health food, but in reality, most fruits are full of carbs and sugar. In fact, studies prove that the produce we consume today is lower in nutrients and much higher in sugar than it was in Paleolithic times. In general, high-sugar fruits like grapes, bananas, and mangoes should be avoided during your keto cleanse.

But that doesn't mean you have to avoid all fruits! I once made a keto fruit salad filled with cucumbers, olives, eggplant, and capers, all covered in a Greek vinaigrette. So yes, fruits are certainly allowed. Just seek out those that are low in sugar.

- Avocados
- Cucumbers
- Eggplants

- Lemons
- Limes
- Olives

- Seasonal wild berries (in moderation)
- Tomatoes

# the pantry

In addition to the whole foods discussed in the previous pages, some pantry items are essential for making the recipes in this book.

## baking products

See page 79 for recommended sweeteners.

- Baking soda
- Blanched almond flour
- Cocoa butter
- Coconut flour
- Egg white protein powder (check carbs and added ingredients—I recommend Jay Robb brand)

- Extracts and essential oils, including pure vanilla extract, for flavoring
- Pecan meal
- Unsweetened baking chocolate
- Unsweetened cocoa powder

- Whey protein powder (check carbs and added ingredients; do not use if dairy sensitive)
- Xanthan gum and guar gum

## sauces and flavor enhancers

- Coconut aminos
- Coconut vinegar
- Fish sauce

## egg replacer

*The only keto egg replacer that I recommend is gelatin. Chia and flax seeds are not recommended because of their estrogenic properties as well as their high total carb count.*

## canned and jarred pantry foods

It is always better to buy fresh, but here are some keto-friendly foods that are also great jarred or canned:

- Banana peppers
- Bell peppers
- Boxed beef and chicken broth
- Canned coconut milk
- Canned salmon
- Canned tuna
- Capers
- EPIC bars (made from grass-fed meat—but check for added sugars)

- Fermented pickles*
- Fermented sauerkraut*
- Mikey's English Muffins
- Nori wraps
- Olives (choose jar over can)
- Organic dried spices
- Paleo mayo
- Pickled eggs
- Pickled herring

- Pizza sauce (check for oils and added sugar)
- Pure Wraps
- Quality marinara sauce (check for oils and added sugar)**
- Sardines
- Tomato paste**
- Tomato sauce**

*Not only is fermenting a great way to preserve food, but it also creates beneficial gut bacteria and helpful digestive enzymes. Fermented sauerkraut is particularly rich in B vitamins.*

**Make sure to buy jarred, not canned, tomato products. The lining of cans contains BPA, a chemical that's associated with several health problems and may affect children's development, and tomatoes' high acidity can cause more BPA to leach into the food.*

# natural sweeteners

| | |
|---|---|
| Stevia with no additives | 0 |
| Stevia glycerite | 0 |
| Swerve | 0 |
| Erythritol | 0 |
| Monk fruit | 0 |
| Yacón syrup | 1 |
| Xylitol | 7 |
| Agave | 13 |
| Maple syrup | 54 |
| Honey | 62 |
| Table sugar | 68 |
| Splenda | 80 |
| HFCS | 87 |

In my recipes, I always use natural sweeteners. Just as sugarcane and honey are found in nature, so are erythritol and the stevia herb.

However, I prefer not to use sweeteners such as honey, maple syrup, and agave in my recipes because, even though they're natural, they raise blood sugar, which not only causes inflammation but will also take you out of ketosis. (A list of where common sweeteners fall on the glycemic index is at right.)

Fructose is particularly problematic. More than glucose, it promotes a chemical reaction called glycation, which results in advanced glycation end products (AGEs). AGEs form a sort of crust around cells that has been linked with a wide range of diseases, from diabetes and heart disease to asthma, polycystic ovary syndrome, and Alzheimer's. Fructose also contributes to nonalcoholic fatty liver disease. For these reasons, I avoid sweeteners high in fructose: table sugar, high-fructose corn syrup, honey, agave, and fruit.

The following is a list of the natural sweeteners that I recommend, all of which have little effect on blood sugar. I'll talk in more detail about each below.

- Erythritol, such as Sukrin brand
- Swerve brand sweetener
- Stevia, liquid or powdered (with no additives)
- Stevia glycerite (thick liquid stevia)
- Monk fruit
- Xylitol
- Yacón syrup

## erythritol

Despite its chemical-sounding name, erythritol is not an artificial sweetener. It's a sugar alcohol that is found naturally in some fruits and fermented foods. Erythritol is a calorie-free sweetener that doesn't raise blood sugar or insulin, and because it's almost completely absorbed before it reaches the colon, it doesn't cause digestive upset the way other sugar alcohols can.

Erythritol is generally available in granulated form, though sometimes you can find it powdered. If you purchase granulated erythritol, I recommend grinding it to a powder before using. In its granulated form, erythritol doesn't dissolve well and can give dishes a grainy texture.

## monk fruit

Also known as lo han kuo, monk fruit is cultivated in the mountains of southern China. Similar to stevia, it's 300 times sweeter than sugar, but unlike stevia, it doesn't have a bitter aftertaste. Monk fruit comes in pure liquid form and in powdered form.

Since it is so much sweeter than sugar, the powdered form of monk fruit is typically bulked up with another sweetener so that it measures cup for cup like sugar. Check the ingredients for things like maltodextrin and only buy brands that use keto-friendly sweeteners, such as erythritol.

### stevia

Stevia is available as a powder or a liquid. Because stevia is so concentrated, many companies add bulking agents like maltodextrin to powdered stevia so that it's easier to bake with. Stay away from those products. Table sugar has a glycemic index of 52, whereas maltodextrin has a glycemic index of 110!

Look for products that contain just stevia or stevia combined with another natural and keto-friendly sweetener.

### stevia glycerite

Stevia glycerite is a thick liquid form of stevia that is similar in consistency to honey. Do not confuse it with liquid stevia, which is much more concentrated. Stevia glycerite is about twice as sweet as sugar, making it a bit less sweet than pure liquid or powdered stevia. I prefer to use stevia glycerite because, unlike the powdered or liquid forms of stevia, it has no bitter aftertaste.

Stevia glycerite is great for cooking because it maintains flavor that many other sweeteners lose when heated. However, it doesn't caramelize or create bulk, so most baking recipes call for combining it with another sweetener.

### swerve brand sweetener

Swerve is zero-calorie brand of sweetener that combines erythritol (see page 79) and oligosaccharides, which are prebiotic fibers found in starchy root vegetables. Swerve is nonglycemic and therefore does not affect blood sugar. It also measures cup for cup just like table sugar.

I use the powdered form of Swerve (the one labeled "confectioners") because it dissolves particularly well when cooking or baking. Swerve even browns and caramelizes like sugar.

### xylitol

Xylitol is a naturally occurring low-calorie sweetener found in fruits and vegetables. It has a minimal effect on blood sugar and insulin. While it's not as low on the glycemic index as erythritol, erythritol doesn't work well for low-carb hard candies (it doesn't melt properly), so I use xylitol instead.

Xylitol has been known to kick some people out of ketosis, so if you're using it for baking or cooking, monitor your ketones closely and stop using it if you find that you're no longer in ketosis.

### yacón syrup

Yacón syrup is a thick syrup that is pressed from the yacón root and tastes a bit like molasses. It has been consumed for centuries in Peru.

I use yacón syrup sparingly, both because it is very expensive and because it has some fructose in it. A small jar lasts us four to six months. I use a tablespoon here and there to improve the texture and flavor of my sauces; it's ideal for giving sweet-and-sour sauce that perfect mouthfeel or giving BBQ sauce a hint of molasses. Using these small amounts keeps the sugar to 1 gram or so per serving.

## using sweeteners in the recipes in this book

If you're trying keto for the first time on your 30-day keto cleanse, the recipes in this book should have just the right amount of sweetness. But if you continue on with the ketogenic lifestyle, you may find that food naturally begins to taste sweeter, and you may want to reduce the amount of sweetener used in a recipe.

Whenever a recipe requires a powdered sweetener, my go-to choice is the natural sugar replacement called Swerve, which is available in granular and powdered form. I always use the powdered (confectioners') form of Swerve because it gives you a smoother finished product and better overall results. That said, you can always pulverize a granular form of erythritol or Swerve in a blender or coffee grinder to get the powdered texture.

If a specific sweetener or type of sweetener (such as powdered or liquid) is called for, do not substitute any other sweetener; these recipes rely on these particular sweeteners. For example, in recipes where the sweetener has to melt, some sweeteners won't work, so it's important to use exactly what's called for.

If a sweetener in an ingredients list is followed by "or equivalent," such as "¼ cup Swerve confectioners'-style sweetener or equivalent amount of liquid or powdered sweetener," you are free to use any keto-friendly sweetener, liquid or powdered. For example, you could use liquid stevia, stevia glycerite, monk fruit, or xylitol.

I've used Swerve, my favorite keto-friendly sweetener, in many of the recipes in this book. But if you prefer to use another keto-friendly sweetener, here are the conversion ratios:

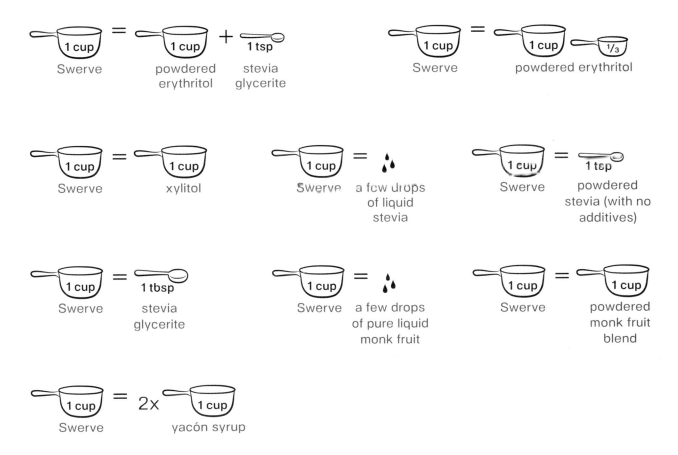

# sweeteners to avoid

### honey

Honey may be less refined than table sugar, but it is still high in calories and fructose. One teaspoon of honey contains 22 calories—more than one teaspoon of sugar, which has 16. The biggest problem with honey, however, is that it is roughly 50 percent fructose (see page 79 for more on fructose).

### agave

Don't be fooled when you see that agave is low on the glycemic index—it's about 90 percent fructose. That makes it a very unhealthy choice (see page 79 for more on the problems with fructose).

### coconut sugar

Even though I see claims all over the Web that coconut sugar is commendably fructose-free, 70 to 80 percent of it is made of sucrose, which is half fructose (and half glucose). This essentially means that, gram for gram, coconut sugar has the same amount of fructose as table sugar.

### sucralose (splenda)

Sucralose, also known as Splenda, is a popular artificial sweetener. Liquid sucralose is so concentrated that you need very small amounts to achieve the desired sweetness. Splenda, however, is bulked up so it can be used in place of table sugar. The first two ingredients in Splenda are dextrose and maltodextrin, which are carbohydrates that are not free of calories. One cup of Splenda contains 96 calories and 32 grams of carbohydrates, which is substantial, especially for those with diabetes.

Even more troubling, sucralose has been found to inhibit the absorption of zinc and iodine, which are essential for proper thyroid function. It is also linked to a decrease in the beneficial bacteria in the gut, which can cause numerous health problems.

### artificial sweeteners

Artificial sweeteners, such as aspartame, acesulfame potassium, neotame, saccharin, sucralose, and advantame, are not good for your health. They reduce the liver's ability to filter out toxins, stress your metabolism, and upset the balance of bacteria in the gut, which is essential for proper immune function. Stay away from all artificial sweeteners.

### other high-sugar sweeteners

Sugar is often hidden in foods, so read the labels! Check for anything ending in "-ose," which indicates a sugar, and for the following: agave nectar, beet sugar, brown rice syrup, brown sugar, cane crystals, corn sweetener, corn syrup, corn syrup solids, dehydrated cane juice, dextrin, dextrose, fructose, fruit juice concentrate, glucose, high-fructose corn syrup, honey, invert sugar, lactose, maltose, malt syrup, maple syrup, molasses, palm sugar, raw sugar, saccharose, sorghum, sorghum syrup, sucrose, syrup, treacle, turbinado sugar, and xylose.

### undesirable sugar alcohols

Although some sugar alcohols, like erythritol, are great keto-friendly sweeteners, others are not keto-friendly at all. Stay away from maltitol and sorbitol, which raise blood sugar and can cause gastrointestinal issues.

**½ cup whole-wheat pasta =**
**noodles from 3 stalks broccoli**
**OR 5 cups zucchini noodles**
**OR 5 cups cabbage noodles**

# tools

For the most part, the recipes in this book require tools that are part of a basic kitchen setup: standard pots, pans, baking sheets, and so on. However, some of the recipes require specialized tools, and there are some tools that will simply make your life in the kitchen easier.

### spiral slicer

*For: vegetable noodles, especially zoodles (page 262)*

A spiral slicer makes it easy to cut vegetables into noodles—see, for instance, the recipe for zucchini noodles on page 262.

I'm often asked what my favorite spiral slicer is. It depends on the thickness of the noodle. For a thicker noodle, I love the Veggetti Pro Table-Top Spiralizer (you can buy it from Amazon through my website under Shop→Maria's Amazon Store). If you prefer a thin, angel hair–type noodle, I recommend the Joyce Chen Saladacco Spiral Slicer (also available from Amazon through my website).

### 8-inch crêpe pan or nonstick pan

*For: wraps (page 254)*

Does such a thing as a healthy nonstick pan exist? Nonstick cookware can be very handy when cooking crêpes, omelets, or the wraps on page 254. But most nonstick pans use Teflon and other chemicals that we want to avoid. Instead, you can try using a well-seasoned cast-iron pan or a stainless-steel pan with lots of oil.

I've also found that the glazed ceramic pans from Ceramcor have a great nonstick surface without chemicals. They can be cleaned as you would any other pan—the surface is very hard to scratch. They are super durable and heavy-duty.

However, there is a little learning curve with these pans. Because they are ceramic, they take longer to heat up. For omelets, I turn my burner on a low setting for 2 or 3 minutes to warm the pan, and then I add my cooking fat; I cook the eggs and turn off the heat when I flip the omelet (it holds heat longer, like a cast-iron pan). The omelet slides right out!

### high-speed blender

*For: pureeing; making shakes, salad dressings, dips, ice cream*

A high-speed blender is perfect for processing liquids. High-powered blenders, such as Blendtec and Vitamix brands, have better performance, durability, and speed—but they're also more expensive.

### ice cream maker
*For: making ice cream and ice cream–based pops and treats*

Ice cream treats are my favorite! You will always find keto ice cream, keto ice pops, and keto push-pops in my freezer. I adore my Conair Cuisinart ICE-21 1.5 Quart Frozen Yogurt/Ice Cream Maker. About ten years ago, I got my first ice cream maker from Cuisinart, and when it broke due to overuse, they sent me a new motor for free!

### immersion blender
*For: pureeing and blending*

I can't believe I went so long without an immersion blender! I'm not a gadget person like my husband is—I like simplicity and I'm not a fan of clutter—so when Craig first asked if I wanted an immersion blender, I politely said, "No, thank you."

But I have to tell you, when I started using one, I was immediately hooked! It is so easy to operate, and I can't believe the power behind this little tool. I love it for making pureed soups, homemade mayonnaise, sauces, and salad dressings, as well as shakes.

### waffle maker
*For: making waffles*

I love to keep grain-free waffles in the freezer for easy breakfasts. My advice is to spend the money on a quality waffle maker. I adore the Waring Pro WMK600 Double Belgian Waffle Maker.

### slow cooker (6-quart)
*For: slow cooking over low heat for several hours*

If you don't have a lot of time for hands-on cooking, a slow cooker is a great tool that can save you time and effort. You can prep the ingredients the night before, turn it on before you leave for work in the morning, and come home to a wonderful home-cooked meal.

### molds
*For: molding items into a desired shape; freezing liquids into individual treats*

Ice pop mold: Chai Ice Lollies (page 386), Bone Broth Ice Pops (page 388)

Silicone mold with twelve 1⅞-ounce cavities: Chai Fat Bombs (page 398), Bone Broth Fat Bombs (page 192), No-Bake Vanilla Bean Petits Fours (page 392), No-Bake Strawberry Petits Fours (page 392). I use one made by World Cuisine, which you can purchase on Amazon: goo.gl/KZ2MFJ

### double boiler
*For: making and reheating sauces*

A double boiler is a great tool for making sure you don't overheat sauces and cause them to separate. I often reheat my Easy Basil Hollandaise (page 136) in a double boiler.

But if you do not have a double boiler, you can use a heat-safe bowl set over a pot of simmering water. I reheated my hollandaise this way when I was camping this summer.

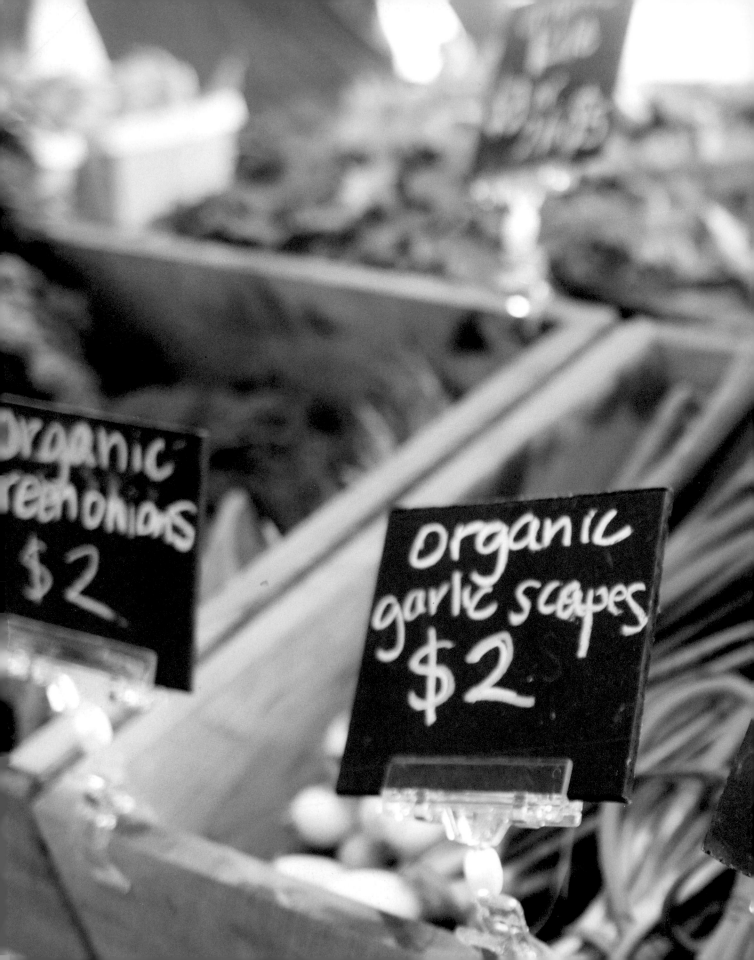

# meal plan and shopping lists

# how to use the 30-day meal plan

In this part of the book, you will find a 30-day meal plan complete with weekly shopping lists. The meals in the plan are made from whole foods and are designed to have the right ratios of fat, protein, and carbs, enabling your body to remove toxins and quickly become keto-adapted.

When following the 30-day meal plan, you may see a dip in energy in the first one to two weeks of the plan. To compensate, add extra water and electrolytes (salt, potassium, magnesium). Also, plan on reducing your workouts in the first week. As your body gets more efficient at burning fat for fuel and you heal leptin and insulin resistance, you will begin to feel full longer and cravings will subside. This can take two to four weeks or longer, depending on your metabolic state. Once fully keto-adapted (after four to six weeks), you will see your energy soar.

During your 30-day cleanse, it's best to stick to the meal plan as closely as you can. If you would like to trade a recipe in the plan for another recipe in this book, make sure that it has similar amounts of carbs and protein (in grams).

The meal plan is designed to feed two people. If you are the only person in your household eating keto, or if you need to feed a whole family ketogenic meals, then you may scale the recipes up or down to suit your needs, keeping in mind what does and does not keep well as leftovers if you are scaling down; just remember to increase or decrease the quantities of the ingredients in the shopping lists accordingly.

If you are new to the ketogenic lifestyle, you may find it a challenge to stick to these meals during the first couple of weeks of the plan, which is the amount of time it takes most people to become keto-adapted. There are no desserts in the meal plan, but I've included dessert recipes in this book to provide you with healthy ketogenic options if irresistible cravings or hunger strike. Most of us rely on sweets in daily life, so I realize that it may be too difficult to cure that sweet tooth while becoming keto-adapted. If you find yourself craving something sweet or feeling extra hungry, use one of my dessert recipes to squelch those cravings and keep yourself from going off the plan by eating sugar or other junk. The keto dessert recipes in this book are also great for what desserts were traditionally reserved for—special occasions such as birthdays, holidays, or having company over. Note that if you are also following the Whole30 plan, no sweeteners of any kind are permitted, so you will need to skip the treats chapter entirely.

The shopping lists include all the ingredients required to make the recipes, including components such as salad dressings and spice blends. When planning your time in the kitchen, remember to account for the time needed to make these components. In some cases, store-bought options for basic components are acceptable; using them will cut down on the total time it takes to prepare the recipes. Note, however, that sea salt and black pepper are not included in the shopping lists; I assume you'll always have those on hand.

If you have food allergies or intolerances, see the individual recipes for ingredient substitutions and/or omissions, and make sure to adjust the shopping lists accordingly.

Finally, read through the recipes in the plan carefully to determine whether special equipment is required; for example, you may need a spiral slicer to make zucchini noodles. You can find my recommendations for special equipment for ketogenic cooking in Part 2.

## the skinny on macros and the ketogenic diet

The three macronutrients, or "macros," in the human diet are fat, protein, and carbohydrates. When you are keto-adapted and burning fat rather than sugar for fuel, there is no dietary need for carbohydrates; your body can generate all the glucose it needs for proper function and health. All you need is a little fiber—10 grams or so a day—to feed your gut microbiome, and if you are eating naturally fermented foods or taking probiotic supplements, you will need even less. The most important thing to focus on when adapting to a ketogenic lifestyle is ensuring that your carb intake is low enough and your protein intake is moderate. If you get those two things right, you will get into ketosis.

Fat helps you feel satiated and keeps cravings at bay. But you should never add fat to your meals if you are not hungry. This is a mistake that many people make with this lifestyle: adding fat to get to some set number. A keto-adapted body can burn body fat and dietary fat equally. So if you are adding extra fat to your diet (in the form of bulletproof coffee, fat bombs, and so on), then your body will use less body fat and more dietary fat for fuel, resulting in less body fat loss.

The most important thing in becoming keto-adapted is to make sure that your total carbs, not net carbs, are below 20 grams a day. Some very active people can consume up to 30 grams of total carbs a day and remain keto-adapted, but 20 grams is a good target.

Moderating protein is another important piece of the puzzle. Too much protein can affect blood sugar (especially in those people who are metabolically damaged with diabetes). A good target is 0.7 times your lean body mass (in pounds) in grams of protein per day. Your lean body mass is your total weight minus your body fat. From the very accurate DEXA body scans to the less

accurate calculations done by some bathroom scales, there are many methods of varying accuracy for determining body fat percentage. I recommend a DEXA scan for the most accurate results.

For example, a woman who weighs 150 pounds and has 30 percent body fat would have 45 pounds of fat (150 x 0.3) and 105 pounds of lean mass (150 − 45), so her protein target would be:

105 x 0.7 = 73.5 grams of protein per day

If you have extreme metabolic damage, you may have to reduce your protein intake to 0.5 times your lean body mass. For a woman with 105 pounds of lean body mass who has metabolic issues, it would be:

105 x 0.5 = 52.5 grams of protein per day

Once you've got your carb and protein levels right, use fat to stay full and satiated. In the first week or two of the 30-day cleanse, you may find this to be a challenge; if that's the case, you can add a bit of extra fat, if needed, with a serving of one of the dessert recipes starting on page 382. My ketogenic desserts, sweetened with a healthy keto sweetener and full of healthy fats, both satisfy a sweet tooth and curb hunger. Keto desserts can be consumed at any time during the eating window.

Once you're keto-adapted, you will easily feel satiated on 1,000 to 1,400 calories a day. The foods you eat when following a ketogenic lifestyle are very nutrient-dense—so much so that even active men seeking to maintain muscle strength can sustain themselves on 1,800 to 2,200 calories a day. So don't add fat just to get to some set percentage of calories or macronutrient ratio if you aren't hungry. Doing so will only hold you back.

# the eating window

The meal plan includes a period of daily intermittent fasting, described in more detail on pages 33 to 35. Intermittent fasting will help you become keto-adapted more quickly, and it has many metabolic advantages, including improved mitochondrial health and regeneration, reduced risk of cancer, and reduced inflammation. Intermittent fasting is beneficial for everyone to practice, whether you are doing a 30-day keto cleanse or are already keto-adapted.

During daily intermittent fasting, you eat all your food within a set window of time; you consume nothing but water outside of this window. A six-hour eating window is preferable for optimal results, but eight hours is acceptable if the shorter window is unrealistic for you. For example, if you eat your first meal of the day at 10:00 a.m., your last meal should ideally be at 4:00 p.m. and definitely no later than 6:00 p.m. You can adjust the timing of this eating window to fit your schedule, but make sure that you stop eating at least three hours before bed. Eating too close to bedtime can inhibit the production of human growth hormone and slow weight loss.

# meal plan comparison: before and after

Sugars are hidden in so much of today's food. Even what most people would consider a healthy diet can be loaded with sugars, which never leaves you feeling full and satiated. A well-formulated keto meal plan removes those sugars and sets you on the path to weight loss and good health. To see how powerful the keto lifestyle is, take a look at the meal plan comparison on the following page.

Meal Plan A represents what one of my clients was eating before she transitioned to a keto diet. Meal Plan B is an example of what she eats now, after becoming keto-adapted. She thought she was eating to lose weight by following Plan A, but she realized that she was way too hungry to sustain that plan. It was filled with diet food, but also with too much sugar—no wonder it didn't work! Even though she consumed lots of food, she never felt satisfied, was often tired during the day, and always felt "on edge."

## Meal Plan A (before becoming keto-adapted)

| Time of Meal | Client's Food/Feeling | Calories | Sugar | My Comments |
|---|---|---|---|---|
| 7:30 a.m. | Coffee with skim milk<br>*I feel hungry.* | 22 | 3 g | *Skim milk has a lot of sugar (lactose).* |
| 8:00 a.m. | Multigrain cereal with skim milk and 8 ounces of grape juice<br>*I feel okay, not full.* | 470 | 64 g | *High-sugar, low-protein food and no fat; this spikes blood sugar and isn't fuel for a productive morning.* |
| 10:00 a.m. | Banana<br>*I am starving.* | 121 | 17 g | *Another blood sugar spike that will keep you hungry. Fructose spikes blood sugar faster than any other type of sugar.* |
| 12:40 p.m. | Meal replacement shake<br>*I am trying to eat "healthy."* | 180 | 18 g | *Meal replacement shakes contain too much sugar, and you don't get the satisfaction of chewing.* |
| 1:15 p.m. | Yogurt with pineapple and fortified water | 332 | 67 g | *Blood sugar spike.* |
| 2:00 p.m. | Two pieces of hard candy | 45 | 7 g | *Another blood sugar spike.* |
| 3:00 p.m. | Diet soda | 0 | 0 g | *You think you are doing good, but cravings persist.* |
| 6:30 p.m. | Small salad with fat-free French dressing, 1 cup spaghetti with marinara sauce, and a piece of garlic bread | 699 | 20 g | *Too low in protein, no fat, and too much carbohydrate and sugar (marinara sauce is notorious for containing added sugars).* |
| 9:45 p.m. | ½ cup fat-free frozen yogurt | 100 | 18 g | *Another blood sugar spike.* |

## Meal Plan B (after becoming keto-adapted)

| Time of Meal | Client's Food/Feeling | Calories | Sugar | Client's Comments |
|---|---|---|---|---|
| 7:30 a.m. | *I wake up energized and not hungry. I drink lots of water.* | | | |
| 10:30 a.m. | Eggs Florentine with Basil Hollandaise (page 166)<br>*I feel full and energized.* | 694 | 0 g | *I ate once I finally got hungry, about 3 hours after waking up. Some days I have to remind myself to eat, as hunger is rarely prevalent.* |
| 2:00 p.m. | *I have lots of energy and I'm in a good mood.* | | | |
| 4:00 p.m. | Keto Greek Avgolemono (page 286) with a side of Lemon Pepper Wings (page 202)<br>*This was good, and I'm full!* | 594 | 0 g | *I finished my food for the day and had no hunger issues through the night.* |

This breakdown of the two meal plans is quite eye-opening. Every 4 grams of carbohydrate equals 1 teaspoon of sugar in your bloodstream. So for Plan A, with its 359 grams of carbs, the result is 90 teaspoons of sugar in your bloodstream over the course of the day! In comparison, Plan B, with its 12 grams of carbs, results in just 3 teaspoons of sugar in the blood. That's much better for insulin sensitivity and weight loss, and because your blood sugar doesn't spike over the course of the day, you don't experience the hunger and cravings that come with Plan A.

| Meal Plan | Calories | Fat | Protein | Carbs | Sugar | Sugar in Bloodstream |
|---|---|---|---|---|---|---|
| A ("Before") | 1,969 | 31 g | 66 g | 359 g | 214 g | 90 teaspoons |
| B ("After") | 1,315 | 111 g | 65 g | 12 g | 0 g | 3 teaspoons |

By shifting from blood-sugar-spiking and hunger-causing carbohydrates to satiating fats and a moderate amount of protein, my client was able to take control of her hunger and get through the day with fewer calories while eating much more nutrient-dense food. The 30-day meal plan in this section will achieve the same result for you.

## should I add carbs or carb up?

*Some people say that adding carbs is necessary for easing sleep problems, hormone irregularities, low energy, and other issues that can occur during a 30-day ketogenic cleanse. But adding carbs in these situations only masks the real problem (such as nutrient deficiency) and will hold you back from your weight-loss and healing goals. Dr. Jacob Wilson recently studied cyclic keto with strength training alongside a ketogenic diet with strength training. The cyclic keto group ate keto during the week and then added carbs on the weekends. The ketogenic group ate keto all week. Both groups lost the same amount of weight, but the group that added carbs lost half as much fat, meaning that they lost a lot of muscle. Losing muscle is the last thing you want, especially as you age.*

*There is no dietary need for carbohydrates. None. That can't be said about any other macronutrient. You need fat and protein to live, but carbs are not needed to sustain life. As long as you are eating a well-formulated, nutrient-dense ketogenic diet, you won't experience issues like poor sleep,*

*imbalanced hormones, or low energy. Low energy, for example, is typically due to dehydration. When you become keto-adapted, your body releases much of the salt and associated water that it holds onto when you eat a higher-carb diet. So you have to add extra electrolytes (salt, potassium, and magnesium) and lots of water to fix the energy issue. Also, the longer you are keto-adapted, the more efficient your body gets at burning fat for fuel; issues with low energy are usually not a problem after a month or two. In fact, most people eating a well-formulated ketogenic diet see their energy soar.*

*But even with a nutrient-dense diet, you sometimes need to supplement to get your levels back to where they should be. Our food and water supply just doesn't contain the nutrients it once did. Water used to be loaded with magnesium (among many other minerals) that today's filtered city water just doesn't have. So adding a magnesium supplement can be a great option to make up for the lack of it in our food and water.*

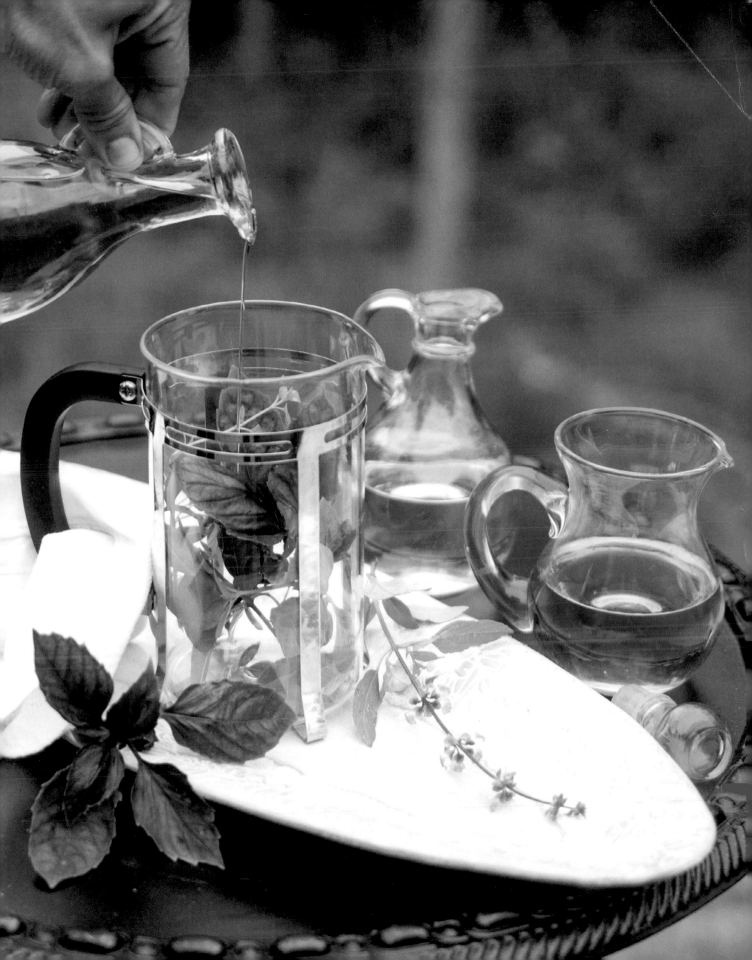

# days 1–7

## meal plan

| | BREAK-YOUR-FAST MEAL | MEAL 2 | | NUTRITION INFO (per person) | |
|---|---|---|---|---|---|
| day 1 | Rosti with Bacon, Mushrooms, and Green Onions **158** | Umami Burgers **296** + | Lemon Pepper Wings **202** | calories (kcal)<br>fat<br>protein<br>carbohydrates | 1304<br>111 g<br>72 g<br>13 g |
| day 2 | Bacon and Eggs Ramen **150** | Reuben Pork Chops **334** + | Italian Marinated Mushrooms **208** | calories (kcal)<br>fat<br>protein<br>carbohydrates | 1324<br>109 g<br>67 g<br>19 g |
| day 3 | Creamiest Keto Scrambled Eggs **154** | California Club Wraps **276** + | Italian Marinated Mushrooms **LEFTOVER** | calories (kcal)<br>fat<br>protein<br>carbohydrates | 1301<br>112 g<br>51 g<br>13 g |
| day 4 | Bacon and Eggs Ramen **LEFTOVER** | Keto Greek Avgolemono **286** + | Warm Spring Salad with Basil Chimichurri and Soft-Boiled Eggs **226** | calories (kcal)<br>fat<br>protein<br>carbohydrates | 1150<br>94 g<br>58 g<br>19 g |
| day 5 | Kimchi Eggs **160** | Umami Burgers **LEFTOVER** + | Warm Spring Salad with Basil Chimichurri and Soft-Boiled Eggs **LEFTOVER** | calories (kcal)<br>fat<br>protein<br>carbohydrates | 1383<br>113 g<br>71 g<br>22 g |
| day 6 | Eggs Florentine with Basil Hollandaise (with English muffin) **166** | Keto Greek Avgolemono **LEFTOVER** + | Lemon Pepper Wings **LEFTOVER** | calories (kcal)<br>fat<br>protein<br>carbohydrates | 1315<br>111 g<br>65 g<br>12 g |
| day 7 | Eggs in a Frame with leftover Easy Basil Hollandaise **168** | California Club Wraps **LEFTOVER** + | Italian Marinated Mushrooms **LEFTOVER** | calories (kcal)<br>fat<br>protein<br>carbohydrates | 1379<br>112 g<br>66 g<br>13 g |

## shopping list

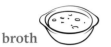

### baking products

Baking soda, 2 pinches

Coconut flour, 4 teaspoons

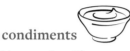

### broth

Chicken bone broth, two 32-ounce boxes (2 quarts)

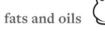

### condiments

Mayonnaise, 1½ cups

### eggs

Eggs, large, 4 dozen (42)

### fats and oils

Coconut oil, 4 ounces (½ cup)

MCT oil, 8 ounces (1 cup)

Paleo fat of choice, 14 to 22 ounces (1¾ to 2¾ cups)

Sesame oil, 1 tablespoon

### fresh herbs

Basil, 3 bunches

Chives, 1 small bunch (2 tablespoons chopped)

Cilantro, 1 small bunch (2 tablespoons chopped)

Ginger, 1 (1-inch-long) piece (1 tablespoon grated)

Thyme, 1 sprig

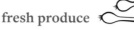

### fresh produce

Asparagus, ½ pound

Avocado, 1 small

Button mushrooms, 2 pounds

Garlic, 1 head

Green cabbage, 1 small head (1 cup shredded)

Green onions, 1 small bunch (¼ cup plus 2 tablespoons, plus more for garnish)

Lemons, 2

Mushrooms, 1 pound

Onions, 2 large (2 cups)

Portobello mushrooms, 1 pound

Romaine lettuce, 1 head (2 cups)

Spinach, 1 pound (4 cups)

Tomatoes, 2 small

Zucchini, 2 medium

### pantry items

Coconut aminos, 2 tablespoons

Coconut vinegar, ½ cup

Egg white protein powder, unflavored, ¼ cup

Fish sauce, 1¼ teaspoons

Kimchi, 16-ounce jar (1 cup)

Pickles, baby, 1 small jar (for garnish)

Sauerkraut, 1 cup

Tomato paste, 6-ounce can (1 tablespoon)

### spices and extracts

Basil, dried, 6½ teaspoons

Chili powder, 1 tablespoon

Red pepper flakes, 1 tablespoon

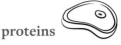

### proteins

Bacon, 8 slices

Chicken thighs, bone-in, skin-on, 6

Chicken wings, 1 pound

Cross-cut beef marrow bones, 7 (each 2 inches long)

Ground beef, 1⅓ pounds

Pork belly, fully cooked, 12-ounce package

Pork chops, bone-in, four 5-ounce

### keto condiments and spice blends

Dairy-Free Thousand Island Dressing (page 118) *(To make, you will need: ¾ cup mayonnaise, ¼ cup chopped dill pickles, ¼ cup tomato sauce, ⅛ teaspoon fish sauce)*

Easy Basil Hollandaise (page 136), 2 heaping tablespoons *(To make, you will need: 1 cup bacon fat, 4 large egg yolks, ½ cup lemon juice, 1 cup (1 ounce) loosely packed fresh basil leaves)*

Herbes de Florence (page 113), 1 teaspoon *(To make, you will need: 2 tablespoons dried basil, 2 tablespoons dried ground marjoram, 2 tablespoons dried oregano leaves, 2 tablespoons dried parsley, 1 tablespoon dried ground rosemary, 1 tablespoon dried thyme leaves, 1 tablespoon red pepper flakes, 2 teaspoons garlic powder, 1 teaspoon onion powder)*

*Looking for Keto Organic Spices? Maria's signature spice blends are available for purchase here:*

http://keto-adapted.com/keto-spices/

# days 8–14

## meal plan

| | BREAK-YOUR-FAST MEAL | MEAL 2 | NUTRITION INFO (per person) | |
|---|---|---|---|---|
| day 8 | Bacon and Mushrooms with Soft-Boiled Eggs 164 | Slow Cooker Ropa Vieja 308 + Simple Crab Salad 236 | calories (kcal) | 1307 |
| | | | fat | 100 g |
| | | | protein | 88 g |
| | | | carbohydrates | 14 g |
| day 9 | Green Eggs and Ham 162 | DOUBLE RECIPE Chiles Rellenos 266 | calories (kcal) | 1225 |
| | | | fat | 109 g |
| | | | protein | 53 g |
| | | | carbohydrates | 9 g |
| day 10 | Steak and Eggs 156 | Poached Salmon with Creamy Dill Sauce 380 | calories (kcal) | 1132 |
| | | | fat | 96 g |
| | | | protein | 62 g |
| | | | carbohydrates | 5 g |
| day 11 | Bacon and Mushrooms with Soft-Boiled Eggs LEFTOVER | Slow Cooker Ropa Vieja LEFTOVER + DOUBLE RECIPE Scotch Eggs 196 | calories (kcal) | 1355 |
| | | | fat | 106 g |
| | | | protein | 90 g |
| | | | carbohydrates | 11 g |
| day 12 | Green Eggs and Ham LEFTOVER | Chiles Rellenos LEFTOVER | calories (kcal) | 1225 |
| | | | fat | 109 g |
| | | | protein | 53 g |
| | | | carbohydrates | 9 g |
| day 13 | Steak and Eggs LEFTOVER | Poached Salmon with Creamy Dill Sauce LEFTOVER | calories (kcal) | 1132 |
| | | | fat | 111 g |
| | | | protein | 65 g |
| | | | carbohydrates | 12 g |
| day 14 | Kimchi Eggs 160 | Slow Cooker Ropa Vieja LEFTOVER + Scotch Eggs LEFTOVER | calories (kcal) | 1067 |
| | | | fat | 72 g |
| | | | protein | 61 g |
| | | | carbohydrates | 8 g |

# shopping list

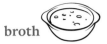

## broth

Beef bone broth or water,
32-ounce box (½ cup)

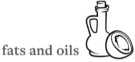

## condiments

Mayonnaise, 30-ounce jar (1 cup)

Mustard, Dijon, 8-ounce bottle
(1½ teaspoons)

Mustard, whole-grain, 8-ounce
bottle (¾ cup)

Salsa, 16-ounce jar (1 cup)

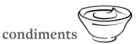

## eggs

Eggs, large, 3 dozen (26)

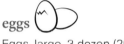

## fats and oils

Coconut oil, 21 ounces (2½ cups
plus 1 tablespoon)

MCT oil, 5½ ounces (½ cup plus
3 tablespoons)

Paleo fat of choice, 1 ounce
(2 tablespoons)

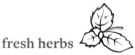

## fresh herbs

Chives, 1 small bunch
(1 tablespoon plus more for
garnish)

Cilantro, 1 bunch (6 tablespoons
plus more for garnish)

Dill, 1 small bunch (1 tablespoon
plus 1 sprig

Tarragon, 1 small bunch
(1 teaspoon)

## fresh produce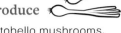

Baby portobello mushrooms,
12 ounces

Celery, 2 stalks (½ cup)

Cucumbers, 2 medium

Garlic, 1 head (1 clove plus
2 teaspoons minced)

Green bell pepper, 1 medium

Jalapeño pepper, 1

Lemon, 1

Limes, 2

Onion, 1 large (¾ cup)

Poblano chiles, 4 medium

Radish, 1 (for garnish)

Red bell pepper, 1 medium

Red onion, 1 small (¼ cup)

Tomato, 1 large

## pantry items

Anchovies, 2-ounce tin

Coconut vinegar, ¼ cup plus
2 teaspoons

Green olives, 12-ounce jar
(3 tablespoons plus more for
garnish)

Kimchi, 16-ounce jar (1 cup)

Tomato sauce, 15-ounce can
(¼ cup)

## proteins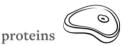

Bacon, ½ pound

Beef brisket, 2 pounds

Chicken thighs, 2 pounds

Crabmeat, two 6-ounce cans

Ground pork, ²/₃ pound

Ham hock steaks, smoked, four
3-ounce

Prosciutto, two 3-ounce
packages (12 slices)

Salmon fillets, six 4-ounce

Venison or beef tenderloins, four
4-ounce

## spices and extracts

Dried oregano leaves,
2 teaspoons

Ground cumin, 2 teaspoons

## keto condiments and
spice blends

Easy Basil Hollandaise (page
136), ½ cup (To make, you will
need: 1 cup bacon fat, 4 large
egg yolks, ½ cup lemon juice,
1 cup (1 ounce) loosely packed
fresh basil leaves)

Easy Dairy-Free Hollandaise
(page 136), 1 cup (To make, you
will need: 1 cup bacon fat, 4 large
egg yolks, ½ cup lemon juice)

*Looking for Keto Organic Spices?
Maria's signature spice blends are
available for purchase here:*

http://keto-adapted.com/keto-spices/

# days 15–21

## meal plan

| | BREAK-YOUR-FAST MEAL | MEAL 2 | | NUTRITION INFO (per person) | |
|---|---|---|---|---|---|
| day 15 | Bacon and Eggs Ramen — 150 | Smothered Bacon and Mushroom Burgers — 294 + | Mixed Green Salad with BLT Deviled Eggs and Bacon Vinaigrette — 232 | calories (kcal) | 1483 |
| | | | | fat | 122 g |
| | | | | protein | 76 g |
| | | | | carbohydrates | 20 g |
| day 16 | Keto Pockets — 170 | Spicy Grilled Shrimp with Mojo Verde — 364 + | Panzanella Salad — 234 | calories (kcal) | 1116 |
| | | | | fat | 94 g |
| | | | | protein | 58 g |
| | | | | carbohydrates | 10 g |
| day 17 | DOUBLE RECIPE Ham and Egg Cups — 172 | Smothered Bacon and Mushroom Burgers — LEFTOVER + | Keto "Fruit" Salad — 224 | calories (kcal) | 1074 |
| | | | | fat | 84 g |
| | | | | protein | 68 g |
| | | | | carbohydrates | 12 g |
| day 18 | Bacon and Eggs Ramen — LEFTOVER | Spicy Grilled Shrimp with Mojo Verde — LEFTOVER + | Mixed Green Salad with BLT Deviled Eggs and Bacon Vinaigrette — LEFTOVER | calories (kcal) | 1278 |
| | | | | fat | 106 g |
| | | | | protein | 62 g |
| | | | | carbohydrates | 19 g |
| day 19 | Keto Pockets — LEFTOVER | Spicy Tuna Stacks — 358 + | Panzanella Salad — LEFTOVER | calories (kcal) | 1328 |
| | | | | fat | 111 g |
| | | | | protein | 71 g |
| | | | | carbohydrates | 12 g |
| day 20 | Ham and Egg Cups — LEFTOVER | Steak au Poivre for Two — 318 + | Keto "Fruit" Salad — LEFTOVER | calories (kcal) | 1136 |
| | | | | fat | 94 g |
| | | | | protein | 54 g |
| | | | | carbohydrates | 8 g |
| day 21 | Keto Pockets — LEFTOVER | Zoodles in Clam Sauce — 378 + | Chicken Tinga Wings — 200 | calories (kcal) | 1117 |
| | | | | fat | 86 g |
| | | | | protein | 70 g |
| | | | | carbohydrates | 16 g |

# shopping list

## broth
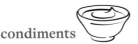

Beef bone broth, 32-ounce box
(¼ cup)

Chicken bone broth, two
32-ounce boxes (4½ cups)

## condiments
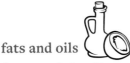

Hot sauce, 5-ounce bottle
(1 teaspoon)

Mayonnaise, 30-ounce jar
(1 cup plus 2 tablespoons)

Mustard, Dijon, 8-ounce bottle
(1 teaspoon)

Mustard, prepared yellow,
8-ounce bottle (2 teaspoons)

## eggs

Eggs, 4 dozen (40 large)

## fats and oils

Coconut oil, 9 to 17 ounces
(1 to 2 cups plus 1 tablespoon)

MCT oil, 14 ounces (1¾ cups)

Paleo fat of choice, 2½ ounces
(⅓ cup)

## fresh herbs
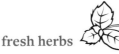

Chives, 1 small bunch (¼ cup plus
more for garnish)

Cilantro, 2 bunches (3 cups)

Ginger, 1-inch piece (1 tablespoon)

Mint, 1 small bunch (1 tablespoon)

Thyme, 1 small bunch (1 sprig)

## fresh produce
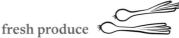

Avocado, 1 medium

Cherry tomatoes, 1 pint (1 cup
plus 12)

Cucumbers, 3 medium (2 plus
¼ cup)

Garlic, 1 head (5 cloves plus
3 tablespoons minced)

Green onions, 1 small bunch
(2 tablespoons plus more for
garnish)

Lettuce, 1 small head (8 leaves)

Limes, 6

Mixed greens, 16-ounce package
(10 cups)

Mushrooms, 1⅔ pounds

Onions, 2 large (2 cups)

Purple cabbage, 1 small head
(¼ cup)

Red onion, 1 small (¼ used)

Tomatillos, 4½ ounces (1 cup)

Tomatoes, 3 medium (3 cups)

Zucchini, 3 medium

## pantry items

Chipotles in adobo sauce,
2 tablespoons

Coconut aminos, 2 tablespoons

Coconut vinegar, ½ cup plus
2 tablespoons

Egg white protein powder,
unflavored, ¼ cup

Swerve confectioners'-style
sweetener, 2 teaspoons

Tomato paste, 6-ounce can
(1 tablespoon)

Tomato sauce, 14-ounce can
(¼ cup)

## proteins
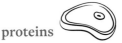

Bacon, 15 slices

Chicken wings, 1 pound

Chorizo, 1 pound

Clams, 6½-ounce can

Ground beef, 1⅓ pounds

Ham, 1 pound (12 slices)

Mortadella, 8 ounces (12 thin
slices)

Pork belly, fully cooked, 12-ounce
package

Rib-eye steak, 8 ounces

Shrimp, 12 jumbo

Tuna, 6-ounce can

## spices and extracts

Black peppercorns, 1 tablespoon

Cayenne pepper, 2 teaspoons

Dried oregano leaves,
½ teaspoon

Ground cumin, 1½ teaspoons

Red pepper flakes, 1 tablespoon
plus more for garnish

## milk

Coconut milk, full-fat, 13½-ounce
can (¼ cup)

# days 22–30

## meal plan

| | BREAK-YOUR-FAST MEAL | MEAL 2 | | NUTRITION INFO (per person) | |
|---|---|---|---|---|---|
| day 22 | Rosti with Bacon, Mushrooms, and Green Onions 158 | Slow Cooker Mole Short Ribs 312 + | Bone Marrow Chili con Keto 242 | calories (kcal) | 1233 |
| | | | | fat | 110 g |
| | | | | protein | 53 g |
| | | | | carbohydrates | 15 g |
| day 23 | Breakfast Chili 148 | Hunan Beef–Stuffed Peppers 322 + | Bok Choy and Mushrooms with Ginger Dressing 250 | calories (kcal) | 1093 |
| | | | | fat | 83 g |
| | | | | protein | 56 g |
| | | | | carbohydrates | 33 g |
| day 24 | Oscar Deviled Eggs 216 | Slow Cooker Mole Short Ribs LEFTOVER + | Bone Marrow Chili con Keto LEFTOVER | calories (kcal) | 1358 |
| | | | | fat | 121 g |
| | | | | protein | 55 g |
| | | | | carbohydrates | 11 g |
| day 25 | Ham and Egg Cups 172 | Hunan Beef–Stuffed Peppers LEFTOVER + | Hot-and-Sour Soup with Pork Meatballs 248 | calories (kcal) | 1228 |
| | | | | fat | 89 g |
| | | | | protein | 80 g |
| | | | | carbohydrates | 28 g |
| day 26 | Breakfast Chili LEFTOVER | Tom Ka Gai (Thai Coconut Chicken) 284 + | Hot-and-Sour Soup with Pork Meatballs LEFTOVER | calories (kcal) | 1306 |
| | | | | fat | 97 g |
| | | | | protein | 84 g |
| | | | | carbohydrates | 25 g |
| day 27 | Oscar Deviled Eggs LEFTOVER | Slow Cooker Mole Short Ribs LEFTOVER + | Bok Choy and Mushrooms with Ginger Dressing LEFTOVER | calories (kcal) | 1165 |
| | | | | fat | 104 g |
| | | | | protein | 46 g |
| | | | | carbohydrates | 13 g |
| day 28 | Breakfast Chili LEFTOVER | Tom Ka Gai (Thai Coconut Chicken) LEFTOVER + | Bone Marrow Chili con Keto LEFTOVER | calories (kcal) | 1284 |
| | | | | fat | 99 g |
| | | | | protein | 76 g |
| | | | | carbohydrates | 22 g |

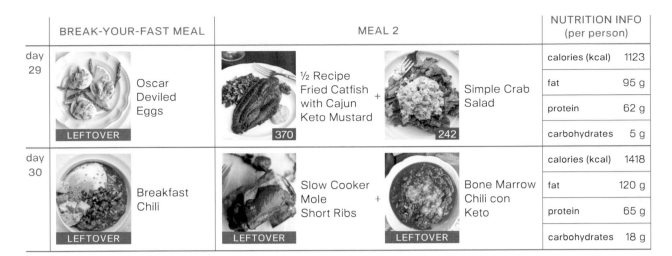

| | BREAK-YOUR-FAST MEAL | MEAL 2 | NUTRITION INFO (per person) | |
|---|---|---|---|---|
| day 29 | Oscar Deviled Eggs LEFTOVER | ½ Recipe Fried Catfish with Cajun Keto Mustard 370 + Simple Crab Salad 242 | calories (kcal) | 1123 |
| | | | fat | 95 g |
| | | | protein | 62 g |
| | | | carbohydrates | 5 g |
| day 30 | Breakfast Chili LEFTOVER | Slow Cooker Mole Short Ribs LEFTOVER + Bone Marrow Chili con Keto LEFTOVER | calories (kcal) | 1418 |
| | | | fat | 120 g |
| | | | protein | 65 g |
| | | | carbohydrates | 18 g |

# shopping list

## baking products

Cocoa powder, unsweetened, 1 tablespoon

## broth

Beef bone broth, 32-ounce box (1½ cups plus 2 tablespoons)

Chicken bone broth, two 32-ounce boxes (6½ cups)

## condiments

Mayonnaise, 30-ounce jar (½ cup)

Mustard, prepared yellow, ¼ cup plus 1 teaspoon

Red curry paste, 4-ounce jar (1½ to 3 teaspoons)

## eggs

Eggs, large, 3 dozen (33)

## fats and oils

Bacon fat or duck fat, ¼ cup plus 2 tablespoons

Coconut oil, 4 ounces (½ cup plus 1 tablespoon)

Paleo fat of choice, 3 tablespoons

MCT oil, 4 ounces (½ cup plus 1 tablespoon)

Sesame oil, toasted, 2 tablespoons

## fresh herbs

Chives, 1 bunch (¼ cup plus 2 tablespoons)

Cilantro, 1 bunch (½ cup plus 1 tablespoon)

Ginger, 2-inch piece

## fresh produce

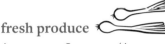

Asparagus, 2 ounces (4 spears)

Avocados, 3 medium

Baby bok choy, 4 heads

Bell peppers, any color, 2 medium

Garlic, 1 head (7 cloves)

Green bell pepper, 1 medium

Green cabbage, 1 small head (1 cup)

Green chiles, 4

Green onions, 9

Limes, 2

Mushrooms, 1½ pounds

Napa cabbage, 1 small head (2 cups)

Onion, 1 large (1¼ cups)

Shallots, 3

## milk

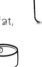

Coconut milk, full-fat, 13½-ounce can

## pantry items

Coconut aminos, 8-ounce bottle (¾ cup plus 1 tablespoon)

Coconut vinegar, 1 tablespoon

Diced green chiles, 4-ounce can

Red chili paste, 1 tablespoon

Rice vinegar, ¼ cup

Tomato sauce, 29-ounce can (3 cups)

Tomatoes, diced, 56-ounce can

## proteins

Bacon, 22 slices

Beef short ribs, 8 (4 pounds)

Catfish fillets, four 4-ounce

Chorizo, 2 pounds

Crabmeat, 6-ounce can (¼ cup)

Cross-cut beef marrow bones, 8 (each 2 inches long)

Flank steak, 1 pound

Ground beef, 2 pounds

Ground pork, ½ pound

Ham, 3 ounces (6 slices)

## spices and extracts

Bay leaves, 2

Cayenne pepper, 1 teaspoon plus more for garnish

Chili powder, ¼ cup

Dried ground oregano, 2 teaspoons

Dried oregano leaves, 2 teaspoons

Dried Thai chiles, 4

Ground cumin, 3 teaspoons

Paprika, 1 teaspoon

## keto condiments and spice blends

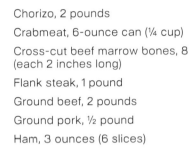

Cajun Seasoning (page 112), 6 tablespoons (To make, you will need: 2½ teaspoons smoked paprika, 2 teaspoons garlic powder, 1¼ teaspoons onion powder, 1¼ teaspoons dried oregano leaves, 1¼ teaspoons dried thyme leaves, 1 teaspoon cayenne pepper, ½ teaspoon red pepper flakes)

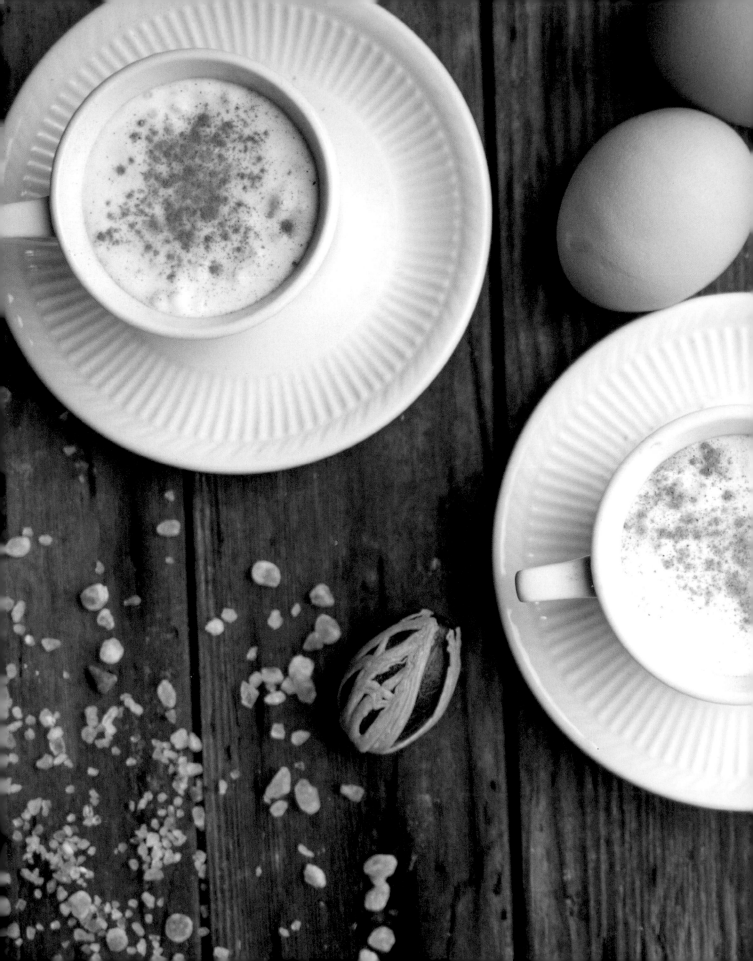

# cleansing ketogenic recipes

## using the recipes

*You'll find a keto meter at the top of each recipe, indicating whether the recipe is high, medium, or low on the keto scale. If a recipe is medium or low and your main goal is weight loss, leave that recipe for when you are closer to your goal. All the recipes are designed for ketosis, but if you are feeling stuck, look for those that rank high on the keto scale.*

*Icons also appear at the top of each recipe to let you know if it is dairy-free, nut-free, egg-free, and/or vegetarian. If a recipe can be made free of dairy, nuts, or eggs by omitting an ingredient or swapping one ingredient for another, the icon will have the word "option" beneath it and you'll find the details within the ingredient list. The number of calories and the amounts and percentages of fat, protein, carbs, and fiber that each recipe contains can be found at the bottom of the recipe.*

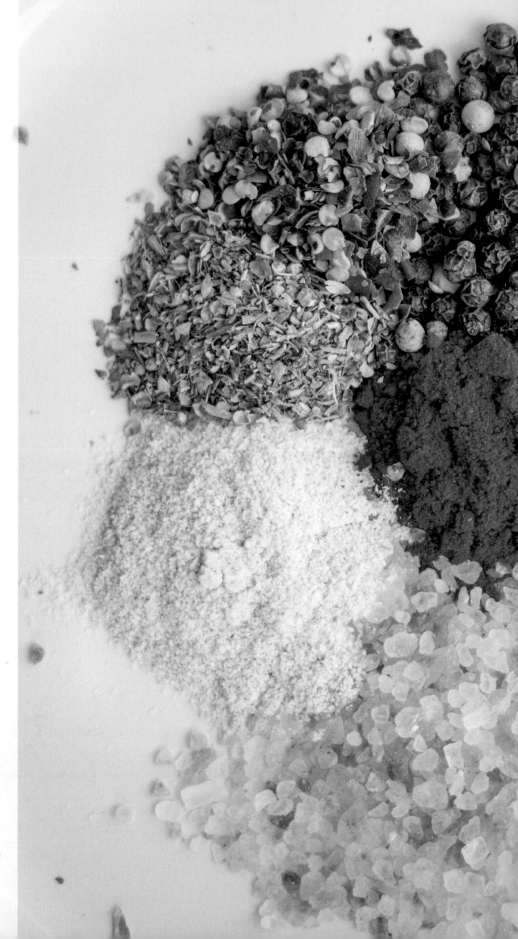

*Many of the sauces, dressings, and spice mixes that I present in this chapter are staples in my fridge and pantry. My refrigerator door is usually stocked with homemade cashew milk and a variety of sauces and salad dressings for easy additions to meals. Plan, plan, plan equals success. I also have my spice mixes premade in labeled jars so they are available when I need them for meals.*

# sauces, dressings, and spice mixes

# homemade cashew milk

L M H KETO ▯ ∅ ⊗ prep time: 2 minutes, plus overnight to soak • yield: 1 quart (1 cup per serving)

This recipe makes a delicious, creamy milk that is free of harmful ingredients and sweeteners.

1½ cups raw cashews, soaked in water overnight

4 cups reverse-osmosis water or spring water

**special equipment:**

high-speed blender and cheesecloth or fine-mesh strainer

**variation:**

Vanilla-Flavored Cashew Milk.

*Add 1 teaspoon of vanilla extract or the seeds scraped from 1 vanilla bean to the blender in Step 1. Then proceed with the recipe as written.*

1. Drain the soaked nuts, then place them in a high-speed blender with the 4 cups of water. Puree until the mixture is completely smooth.

2. To remove the cashew pulp, strain the mixture in a colander lined with cheesecloth or in a fine-mesh strainer. Using your hands, press the pulp to extract all the milk. Discard the pulp. Store the milk in an airtight container in the fridge for up to a week.

NUTRITIONAL INFO (per serving)

| calories | fat | protein | carbs | fiber |
|----------|-----|---------|-------|-------|
| 25 | 2g | 1g | 1g | 0g |
| | 70% | 15% | 15% | |

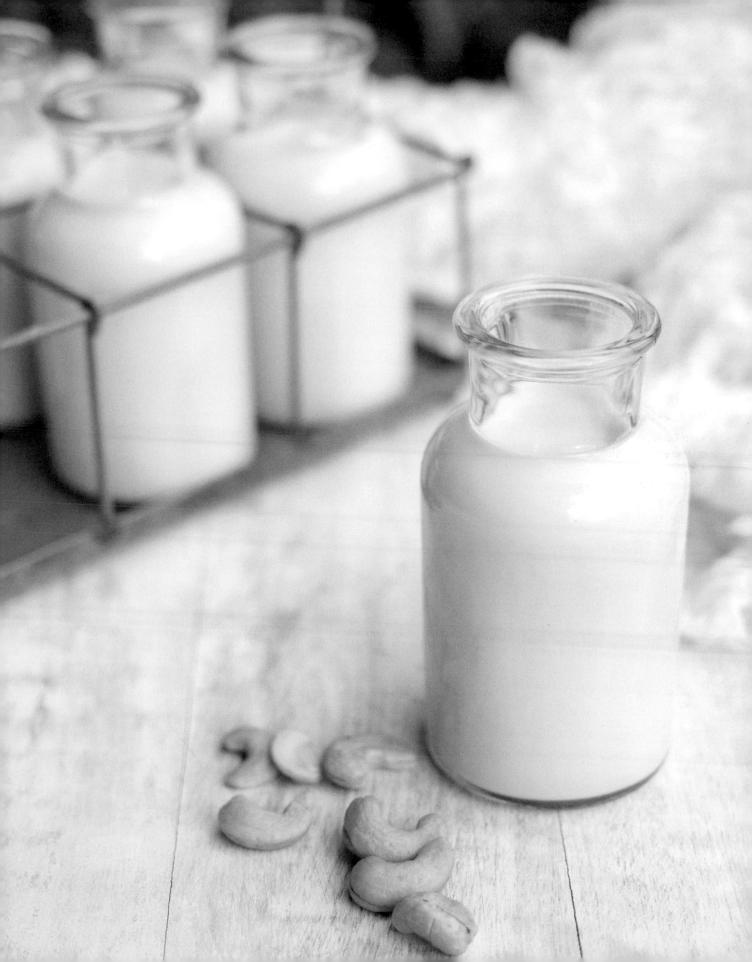

# bone broth—beef, chicken, or fish

L M H KETO | prep time: 10 minutes • cook time: 1 to 3 days • yield: 4 quarts (1 cup per serving)

Nothing could be easier to make than this broth. Once you get all the ingredients in the slow cooker, it does all the work for you. The longer you cook the broth, the thicker it will get. If you roast the beef bones before making the broth, they will create a darker and more flavorful broth (see note below). You can use this broth to make soups and sauces or Bone Broth Fat Bombs (page 192), or drink it as a nourishing beverage.

4 quarts cold water (reverse-osmosis water or filtered water is best)

4 large beef bones (about 4 pounds), or leftover bones and skin from 1 pastured chicken (ideally with the feet, too), or 4 pounds fish bones and head

1 medium onion, chopped

2 stalks celery, sliced ¼ inch thick

2 tablespoons coconut vinegar or apple cider vinegar

2 tablespoons fresh rosemary or other herb of choice

2 teaspoons finely chopped garlic, or cloves from 1 head Garlic Confit (page 142)

2 teaspoons fine sea salt

1 teaspoon fresh or dried thyme leaves

1. Place all the ingredients in a 6-quart slow cooker. Set the heat to high, then, after 1 hour, turn the heat to low. Simmer for a minimum of 1 day and up to 3 days. The longer the broth cooks, the more nutrients and minerals will be extracted from the bones!

2. When the broth is done, pour it through a strainer and discard the solids, but do not skim the fat off the top. The fat makes this broth even more keto-friendly.

3. The broth will keep in the fridge for about 5 days or in the freezer for several months.

note: *For a richer, more deeply flavored beef broth, roast large beef bones in a rimmed sheet pan at 375°F for 50 to 60 minutes and smaller bones for 30 to 40 minutes.*

busy family tip: *Make a double batch with two slow cookers and freeze the broth in large freezer-safe mason jars to have on hand as needed.*

| NUTRITIONAL INFO (per serving) | | | | |
|---|---|---|---|---|
| calories | fat | protein | carbs | fiber |
| 20 | 4g | 1.5g | 1.7g | 0g |
| | 60% | 19% | 21% | |

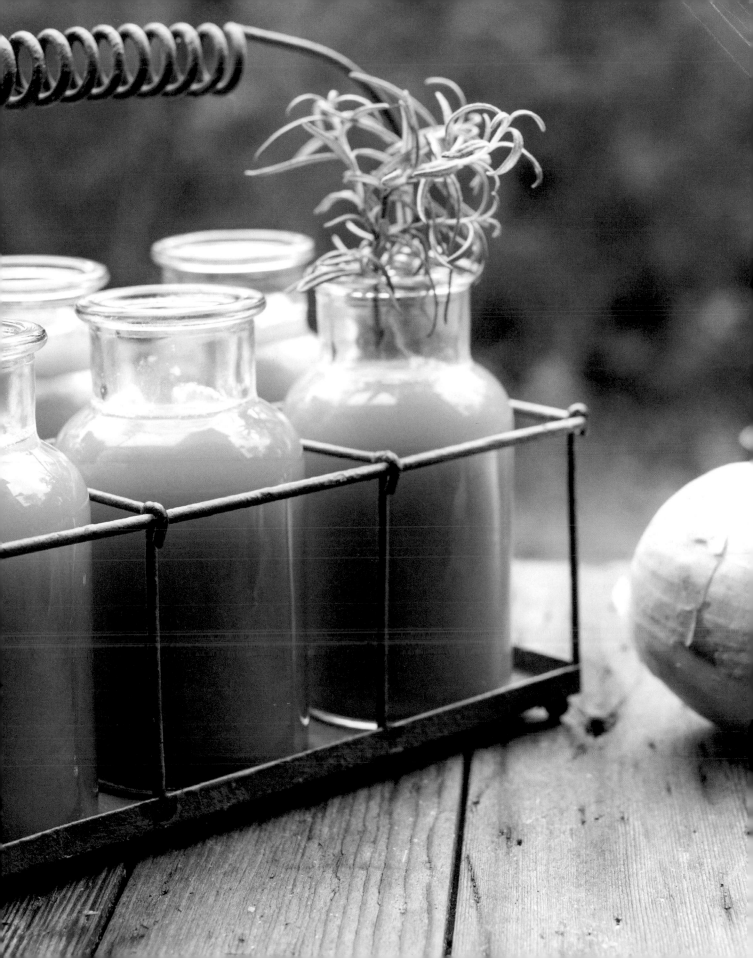

# berbere spice mix

LM H KETO  prep time: 5 minutes • yield: scant ¾ cup (2 teaspoons per serving)

If you crave ethnic food with a touch of spice, try this traditional Ethiopian blend; it tastes amazing on chicken, beef, or pork. Every time I taste it, it takes me back to Ethiopia, where my husband and I adopted our two boys, and special memories fill my mind.

6 tablespoons paprika

3 tablespoons cayenne pepper

1 tablespoon fine sea salt

1 teaspoon garlic powder

1 teaspoon onion powder

1 teaspoon ground coriander

½ teaspoon ginger powder

½ teaspoon ground cardamom

½ teaspoon ground fenugreek

½ teaspoon fresh ground nutmeg

¼ teaspoon ground cloves

Place all the ingredients in a jar with a lid. Cover and shake until well combined. Store in the pantry for up to 2 months.

NUTRITIONAL INFO (per serving)

| calories | fat | protein | carbs | fiber |
|----------|-------|---------|-------|-------|
| 1 | 0.03g | 0.04g | 0.2g | 0.1g |
|  | 13% | 7% | 80% |  |

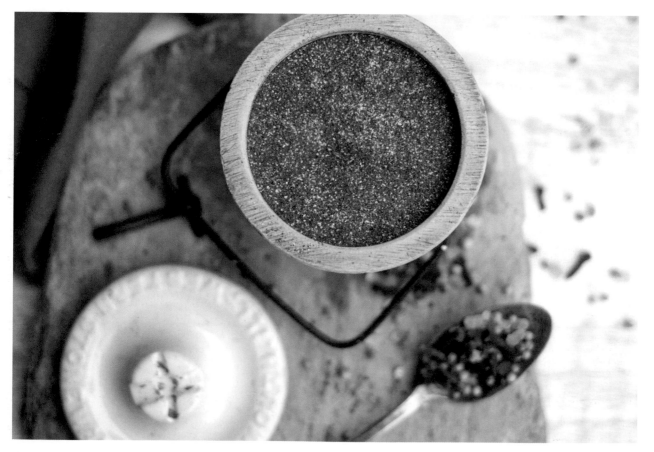

# spicy and sweet hamburger seasoning

**KETO** L-M-H · prep time: 5 minutes · yield: ½ cup plus 3 tablespoons (2 teaspoons per serving)

¼ cup paprika

1 tablespoon plus 2 teaspoons fine sea salt

1 tablespoon plus 1 teaspoon fresh ground black pepper

1 tablespoon plus 1 teaspoon Swerve confectioners'-style sweetener or equivalent amount of powdered erythritol or monk fruit (see page 81)

1 tablespoon plus 1 teaspoon garlic powder

1 tablespoon plus 1 teaspoon onion powder

1 teaspoon cayenne pepper

Place all the ingredients in a large airtight container and shake until well combined. Store in the pantry for up to 2 months.

NUTRITIONAL INFO (per serving)

| calories | fat | protein | carbs | fiber |
|----------|------|---------|-------|-------|
| 11 | 0.2g | 0.4g | 2g | 0.9g |
| | 15% | 13% | 72% | |

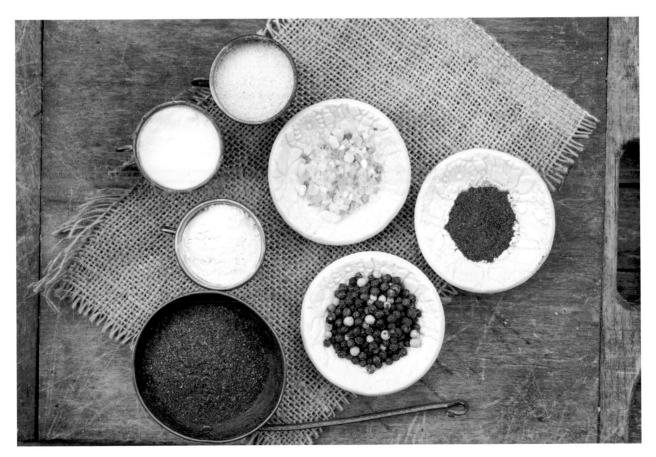

# cajun seasoning

KETO L—M—H · prep time: 5 minutes · yield: about ¼ cup (1 teaspoon per serving)

If you are a fan of spicy food, you must try this seasoning. My son Kai adores this seasoning on catfish (see page 370).

2½ teaspoons smoked paprika

2 teaspoons fine sea salt

2 teaspoons garlic powder

1¼ teaspoons onion powder

1¼ teaspoons dried oregano leaves

1¼ teaspoons dried thyme leaves

1 teaspoon fresh ground black pepper

1 teaspoon cayenne pepper

½ teaspoon red pepper flakes

Place all the ingredients in a jar with a lid. Cover and shake until well combined. Store in the pantry for up to 2 months.

| NUTRITIONAL INFO (per serving) | | | | |
|---|---|---|---|---|
| calories 6 | fat 0.1g | protein 0.2g | carbs 1.1g | fiber 0g |
| | 15% | 13% | 72% | |

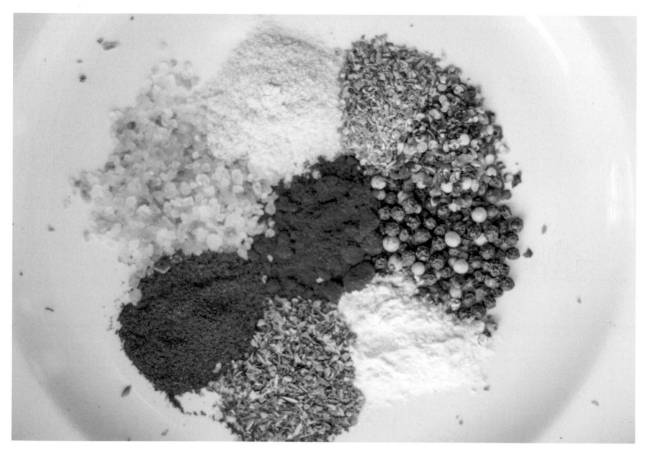

# herbes de florence

prep time: 5 minutes • yield: ¾ cup (2¼ teaspoons per serving)

This herb blend is an Italian twist on herbes de Provence. I love using this blend in salad dressings, adding it to homemade mayo, and rubbing it on poultry for a tasty addition to meals.

2 tablespoons dried basil

2 tablespoons dried ground marjoram

2 tablespoons dried oregano leaves

2 tablespoons dried parsley

1 tablespoon dried ground rosemary

1 tablespoon dried thyme leaves

1 tablespoon red pepper flakes

2 teaspoons garlic powder

1 teaspoon onion powder

Place all the ingredients into a jar with a lid. Cover and shake until well combined. Store in the pantry for up to 2 months.

NUTRITIONAL INFO (per serving)

| calories | fat | protein | carbs | fiber |
|---|---|---|---|---|
| 6 | 0.1g | 0.2g | 1g | 0.4g |
| | 16% | 15% | 69% | |

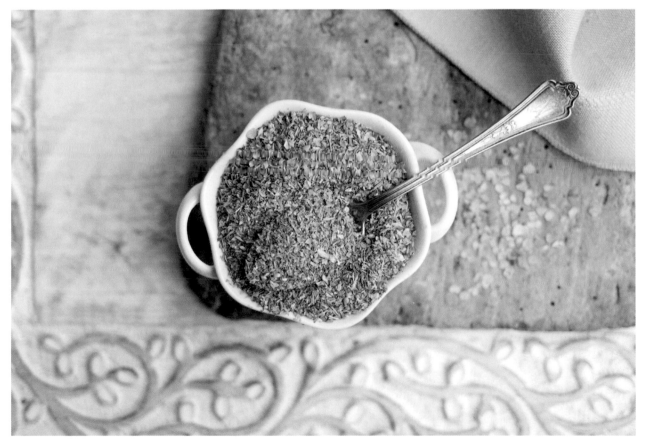

# ranch seasoning

L M H KETO prep time: 5 minutes • yield: ⅓ cup (1¼ heaping teaspoons per serving)

This seasoning tastes great on fish, seafood, and even hamburgers. You can also mix it into homemade mayo to create a tasty keto sauce!

2 tablespoons dried parsley

1 tablespoon plus 1 teaspoon onion powder

2 teaspoons garlic powder

1½ teaspoons dried dill weed

1 teaspoon dried chives

1 teaspoon fine sea salt

1 teaspoon fresh ground black pepper

Place all the ingredients in a jar with a lid. Cover and shake until well combined. Store in the pantry for up to 2 months.

NUTRITIONAL INFO (per serving)

| calories | fat | protein | carbs | fiber |
|----------|-----|---------|-------|-------|
| 5 | 0g | 0.2g | 1.1g | 0.2g |
| | 0% | 15% | 85% | |

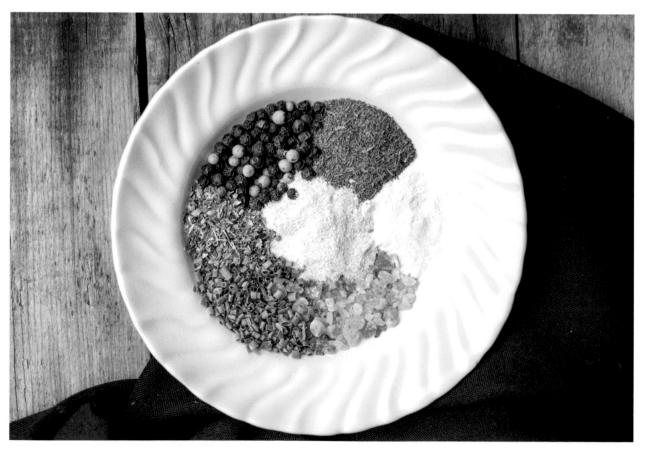

# dairy-free ranch dressing

prep time: 5 minutes, plus 2 hours to chill

yield: 1¾ cups (2 tablespoons plus 1 teaspoon per serving)

1 cup mayonnaise, homemade (page 124) or store-bought (or Egg-Free Keto Mayo, page 125, for egg-free)

¾ cup chicken or beef bone broth, homemade (page 108) or store-bought

2½ teaspoons Ranch Seasoning (page 114)

Place all the ingredients in a 16-ounce (or larger) jar and shake vigorously until well combined. Cover and refrigerate for 2 hours before serving (it will thicken as it rests). Store in an airtight container in the fridge for up to 5 days.

NUTRITIONAL INFO (per serving)

| calories | fat | protein | carbs | fiber |
|---|---|---|---|---|
| 128 | 14g | 0.3g | 0.2g | 0.1g |
| | 98% | 1% | 1% | |

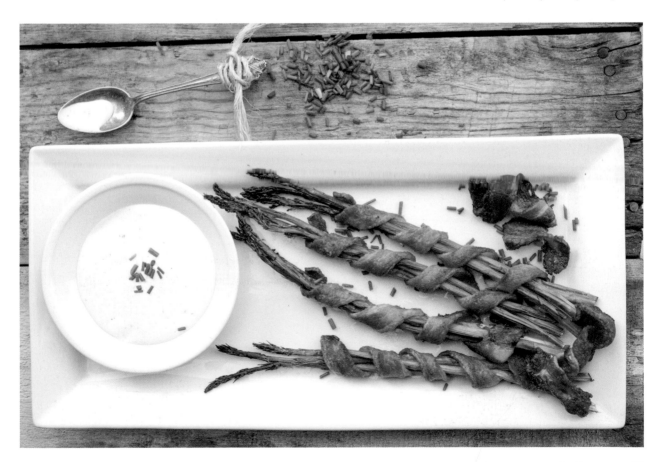

# creamy mexican dressing

L ⌒ M H KETO ▱ ⌀ ⌀ ⌀ option  prep time: 5 minutes • yield: 1½ cups (about 2 tablespoons per serving)

¼ cup MCT oil or extra-virgin olive oil

¼ cup chicken bone broth, homemade (page 108) or store-bought (or vegetable broth for vegetarian)

1 avocado, peeled and pitted

¼ cup fresh cilantro leaves

Juice of 1 lime

1 teaspoon minced garlic

½ teaspoon ground cumin

¼ teaspoon dried oregano leaves

½ to 1 small jalapeño pepper (adjust for desired heat), seeded

Place all the ingredients in a food processor and puree until smooth. Store in a covered jar in the fridge for up to 8 days.

NUTRITIONAL INFO (per serving)

| calories | fat | protein | carbs | fiber |
|----------|-----|---------|-------|-------|
| 72 | 7g | 0.5g | 2g | 1g |
|  | 87% | 2% | 11% |  |

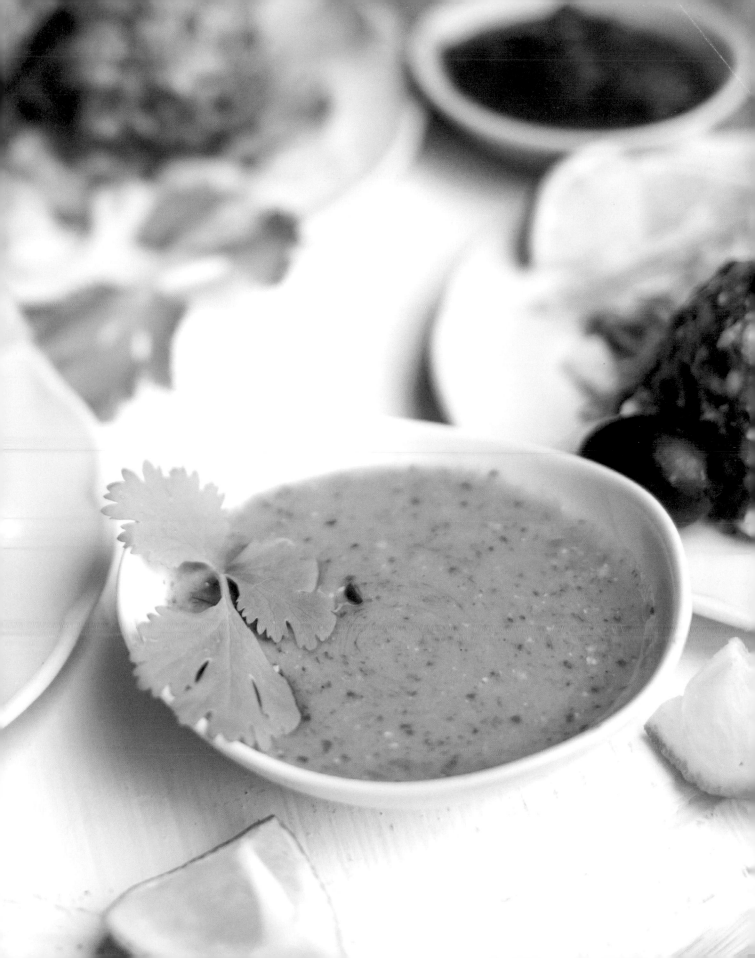

# dairy-free thousand island dressing

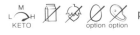 prep time: 5 minutes • yield: 1¼ cups (about 2 tablespoons per serving)

¾ cup mayonnaise, homemade (page 124) or store-bought (or Egg-Free Keto Mayo, page 125, for egg-free)

¼ cup chopped dill pickles

¼ cup tomato sauce

⅛ teaspoon fine ground sea salt

⅛ teaspoon fish sauce (omit for vegetarian)

Place all the ingredients in a jar with a lid, cover, and shake until very smooth. Store in the refrigerator for up to 1 week. Shake well before using.

NUTRITIONAL INFO (per serving)

| calories | fat | protein | carbs | fiber |
|----------|-----|---------|-------|-------|
| 110 | 12g | 0.1g | 0.3g | 0.1g |
| | 98% | 1% | 1% | |

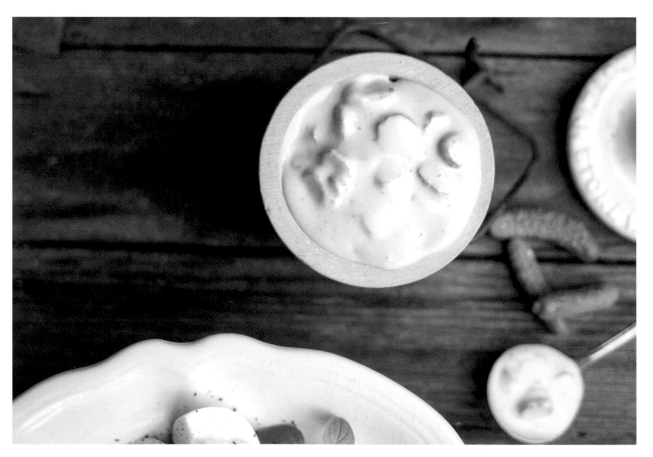

# orange-infused dressing

prep time: 5 minutes, plus 1 day to infuse • yield: 2 cups (2 tablespoons per serving)

This dressing tastes great on leafy greens and Zoodles (page 262), and it pairs amazingly well with Asian Chicken Salad (page 222).

1½ cups MCT oil, extra-virgin olive oil, or avocado oil

Peel from 1 orange

2 tablespoons Swerve confectioners'-style sweetener or equivalent amount of liquid or powdered sweetener (see page 81)

1 teaspoon fine sea salt

¼ teaspoon fresh ground black pepper

3 drops orange oil

½ cup coconut vinegar or apple cider vinegar

Place the oil in a 1-quart jar. Add the orange peel, sweetener, salt, pepper, and orange oil. Cover and let sit at room temperature for 1 day. Discard the peel. Add the vinegar to the jar and shake well before drizzling over greens. Store in the fridge for up to 2 weeks.

NUTRITIONAL INFO (per serving)

| calories | fat | protein | carbs | fiber |
|----------|-----|---------|-------|-------|
| 193 | 21g | 0g | 0g | 0g |
| | 100% | 0% | 0% | |

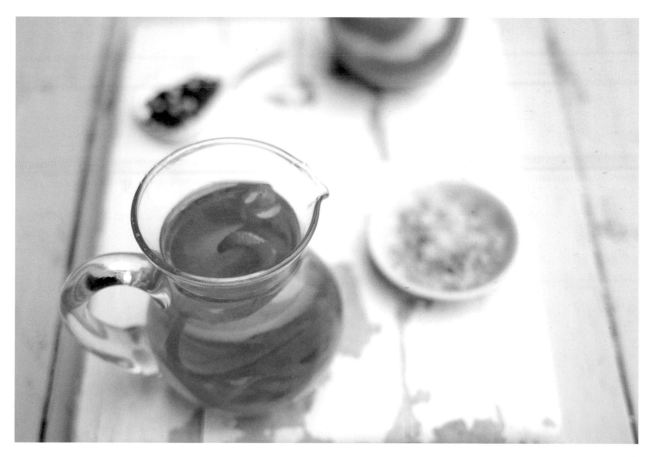

# onion-infused dressing

L→M→H KETO · prep time: 5 minutes, plus 1 day to infuse • yield: 2 cups (2 tablespoons per serving)

1½ cups MCT oil, extra-virgin olive oil, or avocado oil

½ cup sliced onions

2 tablespoons Swerve confectioners'-style sweetener or equivalent amount of liquid or powdered sweetener (see page 81)

1 teaspoon fine sea salt

3 drops food-grade onion oil

½ cup coconut vinegar or apple cider vinegar

1. Pour the oil into a 1-quart jar with a lid. Add the onions, sweetener, salt, and onion oil. Cover and let sit at room temperature for 1 day.

2. Place in the fridge until ready to use. Discard the onion after 1 to 2 days of infusing. Add the vinegar to the jar and shake well before drizzling over greens. Store in the fridge for up to 2 weeks.

| NUTRITIONAL INFO (per serving) | | | | |
|---|---|---|---|---|
| calories | fat | protein | carbs | fiber |
| 164 | 18.4g | 0g | 0.1g | 0g |
| | 100% | 0% | 0% | |

# fat-burning herbes de florence dressing

prep time: 5 minutes • yield: ¾ cup (about 2 tablespoons per serving)

½ cup MCT oil

3 tablespoons coconut vinegar or white wine vinegar

1 tablespoon Herbes de Florence (page 113)

2 tablespoons lemon juice

1 tablespoon minced garlic

Place all the ingredients in a medium jar with a lid. Cover and shake until well combined. Store in the refrigerator for up to 2 weeks, shaking well before serving.

NUTRITIONAL INFO (per serving)

| calories | fat | protein | carbs | fiber |
|----------|-----|---------|-------|-------|
| 175 | 19g | 0.1g | 1g | 0.1g |
| | 98% | 0% | 2% | |

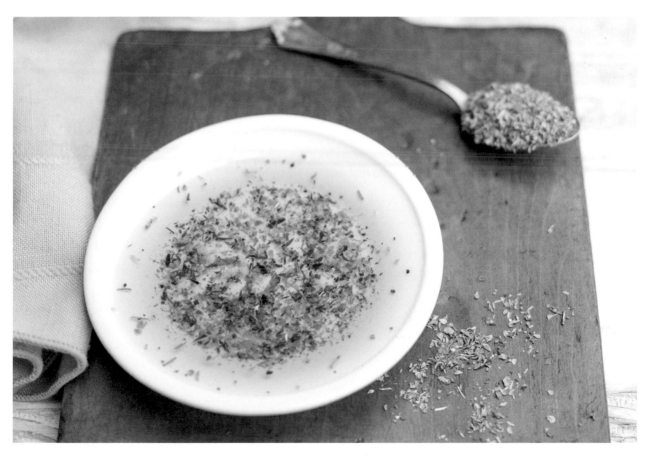

# bacon marmalade

L M H KETO  prep time: 8 minutes • cook time: 25 minutes • yield: 2½ cups (about 2 tablespoons per serving)

1 pound bacon, cut into small dice

1 cup diced onions

2 tablespoons Swerve confectioners'-style sweetener or equivalent amount of liquid or powdered sweetener (see page 81)

2 cups beef bone broth, home-made (page 108) or store-bought

1. Cook the bacon in a large cast-iron skillet over medium-high heat until crisp-tender, about 10 minutes. Add the diced onions and cook for about 5 more minutes.

2. Add the sweetener and broth and bring to a simmer, scraping bits off the bottom of the pan. Increase the heat to high and boil, while stirring, until the liquid has evaporated and the mixture has the texture of a spreadable marmalade, about 10 minutes.

3. Store in a sealed jar in the fridge for up to 6 days.

NUTRITIONAL INFO (per serving)

| calories | fat | protein | carbs | fiber |
|---|---|---|---|---|
| 71 | 6g | 4g | 0.4g | 0.1g |
| | 76% | 22% | 2% | |

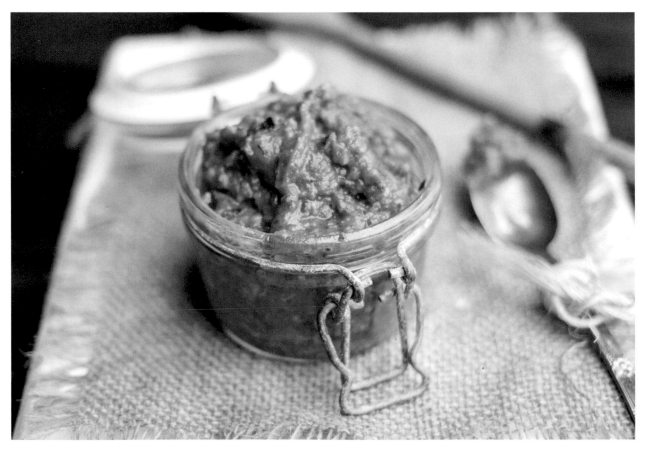

# mole sauce

prep time: 5 minutes • cook time: 15 minutes

yield: 1½ cups (about 2 tablespoons per serving)

If you are a sauce lover like me, make an extra batch of this sauce! You won't regret it. You can use it over Slow Cooker Mole Short Ribs (page 312), Simple Slow Cooker Chicken Thighs (page 290), or grilled chicken thighs.

2 tablespoons MCT oil

¼ cup finely chopped onions

1 clove garlic, minced

1 cup tomato sauce

1 (4-ounce) can diced green chiles

1 tablespoon chopped fresh cilantro

1 tablespoon unsweetened cocoa powder

1 teaspoon ground cumin

1. Heat the oil in a sauté pan over medium heat. Add the onions and fry for 3 minutes, or until translucent. Add the garlic and cook until fragrant, about 1 minute.

2. Add the rest of the ingredients, stir to combine, and simmer for 10 minutes. Remove from heat and puree until smooth, if desired. Store in an airtight container in the fridge for up to 1 week.

NUTRITIONAL INFO (per serving)

| calories | fat | protein | carbs | fiber |
|---|---|---|---|---|
| 14 | 1g | 0.2g | 1g | 0.2g |
|  | 65% | 5% | 29% |  |

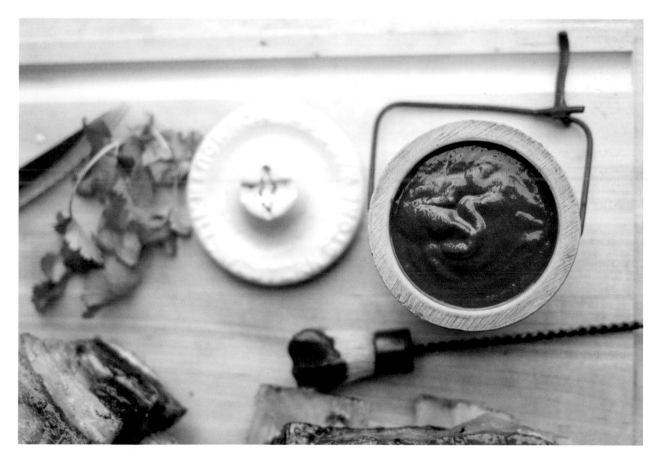

# easy blender mayo

KETO · prep time: 5 minutes · yield: 1½ cups (about 1 tablespoon per serving)

Homemade mayonnaise has a milder and more neutral flavor than store-bought mayo—plus, it's so much healthier! You can personalize this basic mayo to your taste by adding finely chopped or roasted garlic or your favorite herb.

2 large egg yolks

2 teaspoons lemon juice

1 cup MCT oil or other neutral-flavored oil, such as macadamia nut or avocado oil

1 tablespoon Dijon mustard

½ teaspoon fine sea salt

**special equipment:**

Immersion blender

**nut-free option:**

Don't use a nut-based oil

Place the ingredients in the order listed in a wide-mouth, pint-sized mason jar. Place the immersion blender at the bottom of the jar. Turn the blender on and very slowly move it to the top of the jar. Be patient! It should take you about a minute to reach the top. Moving the blender slowly is the key to getting the mayonnaise to emulsify. Voilà! Simple mayo! Store in the fridge for up to 5 days.

**variation: Copycat Baconnaise.**

*Replace the MCT oil with melted, but not hot, bacon fat and omit the ½ teaspoon salt. Taste the mayo and add salt if needed (it may be salty enough from the bacon fat).*

NUTRITIONAL INFO (per serving)

| calories | fat | protein | carbs | fiber |
|---|---|---|---|---|
| 92 | 10g | 0.3g | 0.1g | 0g |
| | 98% | 1.5% | 0.4% | |

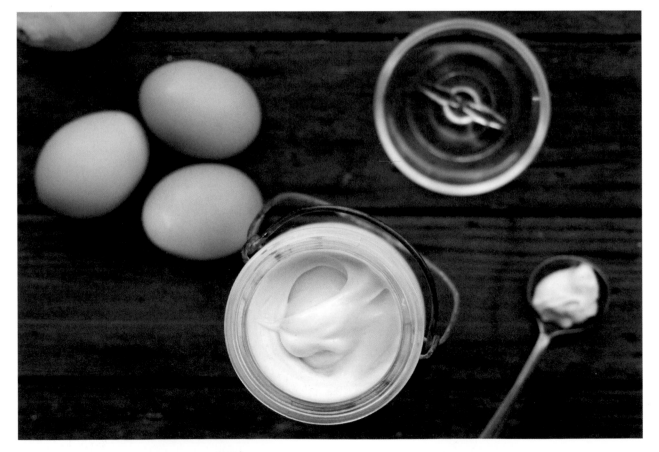

# egg-free keto mayo

prep time: 5 minutes • yield: 1½ cups (2 tablespoons per serving)

3 tablespoons lemon juice

2 tablespoons coconut vinegar or apple cider vinegar

1 tablespoon Swerve confectioners'-style sweetener or equivalent amount of liquid or powdered sweetener (see page 81)

1½ teaspoons Dijon mustard

1¼ teaspoons fine sea salt

½ cup cold-pressed extra-virgin olive oil

½ cup expeller-pressed coconut oil, softened but not melted (see note)

1. Place the lemon juice, coconut vinegar, sweetener, mustard, and salt in a blender or food processor and combine well.

2. Turn the blender to low speed and slowly drizzle in the olive oil drop by drop at first; once ¼ cup of the oil has been incorporated, you can increase the rate of the drizzle.

3. Add the softened coconut oil to the blender and puree just until combined. Place in a jar, cover, and store in the fridge for up to 1 week.

note: *Expeller-pressed coconut oil has the least coconut-y taste of all the coconut oils, so it's a good choice when you want a more neutral flavor, as here. If you'd like an even more neutral taste, palm oil is a good alternative.*

NUTRITIONAL INFO (per serving)

| calories | fat | protein | carbs | fiber |
|----------|-----|---------|-------|-------|
| 228 | 25g | 0.1g | 0.2g | 0g |
|  | 98% | 1% | 1% |  |

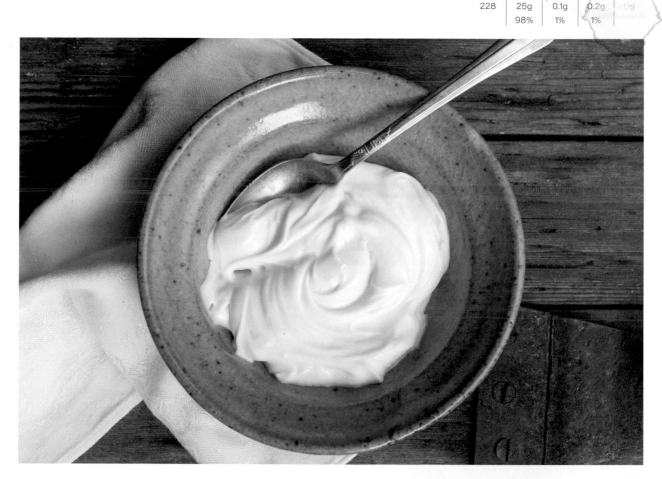

# berbere mayo

L M H KETO · option · prep time: 5 minutes • yield: ½ cup (2 tablespoons per serving)

This mayo tastes great with Doro Watt Chicken Salad Wraps (page 272).

2 tablespoons Berbere Spice Mix (page 110)

½ cup mayonnaise, homemade (page 124) or store-bought (or Egg-Free Keto Mayo, page 125, for egg-free)

Whisk the spice blend and mayo together until well combined. Store in an airtight container in the fridge for up to 1 week.

NUTRITIONAL INFO (per serving)

| calories | fat | protein | carbs | fiber |
|---|---|---|---|---|
| 205 | 23g | 0g | 0.1g | 0g |
| | 100% | 0% | 0% | |

# basil mayonnaise

prep time: 5 minutes • yield: 1 cup (2 tablespoons per serving)

1 cup coarsely chopped fresh basil leaves

¾ cup mayonnaise, homemade (page 124) or store-bought (or Egg-Free Keto Mayo, page 125, for egg-free)

1 clove garlic, crushed to a paste

¼ teaspoon fine sea salt

Place the basil in a food processor or blender and puree until smooth. Add the mayo, garlic, and salt and pulse until well combined. Place in a jar, cover, and store in the fridge for up to 1 week.

| NUTRITIONAL INFO (per serving) | | | | |
|---|---|---|---|---|
| calories | fat | protein | carbs | fiber |
| 155 | 1/g | 0g | 0.1g | 0g |
| | 99% | 0% | 1% | |

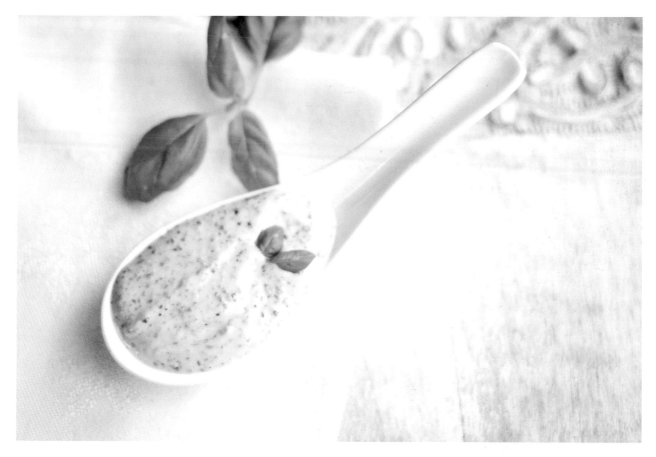

# garlic and herb aioli

L M>H KETO · prep time: 5 minutes · yield: 1 cup (2 tablespoons per serving)

1 cup mayonnaise, homemade (page 124) or store-bought (or Egg-Free Keto Mayo, page 125, for egg-free)

4 cloves garlic, minced

1 teaspoon dried thyme leaves or other herb of choice

½ teaspoon fine sea salt

Place all the ingredients in a food processor and process until the mixture is smooth and the thyme leaves are finely minced. Store in an airtight container in the fridge for up to 8 days.

note: *If making this aioli for the Hawaiian Delight on page 362, use chopped chives instead of thyme leaves for more of an Asian flair.*

NUTRITIONAL INFO (per serving)

| calories | fat | protein | carbs | fiber |
|----------|-----|---------|-------|-------|
| 208 | 23g | 0.1g | 1g | 0.1g |
| | 99% | 0% | 1% | |

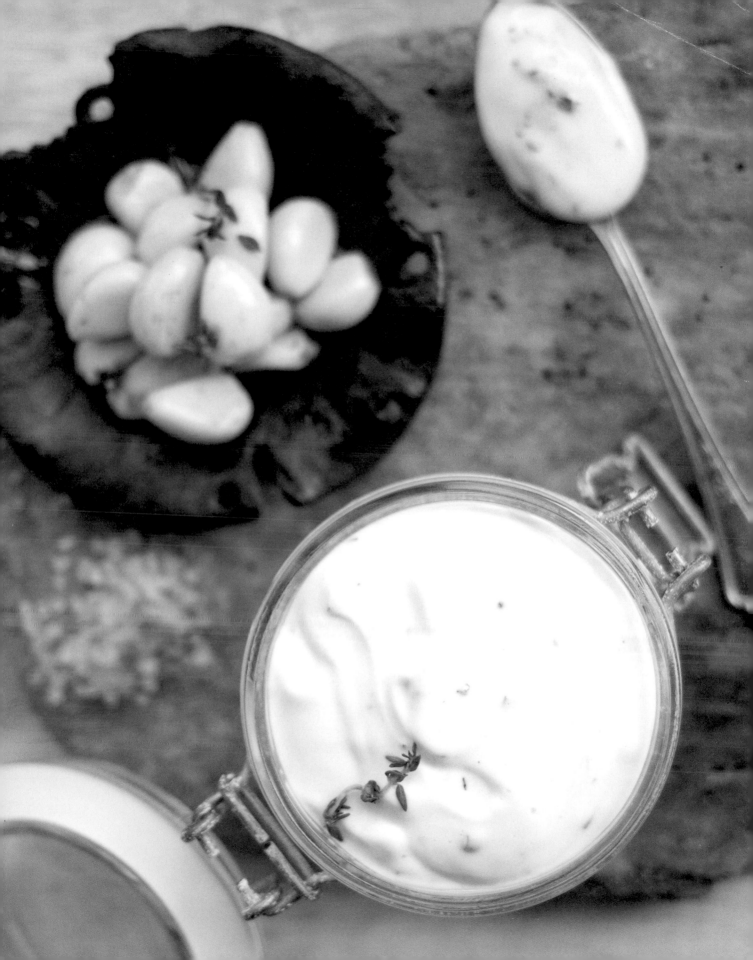

# herbes de florence red sauce

L M H KETO · prep time: 7 minutes • cook time: 30 minutes • yield: 4 cups (about ½ cup per serving)

This recipe utilizes two great tips that I learned from an Italian chef: (1) sautéing onions helps to bring out their sweetness so you don't need to add sugar (which appears in far too many recipes); and (2) adding extra-virgin olive oil and fresh herbs at the very end of cooking gives the sauce a whole new layer of flavor!

¼ cup MCT oil or avocado oil

¼ cup grated onions

4 cloves garlic, minced

3½ pounds fresh, garden-ripened tomatoes or 2 (28-ounce) cans crushed tomatoes

2 tablespoons Herbes de Florence (page 113)

**for garnish:**

2 tablespoons extra-virgin olive oil, for drizzling

2 tablespoons chopped fresh basil or parsley

1. Heat the oil in a deep skillet over medium heat. Add the onions to the pan and sauté for 5 to 8 minutes, until lightly golden. Add the garlic and sauté for an additional 3 minutes.

2. If using fresh tomatoes, remove the skins by slicing an X on the bottom of each tomato and blanching them in boiling water for 30 seconds; rinse in cold water and remove the skins (they will slide right off). Using your hands and working over a bowl to catch the juices, crush the tomatoes into small pieces.

3. Add the crushed tomatoes and juices and Herbes de Florence to the skillet. Reduce the heat and simmer, uncovered, for 30 minutes to 2 hours. The longer the sauce simmers, the more the flavors will open up.

4. Just at the end, add the olive oil and fresh herbs. Store in an airtight container in the fridge for up to 8 days, or freeze for up to 2 months.

NUTRITIONAL INFO (per serving)

| calories | fat | protein | carbs | fiber |
|----------|-----|---------|-------|-------|
| 129 | 9.7g | 9.7g | 8.6g | 2.5g |
| | 68% | 6% | 26% | |

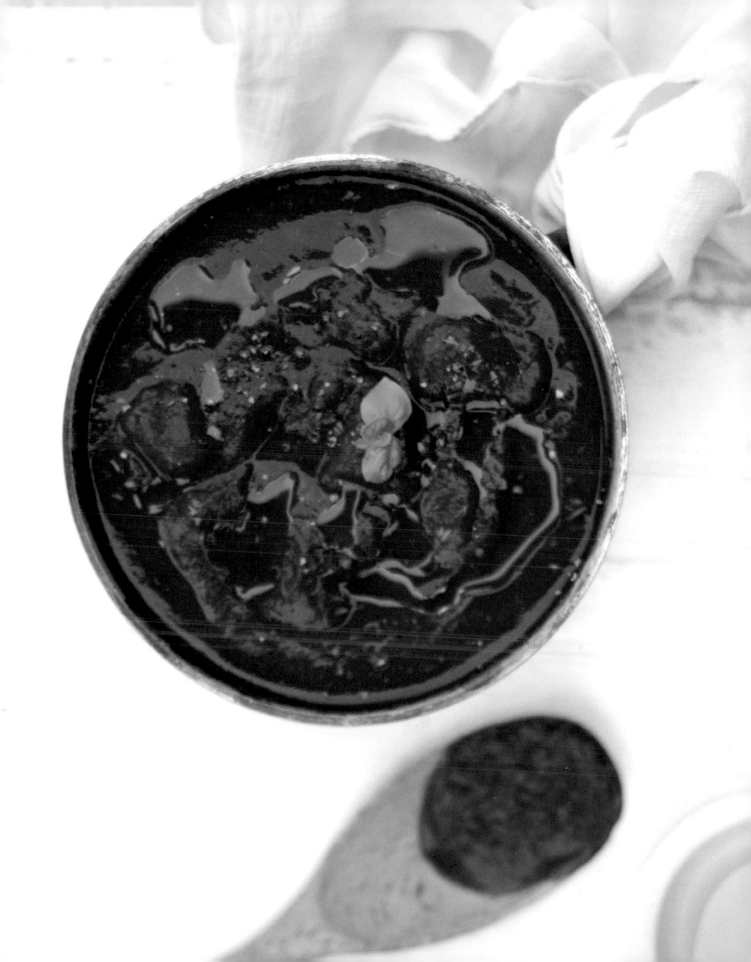

# worcestershire sauce

L M H
KETO

prep time: 8 minutes • cook time: 5 minutes
yield: 2½ cups (3 tablespoons plus 1 teaspoon per serving)

½ cup coconut vinegar

½ cup apple cider vinegar

½ cup Swerve confectioners'-style sweetener or equivalent amount of liquid or powdered sweetener (see page 81)

¼ cup fish sauce

2 tablespoons tamarind paste

1 tablespoon coconut aminos or wheat-free tamari

1 teaspoon onion powder

1 teaspoon fresh ground black pepper

½ teaspoon ground cinnamon

½ teaspoon ground cloves

¼ teaspoon cayenne pepper

2 tablespoons MCT oil or coconut oil

2 shallots, finely minced

4 cloves garlic, minced

1 teaspoon freshly grated ginger

8 anchovies, minced

Juice of 1 lime

1. In a small bowl, combine the vinegars, sweetener, fish sauce, tamarind paste, coconut aminos, and onion powder. Set aside.

2. Heat a dry saucepan over medium heat. Add the black pepper, cinnamon, cloves, and cayenne pepper and toast until fragrant, about 1 minute. Pour the spices into a small bowl and set aside.

3. Heat the oil over medium heat in the same saucepan you used to toast the spices. Add the shallots and sauté for 3 minutes, or until transparent and beginning to brown. Add the garlic, ginger, anchovies, and toasted spices and continue to sauté just until fragrant, about 30 seconds.

4. Pour the vinegar mixture into the saucepan and scrape up any bits on the bottom of the pan. Bring to a boil, then remove from the heat and let cool completely.

5. Strain through a fine-mesh strainer into a bowl and stir in the lime juice. Store in an airtight container in the refrigerator for up to 2 weeks, or freeze for up to 2 months.

NUTRITIONAL INFO (per serving)

| calories | fat | protein | carbs | fiber |
|---|---|---|---|---|
| 48 | 3g | 2g | 3g | 1g |
| | 51% | 26% | 23% | |

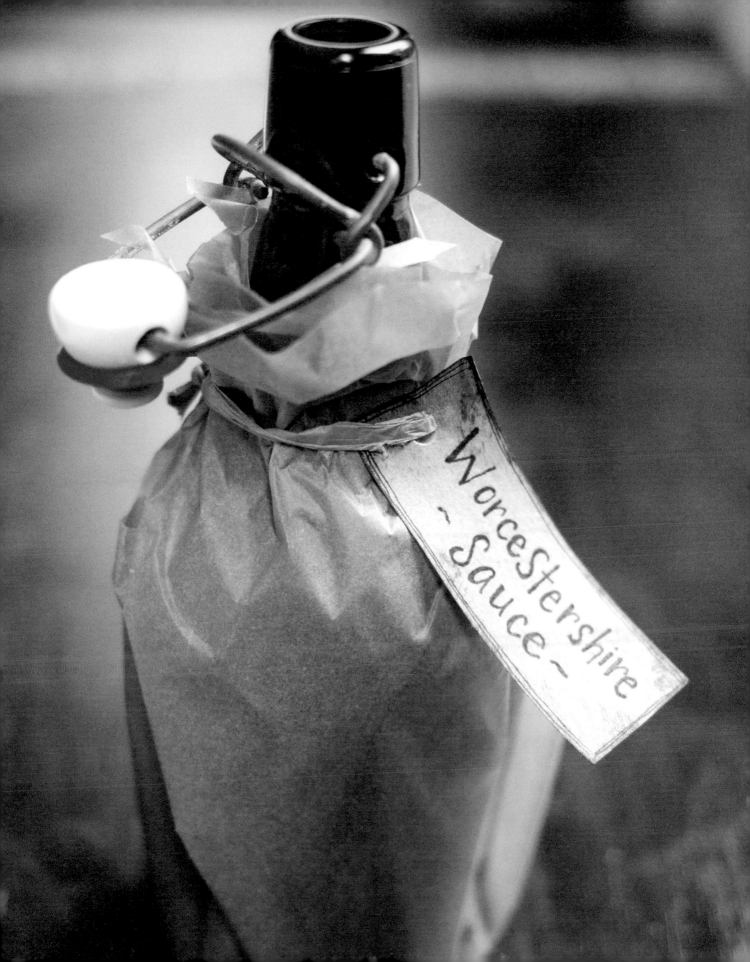

# hot sauce

L M H KETO · option    prep time: 5 minutes • cook time: 5 minutes • yield: 4 cups (1 teaspoon per serving)

I am a true German: I do not like spicy food. But I've learned to appreciate hot sauce because of its great thermogenic properties and its ability to increase metabolic rate.

2 tablespoons MCT oil or coconut oil

15 medium serrano chiles, stemmed and cut crosswise into small pieces (see note)

½ cup diced onions

1 tablespoon minced garlic (about 3 cloves)

2 cups chicken bone broth, homemade (page 108) or store-bought, or water (add ¼ teaspoon salt if using water)

1 cup coconut vinegar or apple cider vinegar

Fine sea salt

1. Heat the oil in a large cast-iron skillet over low heat. Add the chiles, onions, and garlic and cook for 5 minutes, or until the onions are translucent and the chiles are soft. Add the broth.

2. Transfer the sautéed veggies and broth to a high-speed blender or food processor and puree until smooth. With the machine running on low speed, add the vinegar in a slow, steady stream. Add salt to taste.

3. Strain the hot sauce and place in a jar. Cover and store in the fridge for up to 6 months. I recommend that you let the sauce sit for 2 weeks before using to allow the flavors to open up.

note: *When working with this number of chiles, wear food-safe gloves and do not touch your eyes.*

NUTRITIONAL INFO (per serving)

| calories | fat | protein | carbs | fiber |
|----------|------|---------|-------|-------|
| 2 | 0.1g | 0.1g | 0.2g | 0g |
| | 42% | 20% | 38% | |

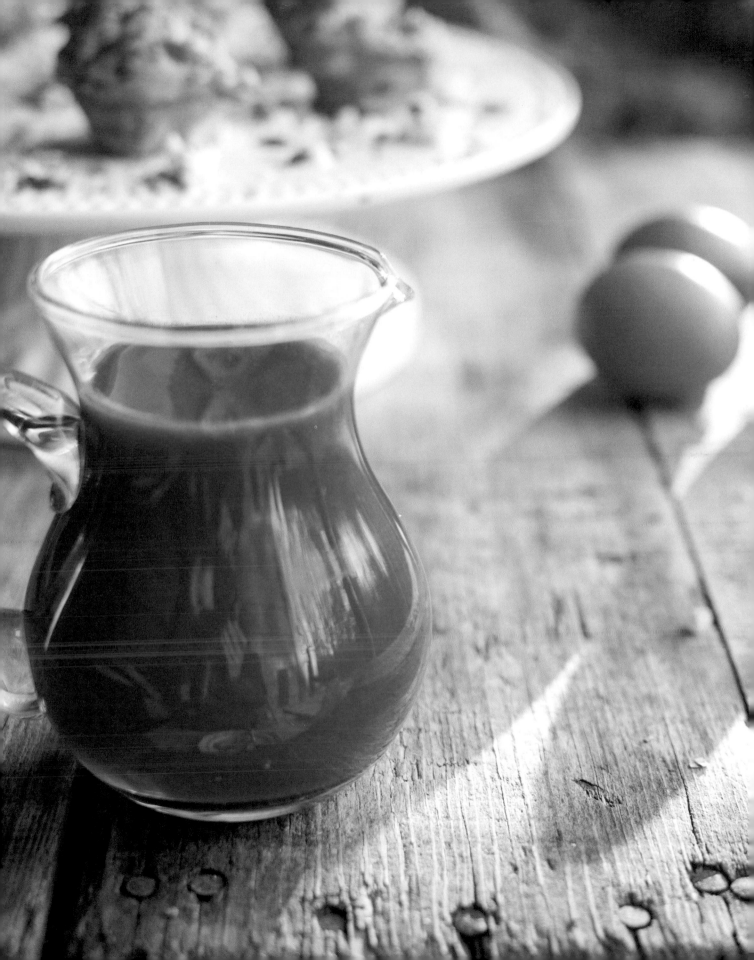

# easy dairy-free hollandaise

This sauce tastes great with my Eggs Florentine (page 166), Florentine Breakfast Burgers (page 152), steak, fish, or chicken.

1 cup bacon fat, beef tallow, or leaf lard

4 large egg yolks

½ cup lemon juice

½ teaspoon fine sea salt

¼ teaspoon fresh ground black pepper

**vegetarian option:**

Use warmed MCT oil, avocado oil, or extra-virgin olive oil.

**variation:**

Easy Basil Hollandaise.

*In Step 2, add 1 cup (1 ounce) loosely packed fresh basil leaves to the blender with the egg yolks and lemon juice. Continue with the recipe as written.*

1. Heat the fat in a small saucepan over high heat (or in the microwave) until very hot and melted. Set aside.

2. Combine the egg yolks and lemon juice in a blender and puree until very smooth. With the blender running on low speed, drizzle in the hot melted fat until a thick, creamy mixture forms. Add the salt and pepper and pulse to combine; adjust the seasoning to taste.

3. Use immediately or keep warm for up to 1 hour in a heat-safe bowl set over warm water. Store in a covered jar in the fridge for up to 5 days. Reheat the sauce in a double boiler or a heat-safe bowl set over a pot of simmering water, whisking often, until the sauce is warm and thick.

NUTRITIONAL INFO (per serving)

| calories | fat | protein | carbs | fiber |
|---|---|---|---|---|
| 101 | 11g | 0.5g | 0.1g | 0g |
|  | 97% | 2% | 1% |  |

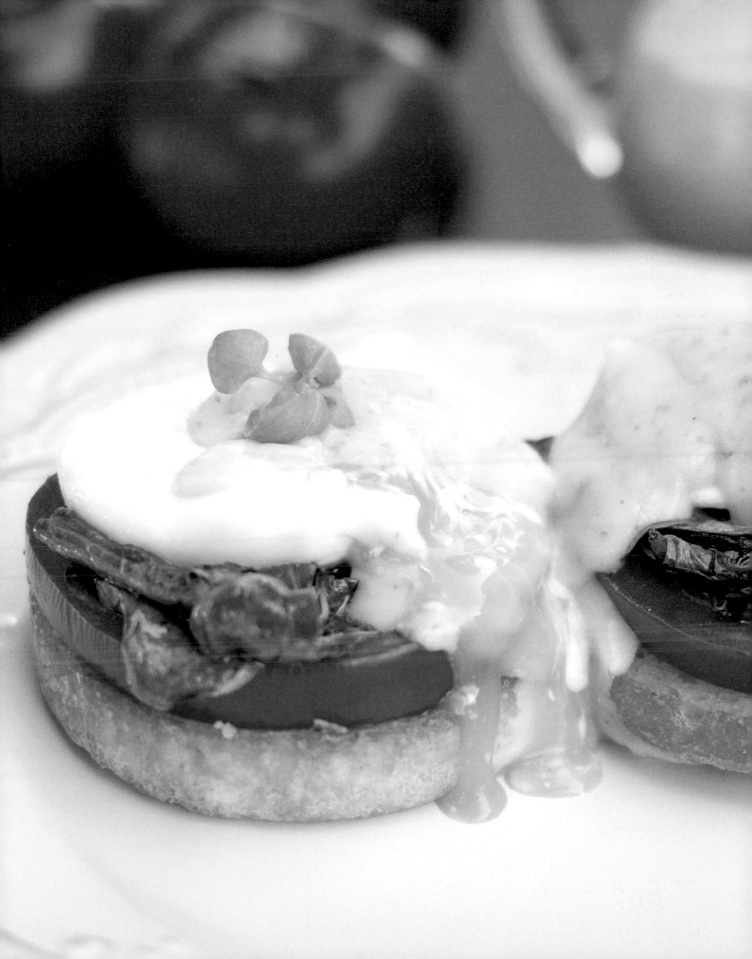

# keto lemon mostarda

L M H KETO · prep time: 5 minutes · yield: ¾ cup (about 2 tablespoons per serving)

Mostarda is traditionally made with candied fruit and mustard, but my Keto Lemon Mostarda is free of sugar! It tastes great with seafood sausage (page 366).

2 tablespoons lemon juice

2 tablespoons Dijon mustard

1 tablespoon coconut vinegar or red wine vinegar

1 clove garlic, minced

½ cup MCT oil

Fine sea salt and fresh ground black pepper

¼ cup Swerve confectioners'-style sweetener or equivalent amount of liquid or powdered sweetener (see page 81) (optional)

In a small bowl, whisk together the lemon juice, mustard, vinegar, and garlic. While whisking, slowly drizzle in the oil until emulsified. Season with salt and pepper to taste and add sweetener, if desired. Store in a covered jar in the fridge for up to 5 days.

| NUTRITIONAL INFO (per serving) | | | | |
|---|---|---|---|---|
| calories | fat | protein | carbs | fiber |
| 81 | 9g | 0g | 0.1g | 0g |
| | 100% | 0% | 0% | |

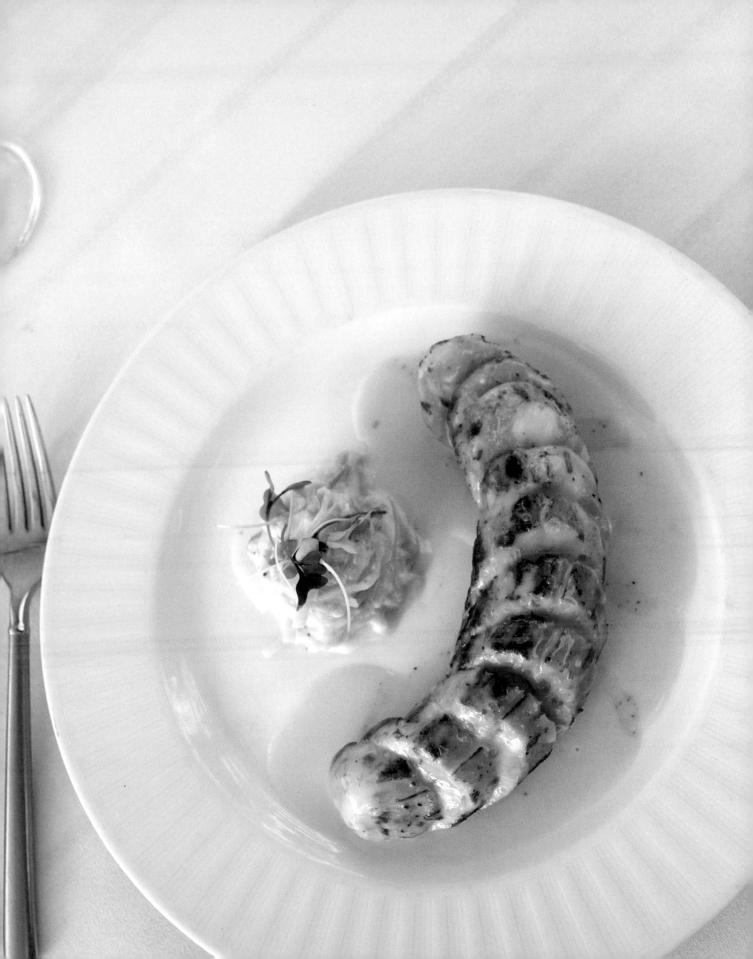

# guacamole

L Ṁ H / KETO    prep time: 15 minutes • yield: 3 cups (½ cup per serving)

Guacamole is an amazing creamy dip, but I have to admit that it becomes unappealing when it turns brown. But there is a solution: you simply need to use the pit and keep the guacamole sealed as airtight as possible! Place the pit in the middle of your bowl of guacamole, then cover the guacamole with large chunks of onion. The onion releases gases to inhibit the oxidation of polyphenol, which causes the fruit to turn brown. Cover tightly with plastic wrap, pressing the wrap directly onto the surface of the onions, and refrigerate until ready to serve. Just before serving, remove the chunks of onion. You can use this same technique with unused avocado. If you use only half an avocado, keep the pit in the other half and place it in a resealable bag. Slice an onion into chunks and place the onion in the bag with the avocado half. Then get as much air as possible out of the bag, seal it, and place it in the fridge.

3 avocados, peeled and pitted

3 to 4 tablespoons lime juice

½ cup diced yellow onions

2 plum tomatoes, diced

2 cloves Garlic Confit (page 142) or raw garlic, crushed to a paste

3 tablespoons chopped fresh cilantro leaves

1 teaspoon fine sea salt

½ teaspoon ground cumin

1. Place the avocado and 3 tablespoons of lime juice in a large bowl and mash until it reaches your desired consistency.

2. Add the rest of the ingredients and stir until well combined. Taste and add more lime juice if you like.

3. Cover tightly and refrigerate for 1 hour for best flavor, or serve immediately. The guacamole will keep in the fridge for 3 days when stored as described above.

NUTRITIONAL INFO (per serving)

| calories | fat | protein | carbs | fiber |
|---|---|---|---|---|
| 175 | 14g | 2g | 11g | 7g |
|  | 72% | 4% | 24% |  |

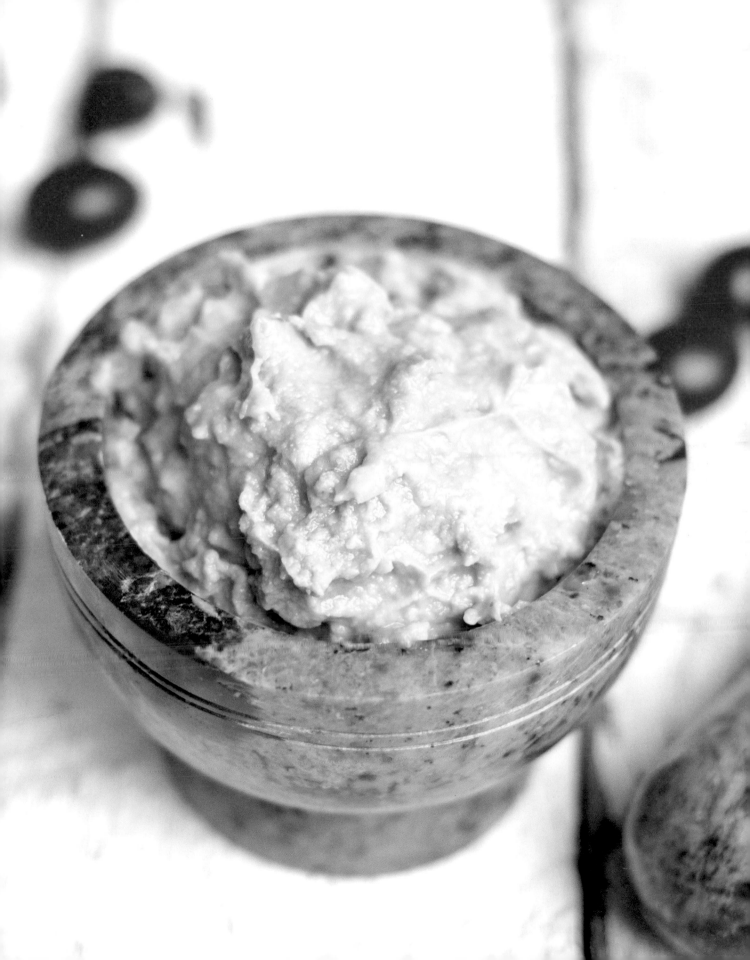

# garlic confit

KETO · L M H · prep time: 5 minutes • cook time: 45 to 60 minutes • yield: 40 servings

1 cup MCT oil or extra-virgin olive oil

20 cloves garlic, peeled

4 sprigs fresh thyme or other herb of choice

busy family tip: *Store garlic confit in the fridge for easy, flavorful additions to meals. You can experiment with different herbs and spices.*

Place the oil, garlic, and herbs in a small saucepan. Poach on low heat until the garlic is very soft, 45 to 60 minutes. Store in an airtight container in the fridge for up to 1 month.

NUTRITIONAL INFO (per serving)

| calories | fat | protein | carbs | fiber |
|---|---|---|---|---|
| 58 | 6g | 0.1g | 1g | 0.1g |
| | 93% | 1% | 7% | |

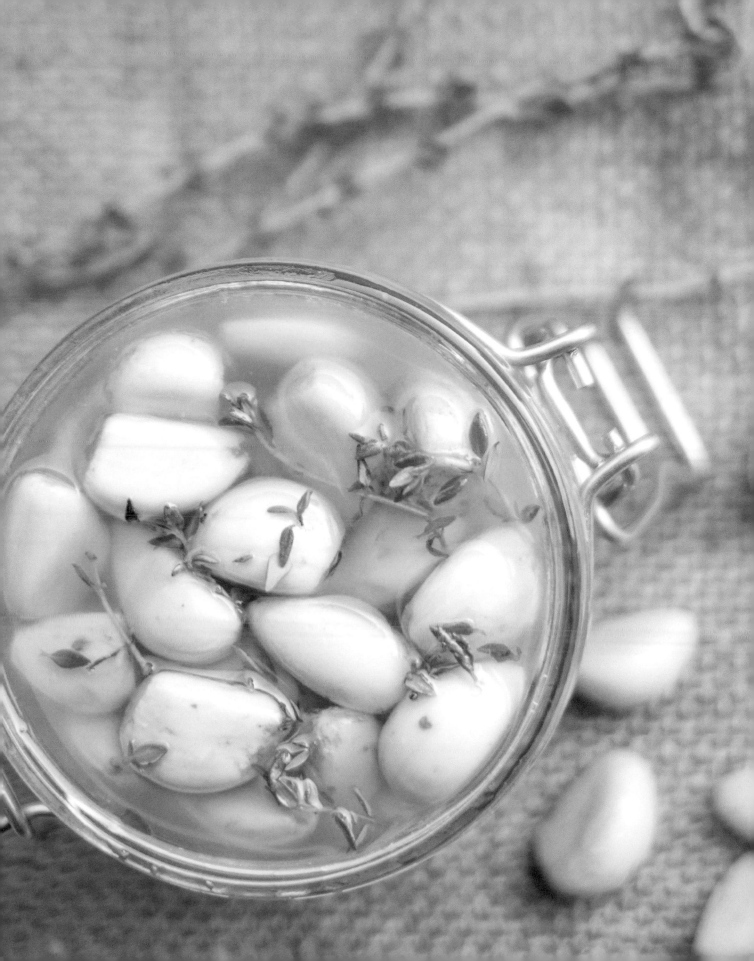

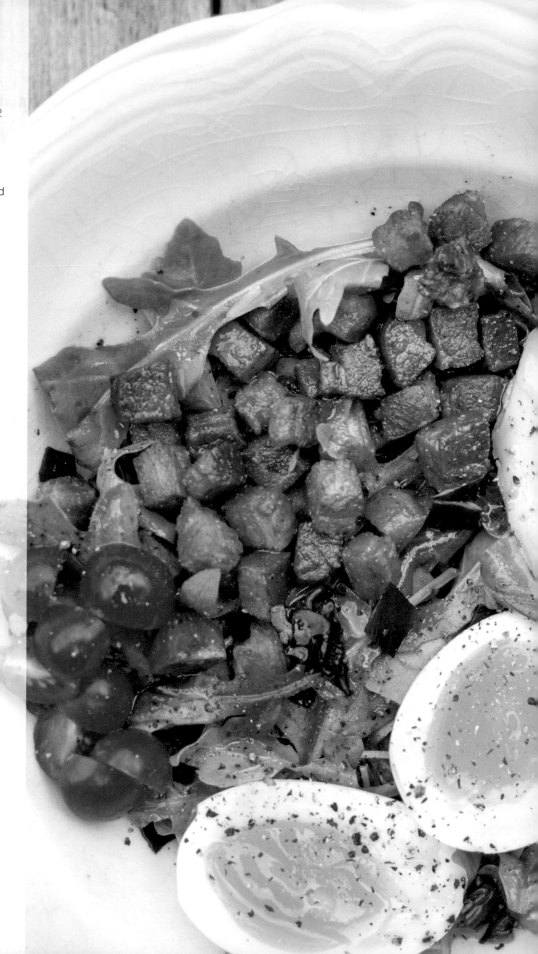

# break-your-fast
# meals

# keto chai

L M H KETO · option · prep time: 3 minutes · cook time: 10 to 15 minutes · yield: 7 (8-ounce) servings

I'm not a fan of drinking your calories if you are eating keto for weight loss. But since keto is more than a weight-loss diet, here is a tasty drink for those of you who are eating keto for healthy healing.

I was saddened to learn how many teabags and loose teas contain added sweeteners. I often take my boys to tea at a local tea shop and play cards with them. One day I asked Lauren, the tea expert there, if she thought that the fruity teas have any sugar, even "natural" sugar. She said, "Most likely. A lot of the loose teas even have tiny marshmallows in them. The Chocolate Safari Tea you often get has marshmallows in it." I was so disturbed by this! She recommended that we purchase organic teas to avoid cheap sweeteners. "But what about organic coconut sugar?" I asked. She said yeah, even organic teas definitely could have some organic natural sugars added. So the big lesson here is: make your own chai!

8 whole cloves

7 cardamom pods

2 cinnamon sticks

1½ teaspoons black peppercorns

1 (2-inch) piece fresh ginger, sliced into thin rounds

5 cups cold water

5 bags black tea

2 cups unsweetened (unflavored or vanilla-flavored) cashew milk, homemade (page 106) or store-bought, or almond milk (or hemp milk for nut-free)

2 to 4 tablespoons Swerve confectioners'-style sweetener or equivalent amount of liquid or powdered sweetener (see page 81)

1 tablespoon coconut oil per cup of tea

1. Place the spices and ginger in a medium saucepan. Toast on low heat while lightly crushing the spices with the back of a spoon.

2. Add the water and bring to a boil. Once boiling, cover the pan, lower the heat, and simmer for 5 to 10 minutes (the longer time will create a stronger chai flavor). Remove from the heat.

3. Place the teabags in the saucepan and steep for 4 minutes. Remove the teabags and add the cashew milk and 2 tablespoons of the sweetener. Stir, taste, and add more sweetener if desired.

4. Bring the chai to a bare simmer over medium heat, then strain it into a teapot. Just before serving, place a tablespoon of coconut oil in each teacup, pour the hot tea over it, and whisk to blend the coconut oil into the tea. Store extra tea in an airtight container in the fridge for up to 1 week.

NUTRITIONAL INFO (per serving)

| calories | fat | protein | carbs | fiber |
|----------|-----|---------|-------|-------|
| 35 | 3g | 1g | 1g | 0.3g |
|  | 78% | 11% | 11% |  |

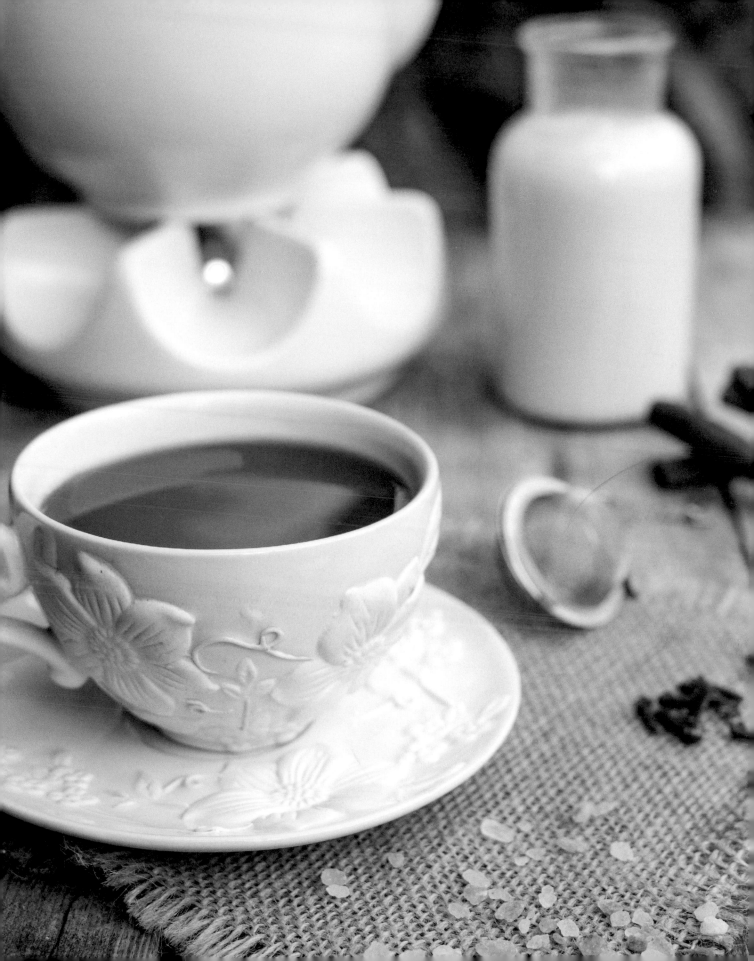

# breakfast chili

LOW KETO M H · prep time: 10 minutes · cook time: 2 hours 15 minutes · yield: 12 servings (1 cup per serving)

4 slices bacon, diced

1 pound 80% lean ground beef

1 pound Mexican-style fresh (raw) chorizo, removed from casings

1 (28-ounce) can diced tomatoes with juices

1 cup tomato sauce

¼ cup chopped onions

1 red bell pepper, chopped

2 green chiles, chopped

½ cup beef bone broth, home-made (page 108) or store-bought

2 tablespoons chili powder

2 teaspoons dried ground oregano

2 teaspoons minced garlic

1 teaspoon ground cumin

½ teaspoon cayenne pepper

½ teaspoon paprika

½ teaspoon fine sea salt

½ teaspoon fresh ground black pepper

2 tablespoons Swerve confectioners'-style sweetener or equivalent amount of liquid or powdered sweetener (see page 81) (optional)

## toppings (per serving):

1 large egg, fried sunny side up (omit for egg-free)

¼ avocado, cut into ½-inch dice

2 tablespoons diced cooked bacon (about 1 strip)

1 teaspoon chopped fresh chives

1. In a stockpot over medium-high heat, fry the diced bacon until crisp, then remove from the pot with a slotted spoon and set aside. Crumble the ground beef and chorizo into the hot pot and cook, stirring often to break up the meat, until evenly browned, about 7 minutes.

2. Pour in the diced tomatoes and tomato sauce. Add the onions, bell pepper, chiles, cooked bacon, and beef broth and stir to combine. Season with the chili powder, oregano, garlic, cumin, cayenne, paprika, salt, black pepper, and sweetener, if using. Stir to blend, then cover and bring to a simmer over medium heat. Once at a simmer, reduce the heat to low and continue to simmer for at least 2 hours, stirring occasionally. The longer the chili simmers, the better it will taste.

3. After 2 hours, taste and add more salt, pepper, and chili powder, if desired. Remove from the heat and serve each portion with a sunny-side-up egg, diced avocado, diced cooked bacon, and chopped chives. Store extras in an airtight container in the fridge for up to 5 days, or freeze for up to 2 months.

note: *This is one of the recipes featured in week 4 of the 30-day meal plan. It makes four more servings than you will need if you're feeding two people, but it's one of those dishes that is so worthwhile to make in a large batch. I recommend that you make the full recipe and freeze the leftovers in individual portions for easy breakfasts after you've completed the meal plan. Also, to help curb your sweet tooth during the cleanse, I suggest you omit the sweetener from this recipe.*

busy family tip: *Store extras in individual-serving containers for an easy breakfast option.*

| NUTRITIONAL INFO (per serving) | | | | |
|---|---|---|---|---|
| calories | fat | protein | carbs | fiber |
| 440 | 34g | 25g | 8g | 3g |
| | 70% | 23% | 7% | |

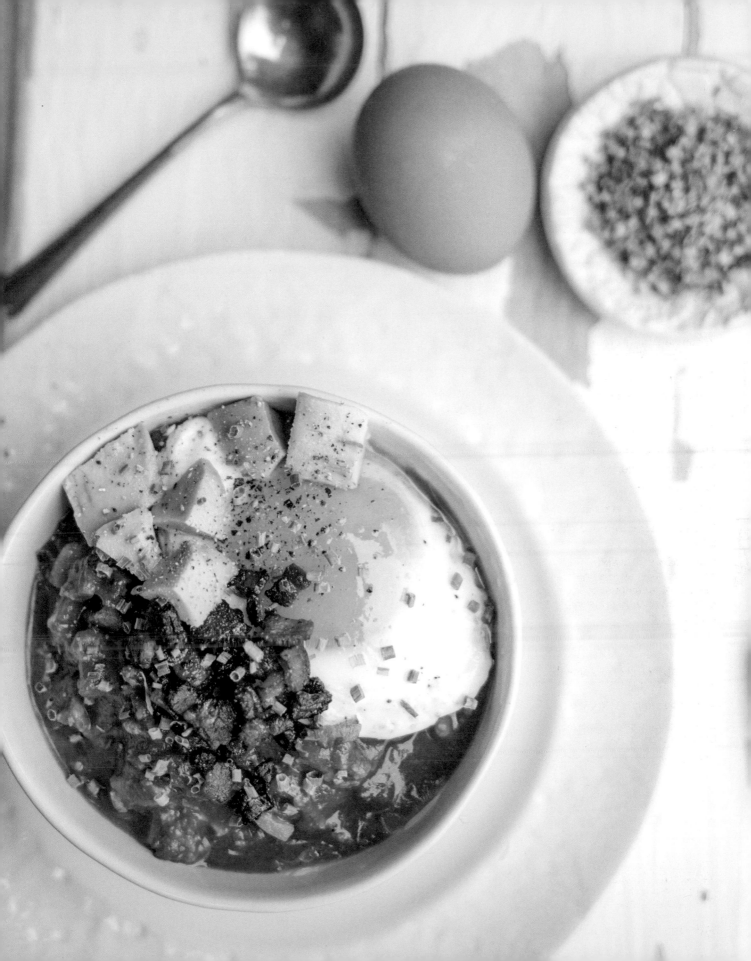

# bacon and eggs ramen

prep time: 5 minutes • cook time: 20 minutes (not including time to make the zoodles and soft-boiled eggs) • yield: 4 servings

Soup, such as ramen, is eaten for breakfast in many cultures. It's a great way to break your fast. This tasty version will keep you nice and warm all day long!

1 tablespoon toasted sesame oil

1 tablespoon coconut oil

1 (12-ounce) package fully cooked pork belly (see note), cut into ¼-inch dice

½ cup minced onions

2 cloves garlic

1 tablespoon red pepper flakes or 1½ teaspoons cayenne pepper

4 cups chicken bone broth, homemade (page 108) or store-bought

2 tablespoons coconut aminos or wheat-free tamari

1 tablespoon coconut vinegar or unseasoned rice vinegar

1 tablespoon grated fresh ginger

1 tablespoon tomato paste

Fine sea salt and fresh ground black pepper

1 recipe Zoodles (page 262), for serving

4 large eggs, soft-boiled (see page 164), for serving (omit for egg-free)

Sliced green onions, for garnish

Red pepper flakes, for garnish

1. Heat the oils in a large soup pot over medium heat. Fry the pork belly in the hot oil until crisp on all sides, about 4 minutes per side.

2. Remove the pork belly from the pot with a slotted spoon, leaving the fat in the pot. Add the onions, garlic, and red pepper flakes and cook over low heat for 4 minutes, or until the onions are translucent.

3. Add the chicken broth, coconut aminos, vinegar, ginger, and tomato paste and bring to a simmer over medium-high heat. Simmer for 8 minutes, then add salt and pepper to taste.

4. Just before serving, divide the zoodles among four bowls. Top each bowl with 1 cup of the broth. Place a soft-boiled egg in each bowl and garnish with green onions and red pepper flakes. This dish is best served freshly made.

note: *Vacuum-sealed packages of fully cooked pork belly are available at Trader Joe's.*

NUTRITIONAL INFO (per serving)

| calories | fat | protein | carbs | fiber |
|---|---|---|---|---|
| 495 | 40g | 24g | 10g | 4g |
| | 73% | 19% | 8% | |

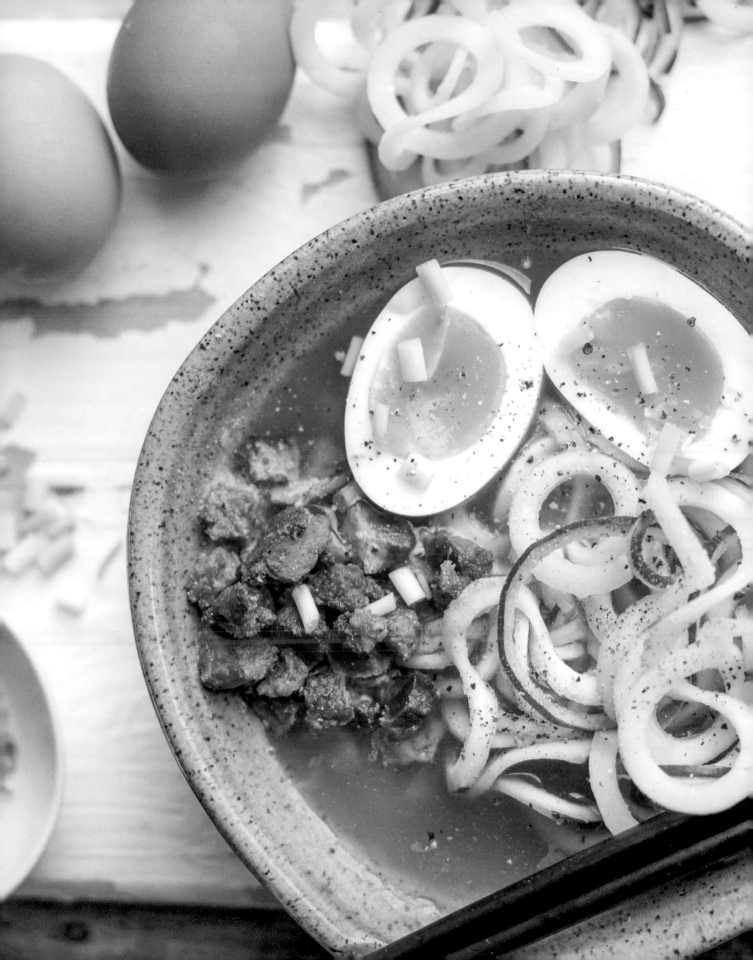

# florentine breakfast burgers

prep time: 5 minutes • cook time: 20 minutes (not including time to make the English muffins and hollandaise) • yield: 4 burgers (1 per serving)

One of the greatest tips for making juicy burgers is dead simple: salt only the outsides of the burgers. Salt removes water from the meat and dissolves some of the meat protein, which causes the insoluble proteins to bind together. This is great for making sausage (when you want a bit of a springy texture) but not for creating tender, juicy burgers. Another tip: handle the meat as little as possible.

1 tablespoon Paleo fat, for frying

1 pound 80% lean ground beef

2½ teaspoons fine sea salt

1½ teaspoons fresh ground black pepper

2 cups spinach or other greens of choice

4 large eggs

4 Keto English Muffins (page 188), split, for serving

1 tomato, cut into ¼-inch-thick slices, for serving

½ cup Easy Basil Hollandaise (page 136), for serving

Fresh basil leaves, for garnish

1. Heat the Paleo fat in a cast-iron skillet over medium-high heat.

2. Using your hands, form the meat into 4 patties. Season the outsides with the salt and pepper. Fry the burgers in the pan on both sides until they reach your desired doneness (see the chart below).

3. Remove the burgers from the pan, leaving the fat in the pan. Add the spinach, season with salt and pepper, and sauté over medium heat until the leaves are softened, about 2 minutes.

4. Poach the eggs (see page 166).

5. Serve each burger on an English muffin, fried in the leftover fat if desired. Top with a slice of tomato, one-quarter of the wilted spinach, a poached egg, and some basil hollandaise. Garnish with fresh basil. These burgers are best served fresh.

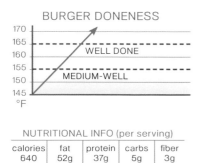

BURGER DONENESS

| °F | |
|---|---|
| 170 | |
| 165 | |
| 160 | WELL DONE |
| 155 | |
| 150 | MEDIUM-WELL |
| 145 | |

NUTRITIONAL INFO (per serving)

| calories | fat | protein | carbs | fiber |
|---|---|---|---|---|
| 640 | 52g | 37g | 5g | 3g |
| | 74% | 23% | 3% | |

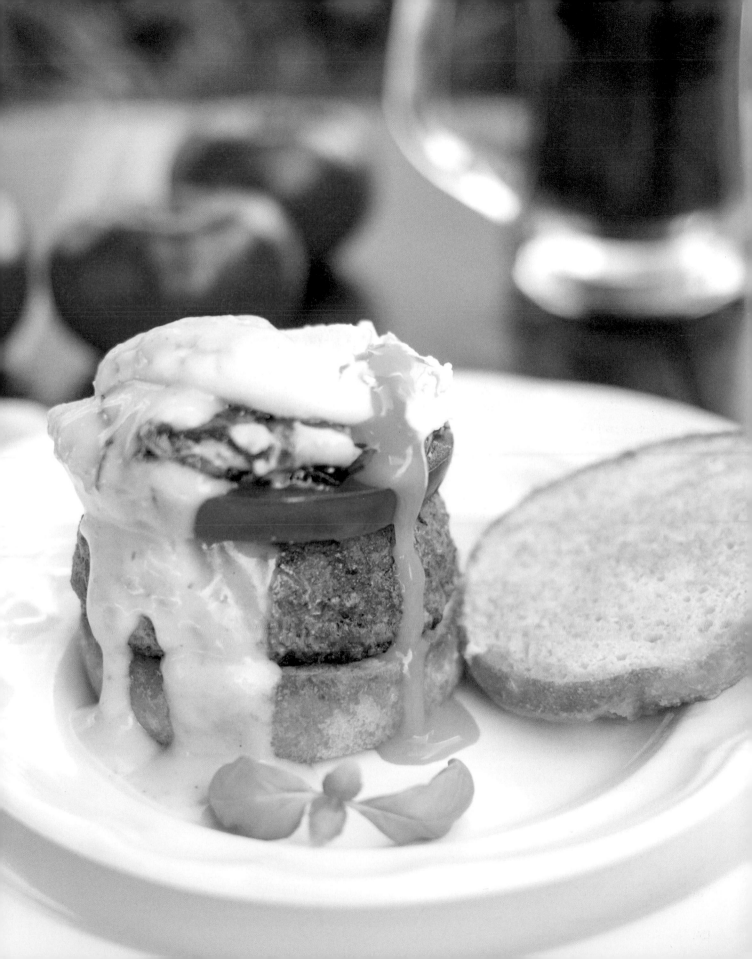

# creamiest keto scrambled eggs

KETO

prep time: 3 minutes • cook time: 25 minutes • yield: 2 servings

If a breakfast of eggs soft-scrambled with roasted bone marrow sounds a little crazy to you, let me list the reasons you should consider starting your day this way:

- Bone marrow is one of the few natural sources of vitamin K2, which helps reverse artery calcification, reverse Alzheimer's, and increase fertility and has anti-aging properties as well as many other healing properties.
- Marrow is also one of the best, densest sources of fat-soluble vitamins.
- Marrow is a great high-fat, moderate-protein food for a keto-adapted diet.

Still not convinced? If the health reasons alone haven't convinced you, then the incredible taste and creamy texture of bone marrow will!

2 (2-inch) cross-cut beef or veal marrow bones, split lengthwise

1 teaspoon fine sea salt, divided

½ teaspoon fresh ground black pepper, divided

5 large eggs

1 teaspoon fresh herbs of choice (whole or chopped leaves, depending on size), for garnish (optional)

1. Preheat the oven to 450°F.

2. Rinse and drain the bones and pat dry. Season them with ½ teaspoon of the salt and ¼ teaspoon of the pepper and place them cut side up in a roasting pan.

3. Roast for 15 to 25 minutes (the exact timing will depend on the diameter of the bones; if they are 2 inches in diameter, it will take closer to 15 minutes), until the marrow in the center has puffed slightly and is warm. To test for doneness, insert a metal skewer into the center of the bone; there should be no resistance when it is inserted, and some of the marrow will have started to leak from the bones.

4. Heat a cast-iron skillet over medium heat. Place some of the liquid from the roasting pan in the skillet. Using a small spoon, scoop the marrow out of the bones into a bowl, then add the eggs and the remaining ½ teaspoon of salt and ¼ teaspoon of pepper and whisk until well combined. Pour the egg mixture into the skillet. Gently scramble the eggs until they are set and creamy. Garnish with fresh herbs.

5. Best served fresh. Store extras in an airtight container in the fridge for up to 3 days.

NUTRITIONAL INFO (per serving)

| calories | fat | protein | carbs | fiber |
|----------|-----|---------|-------|-------|
| 398 | 35g | 18g | 2g | 0.4g |
| | 80% | 18% | 2% | |

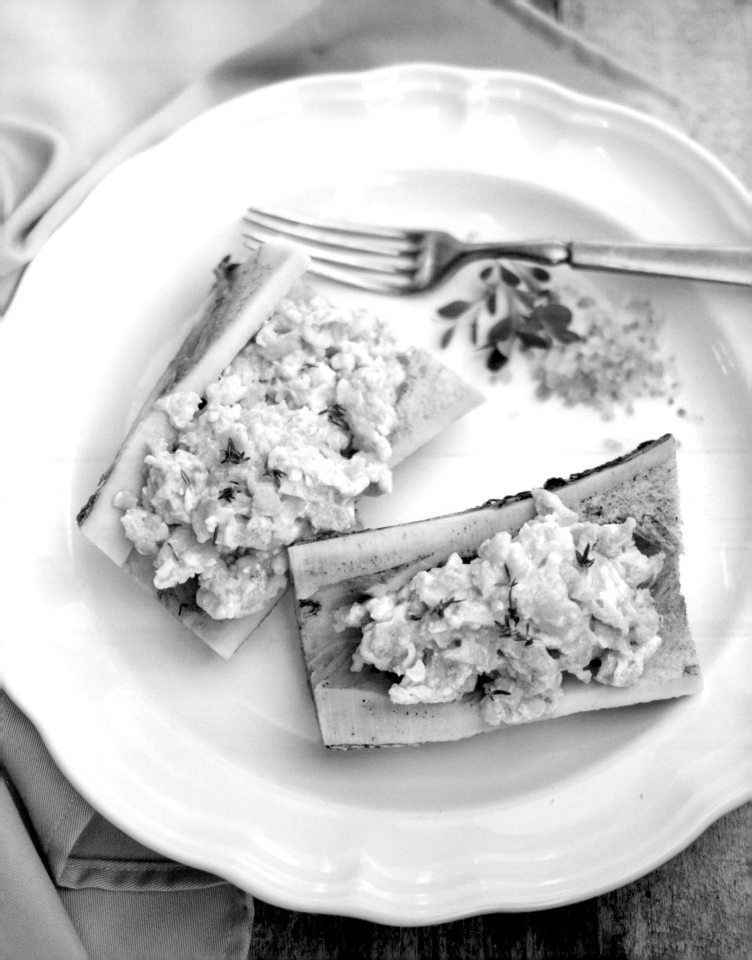

# steak and eggs

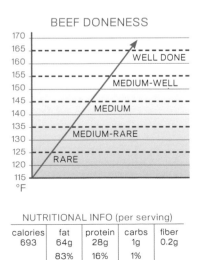

prep time: 2 minutes (not including time to make the hollandaise)
cook time: 10 minutes, plus 10 minutes to rest • yield: 4 servings

4 (4-ounce) venison or beef tenderloins

Fine sea salt and fresh ground black pepper

1 tablespoon Paleo fat, for frying

4 large eggs

1 cup Easy Dairy-Free Hollandaise (page 136)

1. Season the tenderloins generously on all sides with salt and pepper. Heat the Paleo fat in a cast-iron skillet over medium-high heat. Once hot, add the tenderloins and sear in the fat for 3 minutes on each side, or to your desired doneness (see chart below). Remove from the heat and allow to rest for 10 minutes before slicing or serving. Leave the fat in the pan.

2. While the meat is resting, crack the eggs into the hot skillet with the reserved fat. Season with salt and pepper and fry on medium-low heat until the whites are cooked through on top and the yolks are still runny, about 4 minutes.

3. Slice the tenderloin and place on serving plates. Top with the eggs and hollandaise. Best served fresh.

note: *This dish appears in week 2 of the 30-day meal plan. To use as leftovers, the steak and hollandaise can be made ahead and rewarmed, but the eggs should be fried just before serving.*

BEEF DONENESS

```
170
165 - - - - - - - - - - - - - - - - - - - - -
160          WELL DONE
155 - - - - - - - - - - - - - - - - - - - - -
150        MEDIUM-WELL
145 - - - - - - - - - - - - - - - - - - - - -
140       MEDIUM
135 - - - - - - - - - - - - - - - - - - - - -
130    MEDIUM-RARE
125 - - - - - - - - - - - - - - - - - - - - -
120   RARE
115
°F
```

NUTRITIONAL INFO (per serving)

| calories | fat | protein | carbs | fiber |
|----------|-----|---------|-------|-------|
| 693 | 64g | 28g | 1g | 0.2g |
| | 83% | 16% | 1% | |

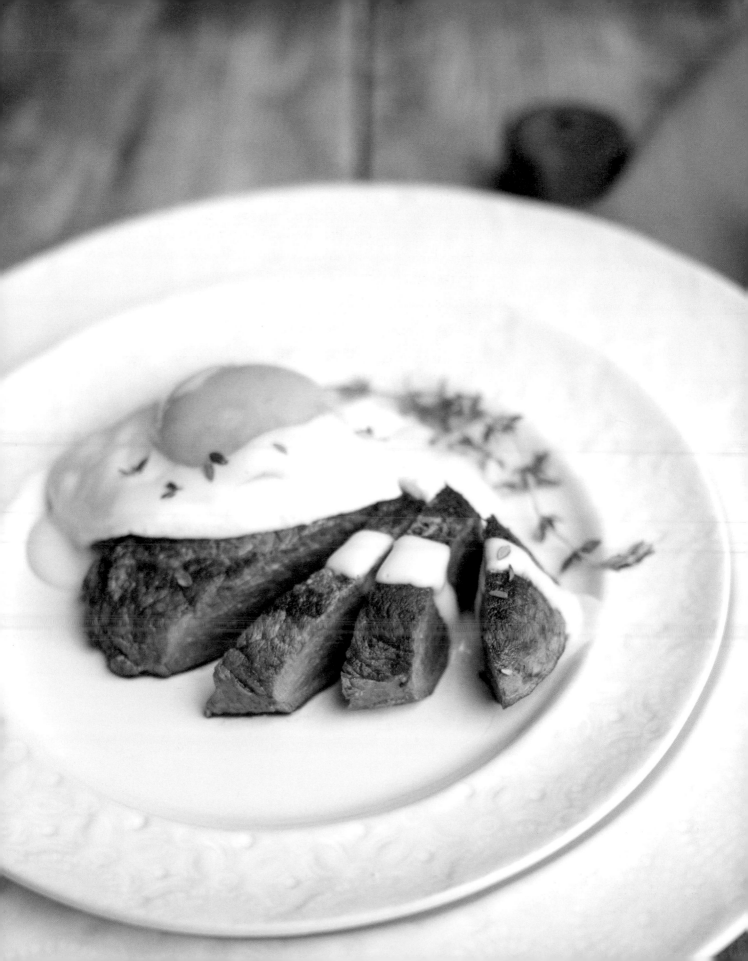

# rosti with bacon, mushrooms, and green onions

L M H KETO  prep time: 10 minutes • cook time: 25 minutes • yield: 2 servings

A rosti is traditionally made of shredded potatoes pressed into pancake-like shapes and fried. Using cabbage instead of potatoes is a great keto adaptation that will not disappoint when it comes to flavor!

2 slices bacon, diced

2 tablespoons coconut oil or lard

1 cup mushrooms, thinly sliced

¼ cup chopped green onions, plus more for garnish (optional)

¼ teaspoon minced garlic

1 cup shredded cabbage

1 large egg

½ teaspoon fine sea salt

⅛ teaspoon fresh ground black pepper

1. Place the bacon in a large skillet over medium heat and fry until cooked and crispy. Reserve a little bit of the cooked bacon for garnish, if desired. Add the coconut oil, mushrooms, green onions, and garlic. Sauté for 5 minutes, or until the mushrooms are golden.

2. In a large bowl, mix the shredded cabbage, egg, salt, and pepper. Transfer to the skillet with the bacon mixture. Spread out the cabbage mixture in the pan and press it down to form a large pancake. Cook over medium heat until the bottom is crispy and golden brown, about 5 minutes. Flip with a large spatula and cook for another 10 minutes, or until the cabbage softens.

3. Remove from the heat and serve. Store extras in an airtight container in the fridge for up to 4 days. To reheat, fry in a skillet with a tablespoon of Paleo fat or coconut oil on both sides until crispy, about 3 minutes a side. Garnish with green onions and/or reserved bacon, if desired.

NUTRITIONAL INFO (per serving)

| calories | fat | protein | carbs | fiber |
|---|---|---|---|---|
| 275 | 24g | 10g | 5g | 2g |
|  | 71% | 15% | 14% |  |

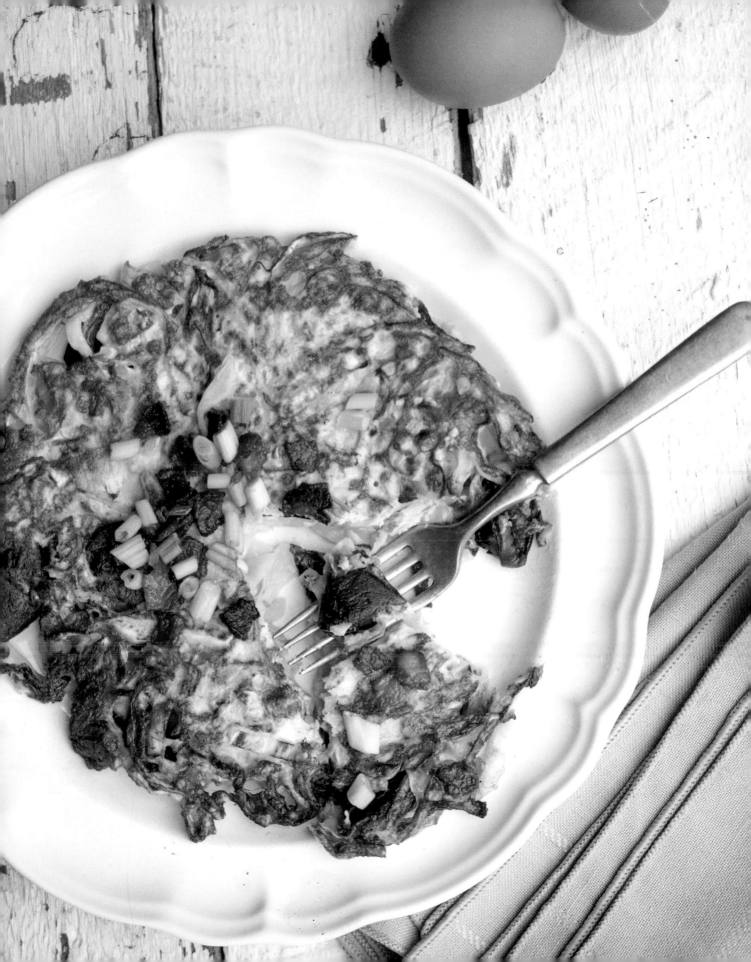

# kimchi eggs

LMH KETO · prep time: 4 minutes • cook time: 5 minutes • yield: 2 servings

If you like spicy foods, this is a perfect breakfast for you!

1 tablespoon Paleo fat

4 large eggs

Fine sea salt and fresh ground black pepper

1 cup kimchi (see note)

## for garnish (optional):

Sliced green onions

Red pepper flakes

1. Heat the fat in a cast-iron skillet over low heat. Crack the eggs into the skillet. Season with salt and pepper. Cover with a lid and cook until the whites are cooked through on top and the yolks are still runny, about 4 minutes.

2. Meanwhile, divide the kimchi between two serving bowls. When the eggs are done, remove them from the heat and place 2 eggs into each bowl. Garnish with green onions and red pepper flakes, if desired.

note: *When buying premade kimchi, check the label to make sure that there are no added sugars or MSG. For instructions on making homemade kimchi, see my Easy Kimchi recipe in my previous cookbook,* Quick & Easy Ketogenic Cooking.

NUTRITIONAL INFO (per serving)

| calories | fat | protein | carbs | fiber |
|----------|-----|---------|-------|-------|
| 240 | 16g | 16g | 8g | 3g |
| | 60% | 27% | 13% | |

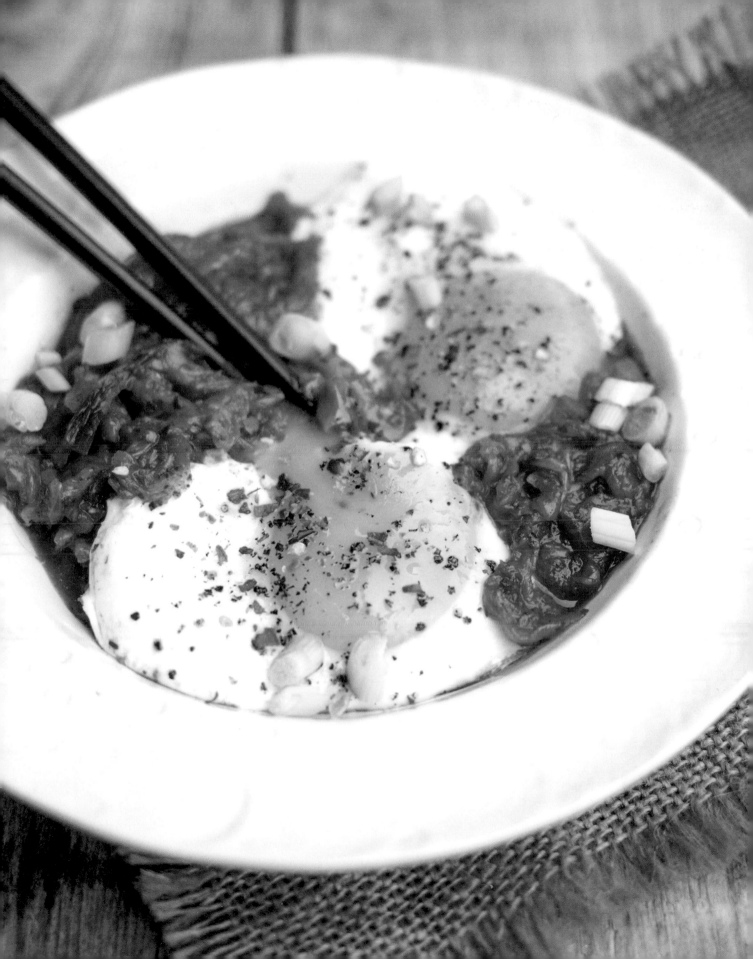

# green eggs and ham

LM KETO H · 🗍 · ⊘  prep time: 5 minutes (not including time to make the hollandaise)
cook time: 10 minutes • yield: 4 servings

Every year on Dr. Seuss's birthday, I make green eggs and ham for my family. Dr. Seuss was an integral part of one of my favorite summer memories: When I was in college, I worked at Camp St. Croix, an environmental camp for kids, and we put on a puppet show of *The Lorax* to teach the kids about healthy environmental practices. I loved that summer job and all the very special people and kids I worked with there. This recipe is in honor of all my amazing camp memories.

To save on cost and time spent running to the market, I get a whole pasture-raised pig from a local farmer to keep in our chest freezer. I love having choices for different cuts of meat readily available in my freezer at all times! When ordering a whole pig, one of the options is smoked ham hocks, which comes from the shank. It is already cooked; all you need to do is heat it up (it tastes great cold, too). You don't need to purchase a whole pig to make this dish, though—just stop by your local butcher to purchase smoked ham hock steaks to store in your freezer for easy breakfasts or dinners.

4 (3-ounce) smoked ham hock steaks

1 tablespoon coconut oil or other Paleo fat

4 large eggs

Fine sea salt and fresh ground black pepper

½ cup Easy Basil Hollandaise (page 136)

1. Preheat the oven 425°F.

2. Place the ham hocks on a rimmed baking sheet. Place in the oven for 10 minutes, or until the skin gets crispy. (*Note:* Smoked ham hocks can be served cold, too.)

3. Fry the eggs: Heat the oil in a cast-iron skillet over low heat. Crack the eggs into the pan. Season with salt and pepper. Cover the pan with a lid and fry until the whites are cooked through but the yolks are still runny, about 4 minutes. Remove the eggs from the pan.

4. Place each ham hock on a plate and top with 1 fried egg and 2 table-spoons of basil hollandaise.

notes: *A toaster oven works great for this recipe!*

*This dish appears in week 2 of the 30-day meal plan. To use it as leftovers, the ham and hollandaise can be made ahead and rewarmed, but the eggs should be fried just before serving.*

NUTRITIONAL INFO (per serving)

| calories | fat | protein | carbs | fiber |
|---|---|---|---|---|
| 640 | 61g | 22g | 1g | 0.1g |
|  | 86% | 14% | 0% |  |

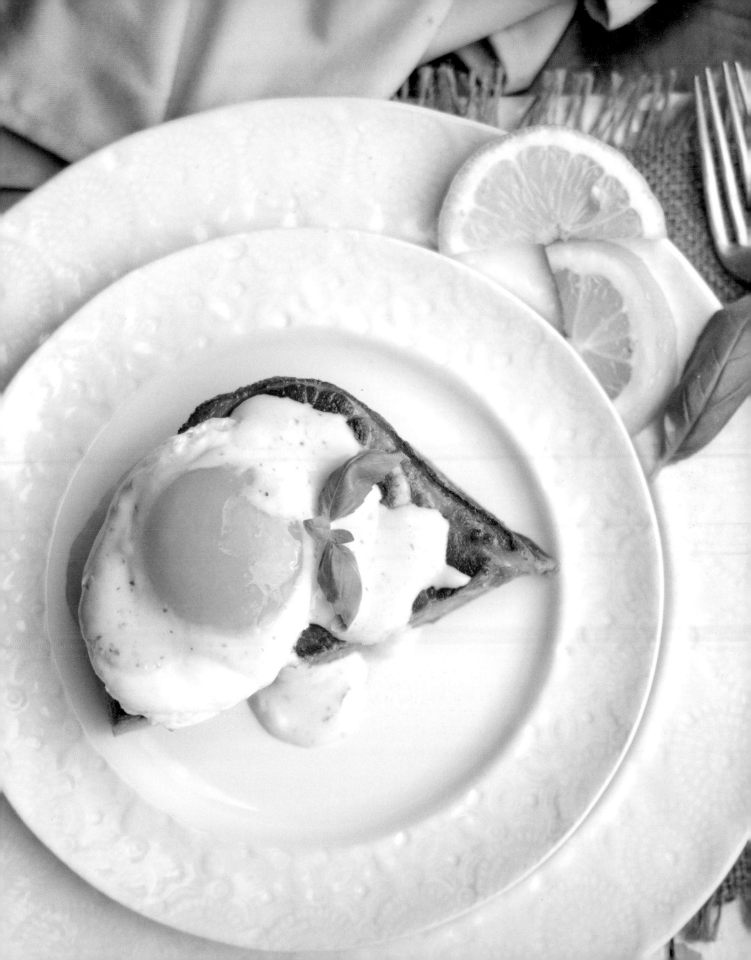

# bacon and mushrooms with soft-boiled eggs

L⟍M⟋H KETO  ▯  ⊘  ⊘ option  prep time: 8 minutes • cook time: 15 minutes • yield: 4 servings

½ pound bacon, diced

12 ounces baby portobello mushrooms, stemmed and quartered

¼ cup diced onions

4 large eggs (omit for egg-free)

3 tablespoons plus 2 teaspoons coconut vinegar or red wine vinegar

3 tablespoons MCT oil or extra-virgin olive oil

1 teaspoon Dijon mustard

½ teaspoon fine sea salt

¼ teaspoon fresh ground black pepper

1 teaspoon Swerve confectioners'-style sweetener or equivalent amount of liquid or powdered sweetener (see page 81) (optional)

Chopped fresh chives, for garnish

1. Place the diced bacon in a skillet and sauté over medium heat until crispy, about 5 minutes. Using a slotted spoon, remove the bacon but leave the drippings in the pan. Add the mushrooms and onions and sauté in the drippings for 10 minutes, or until the mushrooms are golden brown and cooked through.

2. Meanwhile, make the soft-boiled eggs: Place the eggs in a pot of simmering, not boiling, water, cover, and simmer for 6 minutes. Immediately rinse under cold water. Peel and set aside.

3. Add the vinegar, oil, mustard, salt, pepper, and sweetener, if using, to the sauté pan with the mushrooms and stir well. Add the crispy bacon and stir to combine.

4. Place the mushroom mixture on a serving platter. Slice the eggs in half and place them yolk side up on top of the mushroom mixture. Garnish with fresh chives.

5. Store extras in an airtight container in the fridge for up to 4 days. Best served fresh.

note: *This is one of the recipes featured in week 2 of the 30-day meal plan. To help curb your sweet tooth during the cleanse, I suggest that you omit the sweetener from this recipe.*

NUTRITIONAL INFO (per serving)

| calories | fat | protein | carbs | fiber |
|----------|-----|---------|-------|-------|
| 528 | 44g | 28g | 5g | 1g |
| | 75% | 21% | 4% | |

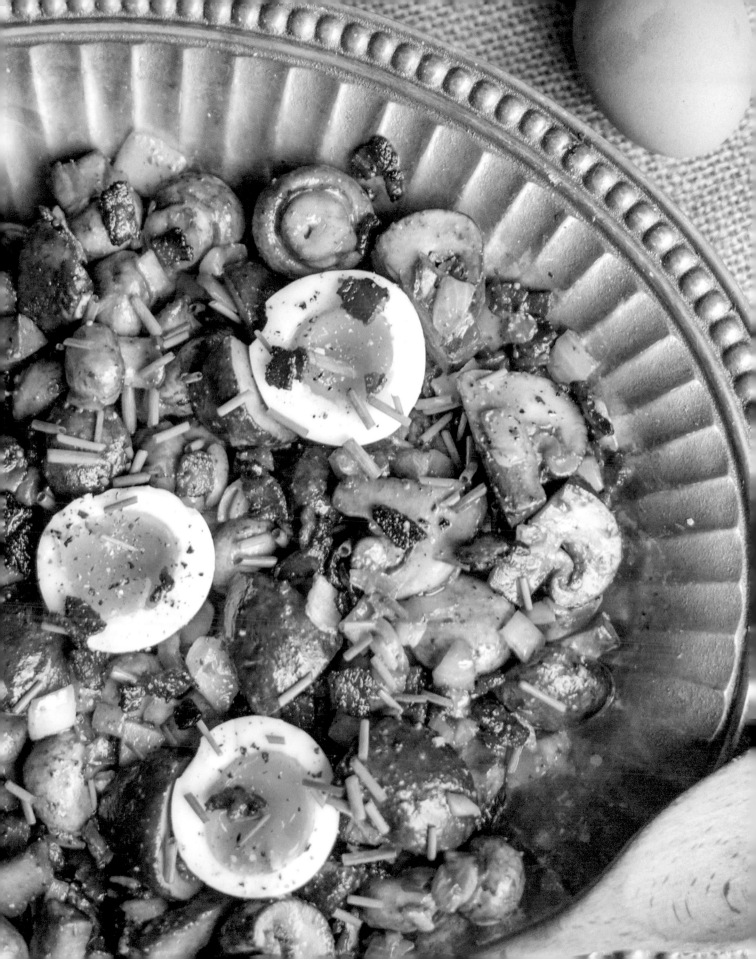

# eggs florentine with basil hollandaise

L→H M KETO  prep time: 8 minutes (not including time to make the hollandaise and muffins/buns)
cook time: 12 minutes • yield: 2 servings

Back in the day, my husband and I frequented a cute French bistro called Salut in St. Paul, Minnesota. In the summer, it was the best—on beautiful days we would sit outside on Grand Avenue with our little dog, Ohana, next to us. I always ordered the eggs Florentine with basil hollandaise, with Parmesan crisps instead of a bun, and they always gave me extra hollandaise. To make this breakfast dairy-free, I used Keto English Muffins (page 188) instead of Parmesan crisps. Another option is to use Keto Buns (page 256).

2 tablespoons Paleo fat, such as lard

2 tablespoons diced onions

1 teaspoon minced garlic

4 cups fresh spinach (frozen not recommended)

½ teaspoon fine sea salt

¼ teaspoon fresh ground black pepper

Pinch of fresh ground nutmeg

1 tablespoon coconut vinegar

4 large eggs

2 Keto English Muffins (page 188) or Keto Buns (page 256), sliced in half and fried

2 (½-inch-thick) slices tomato

2 heaping tablespoons Easy Basil Hollandaise (page 136)

1. Melt the fat in a cast-iron skillet over medium heat. Add the onions and garlic and sauté for 5 minutes, or until the onions are translucent. Add the spinach and sauté for another 2 minutes. Season with the salt, pepper, and nutmeg; taste and adjust the seasoning if desired.

2. Poach the eggs: In a saucepan, bring 3 to 4 inches of water to a boil.

3. While the water is heating, place ½ tablespoon of vinegar in each of two individual ramekins, then crack 2 eggs into each ramekin. The vinegar helps stabilize the egg whites.

4. When the water is boiling, lower the heat to maintain a gentle simmer and swirl the water in a whirlpool fashion. Gently drop each egg into the center of the whirlpool and poach for 4 minutes, or until the whites are totally set but the yolks are still runny. *Note:* If you are new to poaching eggs, cook one ramekin at a time.

5. Remove the eggs with a slotted spoon and rest the spoon on a paper towel for a moment to drain the excess water.

6. Place two fried keto English muffin or keto bun halves on each of two serving plates. Top each bun with a slice of tomato, then the spinach, and then a poached egg. Top each stack with a heaping tablespoon of basil hollandaise.

busy family tip: *The poached eggs can be made up to 3 days ahead. Store in water in an airtight container in the fridge. To reheat, place in very hot water for 30 seconds.*

NUTRITIONAL INFO (per serving)

| calories | fat | protein | carbs | fiber |
|----------|-----|---------|-------|-------|
| 754 | 67g | 27g | 9g | 4g |
| | 80% | 15% | 5% | |

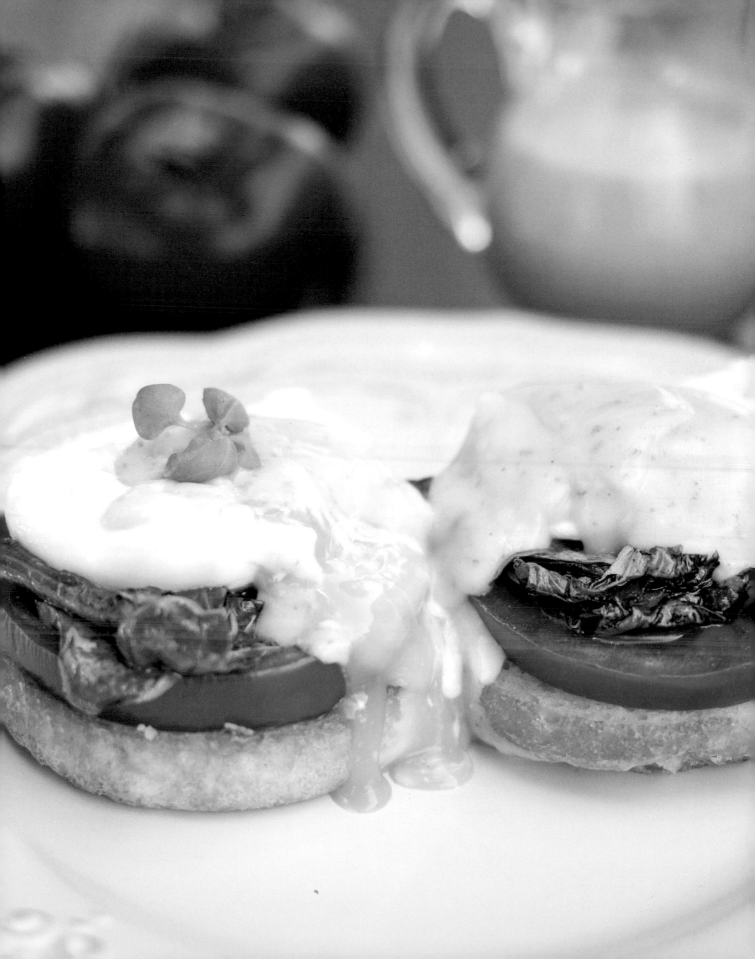

# eggs in a frame

**KETO** ⬜ ⊘ ⊘ option  prep time: 10 minutes (not including time to make the buns)
cook time: 5 minutes • yield: 2 servings

2 tablespoons coconut oil

4 Keto Buns (page 256)

4 large eggs

½ teaspoon fine sea salt

2 slices bacon, fried and crumbled (omit for vegetarian)

2 tablespoons sliced green onions

¼ cup Easy Basil Hollandaise (page 136) (optional)

busy family tip: *I store keto buns in my freezer at all times for easy additions to recipes like this one.*

1. Heat the oil in a skillet over medium-low heat.

2. Cut a 1½-inch circle in the center of each keto bun. Place the buns with the holes as well as the cutouts in the warm skillet. Crack an egg into the middle of the hole in each bun. Sprinkle each egg with salt, bacon crumbles, and green onions.

3. Cover and cook until the eggs are set in the middle, about 5 minutes. Remove from the skillet and serve. To up the keto level of this recipe, serve each portion with 2 tablespoons of basil hollandaise.

NUTRITIONAL INFO
(per serving without hollandaise)

| calories | fat | protein | carbs | fiber |
|----------|-----|---------|-------|-------|
| 345 | 23g | 29g | 1g | 0.5g |
| | 61% | 35% | 4% | |

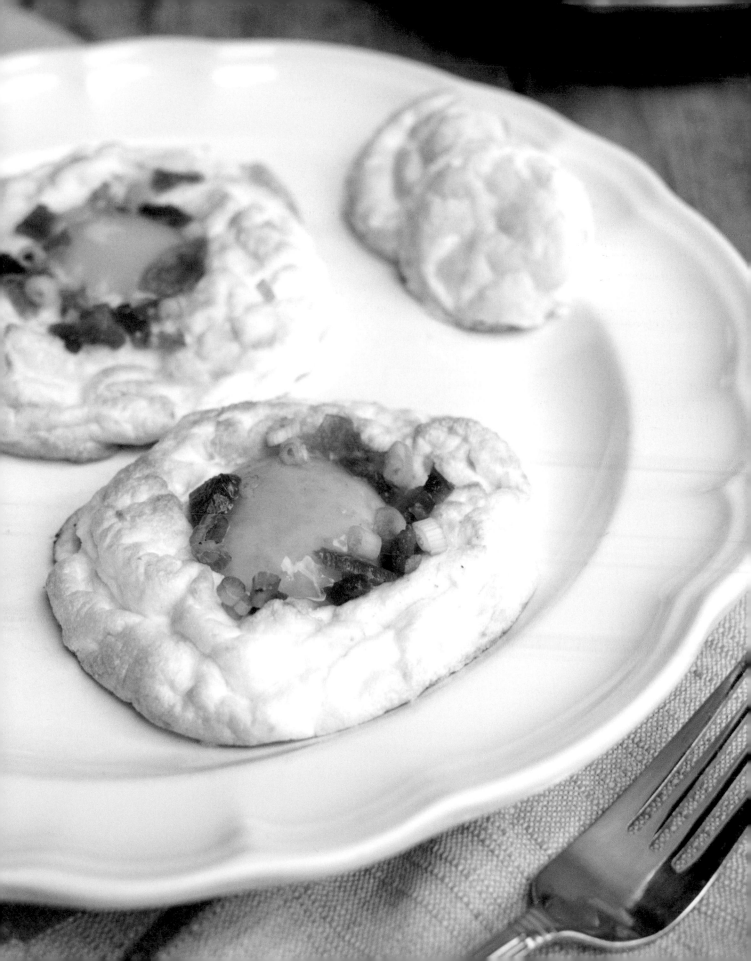

# keto pockets

prep time: 8 minutes • cook time: 4 to 6 minutes • yield: 12 pockets (2 per serving)

12 thin slices mortadella (see note)

6 large eggs, scrambled

6 slices bacon, cooked and crumbled, or 3 ounces ham, chopped

1 tablespoon coconut oil

6 cups arugula, for serving (optional)

½ cup keto dressing of choice (pages 115 to 121) (optional)

1. Lay the slices of the mortadella on a clean, dry work surface. Place 3 tablespoons of the scrambled eggs and 2 tablespoons of crumbled bacon on each slice of mortadella.

2. To make the pocket, fold over the mortadella to form a semicircle and secure with toothpicks. *Note:* The pockets can be made 2 days ahead and stored in the refrigerator, then cooked just before serving.

3. Heat the oil in a large sauté pan over medium-high heat. Fry the mortadella pockets for about 1 minute per side, until they are slightly charred. Remove and discard the toothpicks.

4. Transfer the pockets to a platter. If desired, serve over arugula tossed with your favorite keto salad dressing.

note: *If you don't eat nuts, avoid German-style mortadella, as it often contains pistachios, or choose a good-quality bologna instead.*

NUTRITIONAL INFO (per serving, without arugula or dressing)

| calories | fat | protein | carbs | fiber |
|----------|-----|---------|-------|-------|
| 271 | 22g | 17g | 1g | 0g |
|  | 73% | 26% | 1% |  |

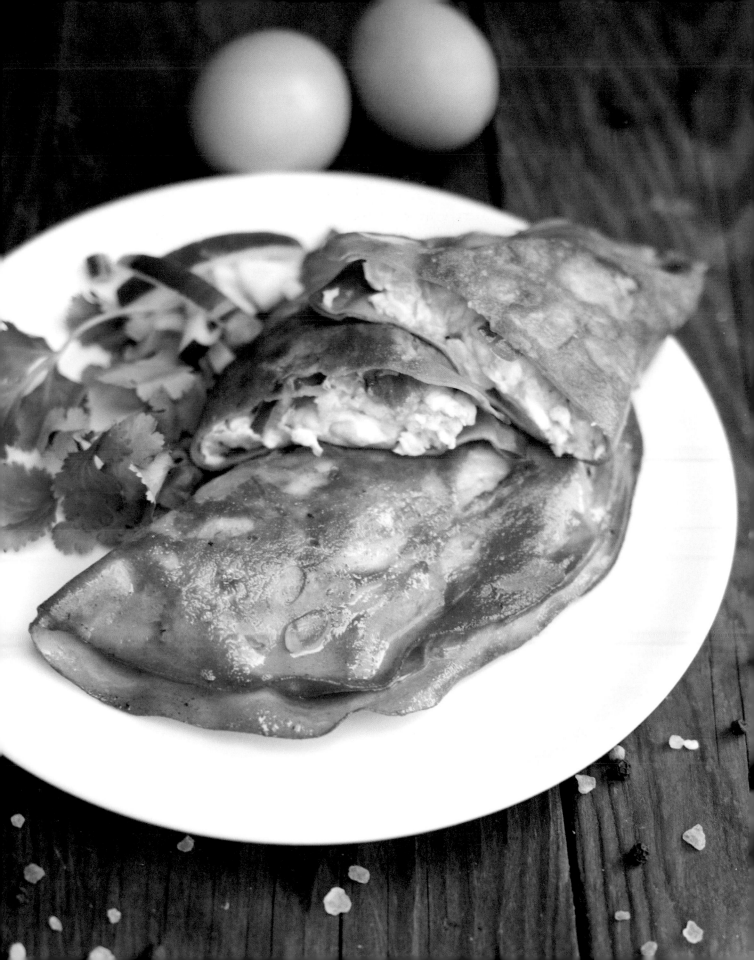

# ham and egg cups

Coconut oil, for the pan

6 slices ham, about 4 inches in diameter

6 large eggs

½ teaspoon fine sea salt

¼ teaspoon fresh ground black pepper

2 tablespoons chopped fresh chives, for garnish

6 tablespoons Easy Basil Hollandaise (page 136) (optional)

1. Preheat the oven to 400°F. Grease a 6-well muffin tin.

2. Place 1 slice of ham in each well. Break an egg into each ham cup. Sprinkle the eggs with the salt and pepper.

3. Bake for 12 minutes, or until the egg whites are set but the yolks are still a bit runny.

4. Serve garnished with chopped chives. To up the keto content, serve each cup with a tablespoon of basil hollandaise, reheated (if necessary) according to the instructions on page 136.

NUTRITIONAL INFO
(per serving, without hollandaise)

| calories | fat | protein | carbs | fiber |
|----------|-----|---------|-------|-------|
| 360 | 25g | 32g | 2g | 0.2g |
| | 62% | 36% | 2% | |

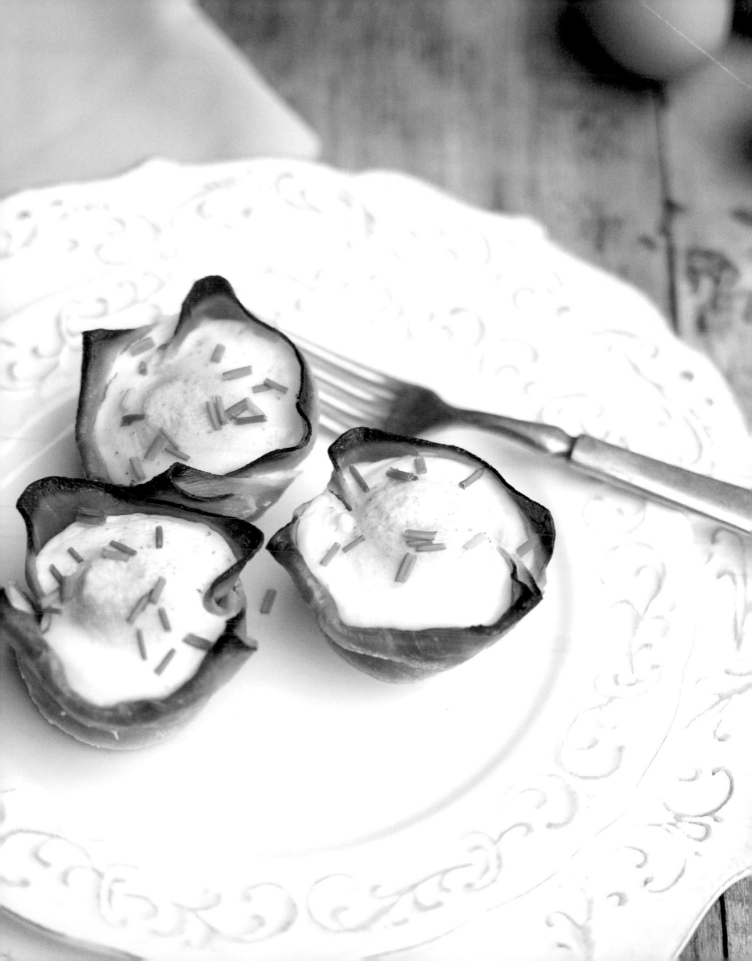

# basil deviled eggs

prep time: 15 minutes (not including time to make the mayo)
cook time: 11 minutes • yield: 24 (2 halves per serving)

12 large eggs

½ cup Basil Mayonnaise (page 127)

1 teaspoon coconut vinegar or apple cider vinegar

½ teaspoon fine sea salt

6 cups mixed greens, for serving

12 cherry tomatoes, halved, for garnish

Fresh basil leaves, for garnish

¾ cup Easy Basil Hollandaise (page 136) (optional)

1. Hard-boil the eggs: Place the eggs in a large saucepan and cover with cold water. Bring the water to a boil, then immediately cover the pan and remove it from the heat. Allow the eggs to cook in the hot water for 11 minutes.

2. After 11 minutes, drain the hot water and rinse the eggs with very cold water for a minute or two to stop the cooking process. Peel the boiled eggs and cut them in half lengthwise. Remove the yolks and place them in a bowl (or a food processor). Mash or blend the egg yolks with a fork (or a food processor) until they are the texture of very fine crumbles.

3. Add the basil mayonnaise, vinegar, and salt to the egg yolks and stir to evenly combine. Fill the egg white halves with the yolk mixture.

4. Divide the mixed greens among 12 plates and place 2 deviled eggs on each plate. Garnish with cherry tomato halves and basil leaves and drizzle each deviled egg with 1½ teaspoons of basil hollandaise, if desired.

5. Keep leftover deviled eggs in an airtight container in the fridge for up to 3 days.

busy family tip: *I keep a dozen hard-boiled eggs in my fridge at all times. My boys, who are five and six, love to help me in the kitchen, and peeling eggs is one of the things they can do without my constant attention so I can prepare other food.*

NUTRITIONAL INFO
(per serving, without hollandaise)

| calories | fat | protein | carbs | fiber |
|---|---|---|---|---|
| 198 | 18g | 7g | 2g | 1g |
| | 82% | 14% | 4% | |

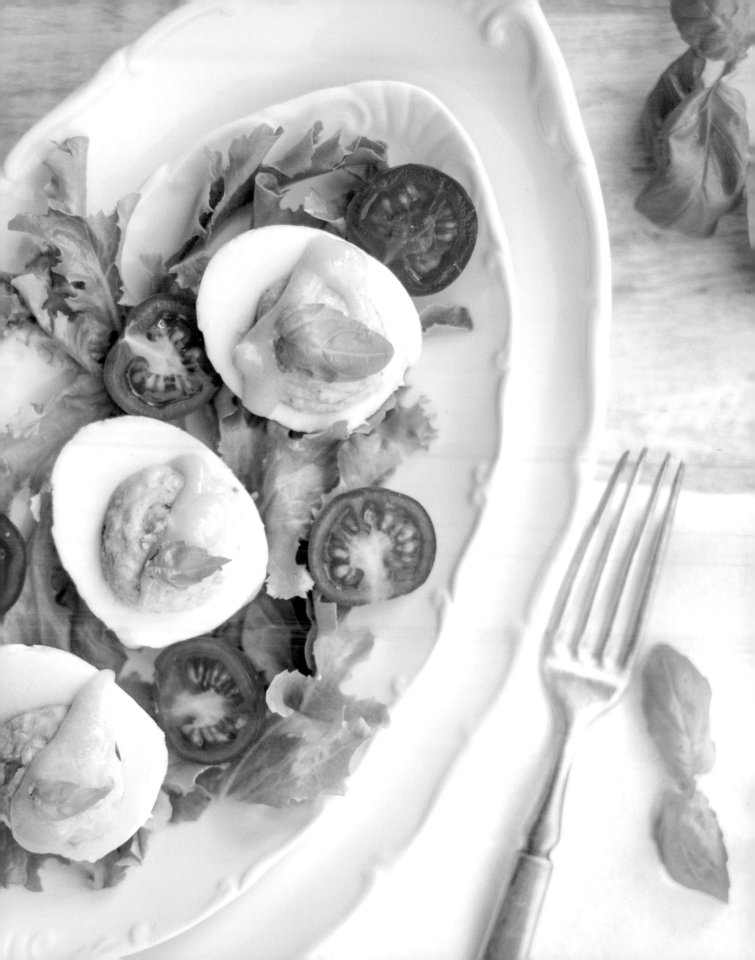

# breakfast salad

 prep time: 10 minutes (not including time to make the croutons, soft-boiled egg, or dressing)
yield: 1 serving

I adore a breakfast salad. The soft-boiled egg, crispy pork belly croutons, and creamy avocado make a tasty meal for breaking your fast!

2 cups arugula

1 tablespoon chopped purple cabbage

2 tablespoons Crispy Pork Belly Croutons (page 260)

1 soft-boiled egg (see page 164)

¼ avocado, sliced

2 cherry or grape tomatoes, quartered

2 tablespoons Onion-Infused Dressing (page 120), Dairy-Free Ranch Dressing (page 115), or keto dressing of choice (pages 115 to 121)

Fine sea salt and fresh ground black pepper

Place the arugula and cabbage in a salad bowl. Top with the pork belly croutons, soft-boiled egg, avocado slices, and tomato quarters. Drizzle with the salad dressing and sprinkle with salt and fresh ground pepper.

tip: *This recipe calls for just one-quarter of an avocado. If you are wondering what to do with the rest of the avocado, try freezing it! All you have to do is sprinkle the peeled avocado with some lemon juice, wrap it tightly in plastic wrap, and place it in the freezer. You'll be amazed at how bright green the frozen avocado is, even after peeling. You can also freeze whole, unpeeled avocados. When I find myself purchasing too many avocados at once, usually because they're on sale, I pop them in the freezer. Both peeled and unpeeled avocado will keep in the freezer for up to 1 month. When you are ready to consume the frozen avocado, just remove it from the freezer and allow it to thaw.*

| NUTRITIONAL INFO | | | | |
| --- | --- | --- | --- | --- |
| calories | fat | protein | carbs | fiber |
| 375 | 34g | 11g | 7g | 4g |
| | 81% | 12% | 7% | |

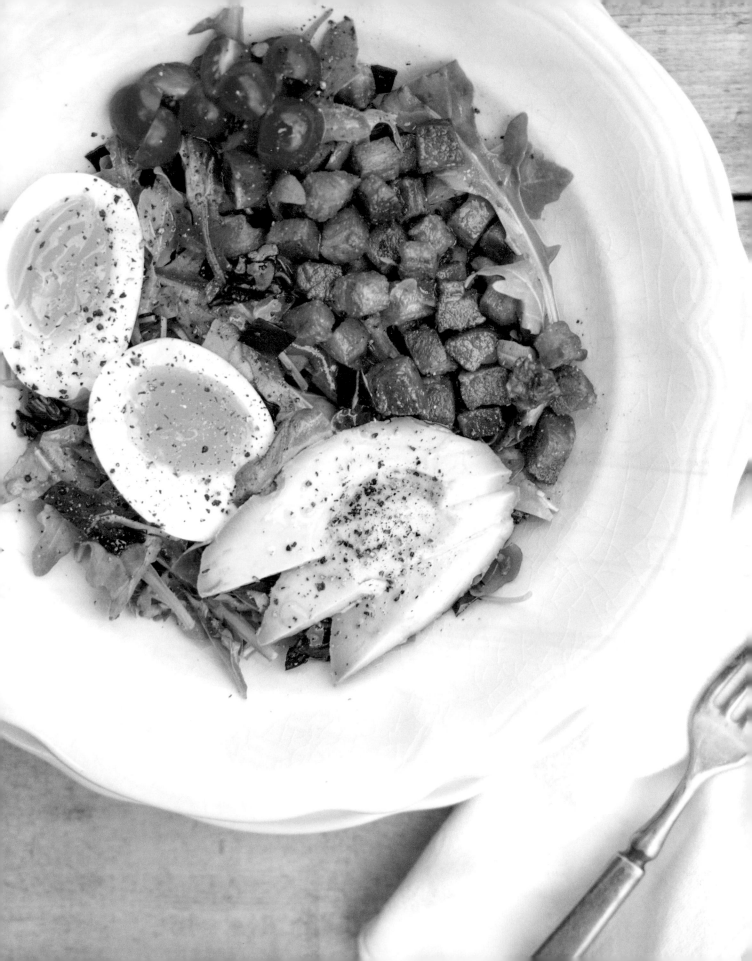

# dairy-free yogurt

L M H KETO

prep time: 10 minutes, plus 16 to 24 hours to culture
cook time: 10 minutes • yield: 4 cups (1 cup per serving)

Dairy-free yogurt is often quite thin. To thicken it, I add 1 teaspoon of gelatin per 2 cups of homemade yogurt.

1 (13½-ounce) can full-fat coconut milk

2 cups unsweetened (unflavored or vanilla-flavored) cashew milk, homemade (page 106) or store-bought, or almond milk

¼ cup Swerve confectioners'-style sweetener or equivalent amount of liquid or powdered sweetener (see page 81) (optional)

2 teaspoons grass-fed powdered gelatin

1 teaspoon probiotic powder (must contain one of these strains: *Lactobacillus bulgaricus*, *Streptococcus thermophilus*, *Bifidobacterium lactis*, or *Lactobacillus acidophilus*)

1. Place the coconut milk, cashew milk, and sweetener in a saucepan and bring to a gentle boil, then remove from the heat and pour into a heatproof glass bowl.

2. Allow the milk mixture to cool to 115°F. While the milk is cooling, dissolve the gelatin in 2 tablespoons of cool water to soften. Once fully dissolved, add it to the warm milk mixture and stir well to combine.

3. Once the milk mixture reaches 115°F, add the probiotic powder and stir well.

4. Pour the mixture into a sterile 1-quart glass jar with a tight-fitting lid. Cover and place in a warm place (around 100°F). I store mine in the oven on the proofing setting. If that is not an option for you, wrap a large towel around the jar and keep it in a warm area so the yogurt stays between 105°F and 115°F for as long as possible.

5. Allow the yogurt to culture for 16 to 24 hours. The longer it cultures, the tangier it will be. Once the yogurt is cultured to your desired taste, cover securely and refrigerate for at least 6 hours. This stops the fermentation process. The yogurt will thicken as it cools. It will keep in the fridge for 1 week.

NUTRITIONAL INFO (per serving)

| calories | fat | protein | carbs | fiber |
|----------|-----|---------|-------|-------|
| 101 | 9g | 2g | 2g | 0.1g |
| | 83% | 10% | 7% | |

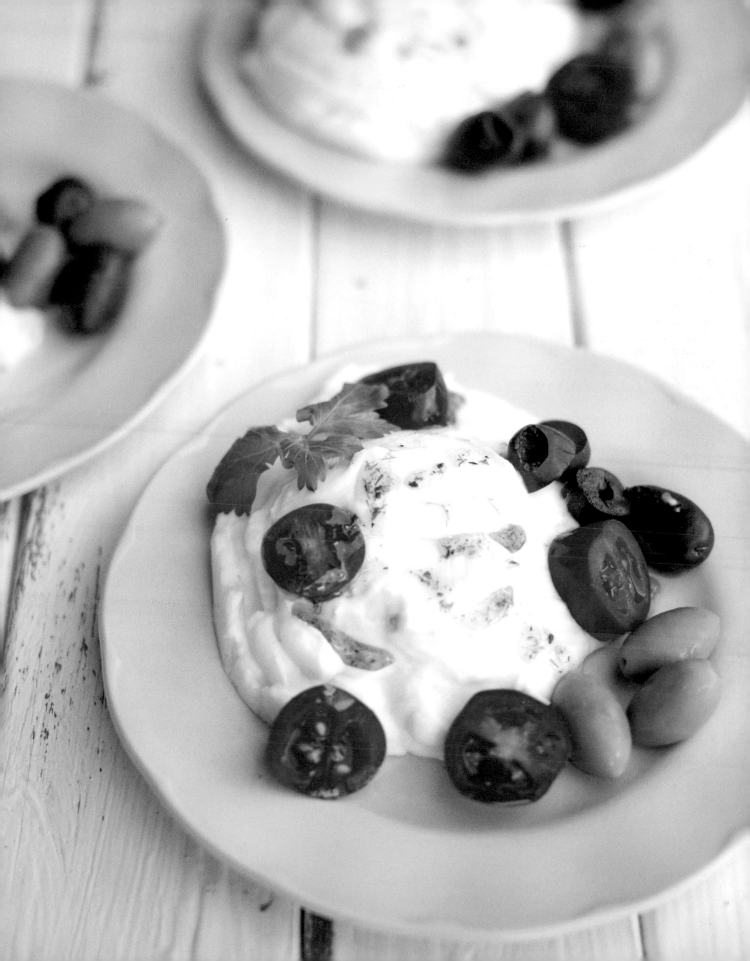

# snickerdoodle waffles

L M H
KETO  prep time: 5 minutes • cook time: 8 minutes • yield: 2 waffles (1 per serving)

This recipe was a thorn in my side! I must have worked on it for a month nonstop. I wanted to create a zero-carb waffle without nuts or nut flours (since nut flours are an often-overeaten keto food that can cause weight gain), and I wanted it to be dairy-free, so creating the perfect keto topping was important. I would lie awake thinking about how to make the batter thick enough without adding too much protein powder, which often made the waffles too dry. Then one evening my son wanted deviled eggs (he always wants deviled eggs). As we sat and chatted while peeling eggs at the sink, I looked over at that waffle maker and thought, "Hard-boiled eggs would thicken the batter!" Sure enough, it worked. Not only that, but they are not dry at all and taste amazing—especially when topped with vanilla bean crème anglaise!

2 large eggs

2 hard-boiled eggs (see page 174)

2 tablespoons Swerve confectioners'-style sweetener or equivalent amount of liquid or powdered sweetener (see page 81)

1 tablespoon vanilla-flavored egg white protein powder

1 tablespoon ground cinnamon

½ teaspoon baking powder

⅛ teaspoon fine sea salt

2 tablespoons coconut oil

1 to 2 teaspoons vanilla extract or 1 teaspoon almond extract

Melted coconut oil or coconut oil spray, for the waffle iron

¼ cup Vanilla Bean Crème Anglaise (page 404), divided, for serving (optional)

1. Preheat a waffle iron to high heat. Place the raw eggs, hard-boiled eggs, sweetener, protein powder, cinnamon, baking powder, and salt in a blender or food processor and combine until smooth and thick. Add the 2 tablespoons of coconut oil and extract and pulse to combine well.

2. Grease the hot waffle iron with melted coconut oil. Place 3 tablespoons of the batter in the center of the iron and close the lid. Cook for 3 to 4 minutes, until golden brown and crisp.

3. Remove from the waffle iron and serve with 2 tablespoons of the vanilla bean crème anglaise, if desired.

4. Repeat with the remaining batter and serve with the remaining 2 tablespoons of crème anglaise, if using.

note: *If you're a visual learner, check out the video I made for this recipe on my website: MariaMindBodyHealth.com/videos/*

NUTRITIONAL INFO
(per serving, without Vanilla Bean Crème Anglaise)

| calories | fat | protein | carbs | fiber |
|----------|-----|---------|-------|-------|
| 275 | 23g | 14g | 3g | 2g |
| | 76% | 20% | 4% | |

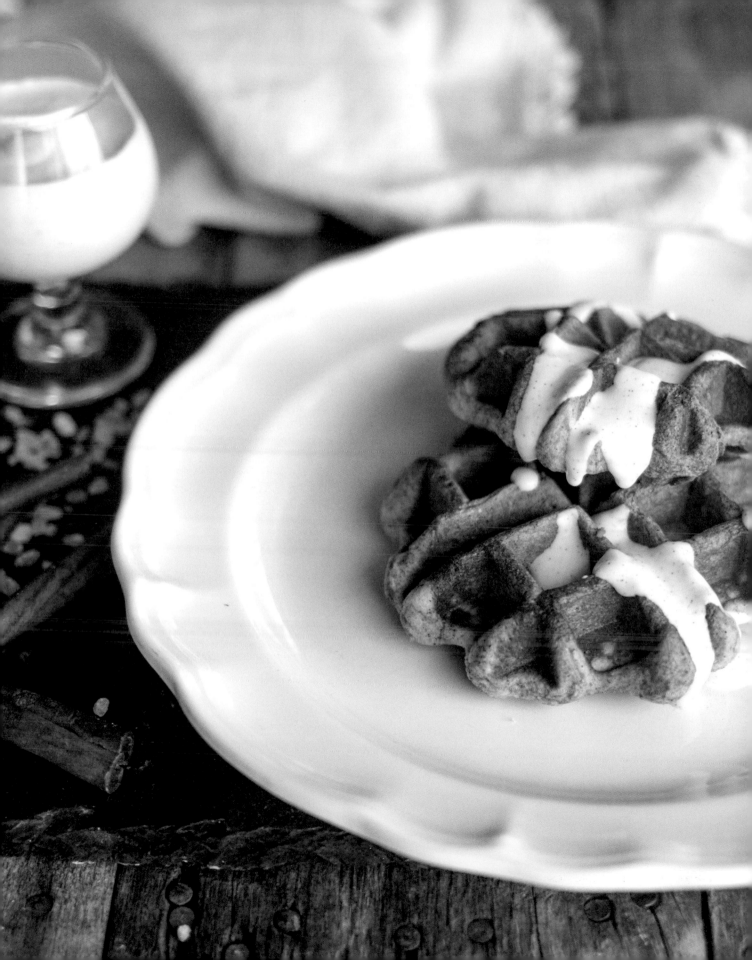

# chocolate waffles

prep time: 5 minutes (not including time to make the hard-boiled eggs or hot fudge sauce)
cook time: 8 minutes • yield: 2 waffles (1 per serving)

2 large eggs

2 hard-boiled eggs (see page 174)

2 tablespoons Swerve confectioners'-style sweetener or equivalent amount of liquid or powdered sweetener (see page 81)

1 tablespoon vanilla-flavored egg white protein powder

2 tablespoons unsweetened cocoa powder

½ teaspoon baking powder

⅛ teaspoon fine sea salt

2 tablespoons coconut oil

1 to 2 teaspoons vanilla extract or 1 teaspoon almond extract

Melted coconut oil or coconut oil spray, for the waffle iron

¼ cup Hot Fudge Sauce (page 403), divided, for serving

1. Preheat a waffle iron to high heat. Place the raw eggs, hard-boiled eggs, sweetener, protein powder, cocoa powder, baking powder, and salt in a blender or food processor and combine until smooth and thick. Add the 2 tablespoons of coconut oil and extract and pulse to combine well.

2. Grease the hot waffle iron with melted coconut oil. Place 3 table-spoons of the batter in the center of the iron and close the lid. Cook for 3 to 4 minutes, until golden brown and crisp.

3. Remove from the waffle iron and serve with 2 tablespoons of the hot fudge sauce, if desired.

4. Repeat with the remaining batter and serve with the remaining 2 tablespoons of hot fudge sauce.

note: *You can make these waffles extra chocolaty by using chocolate-flavored egg white protein powder and/or chocolate extract instead of vanilla or almond extract.*

NUTRITIONAL INFO
(per serving, with hot fudge)

| calories | fat | protein | carbs | fiber |
|----------|-----|---------|-------|-------|
| 305 | 24g | 19g | 3g | 1g |
| | 71% | 25% | 4% | |

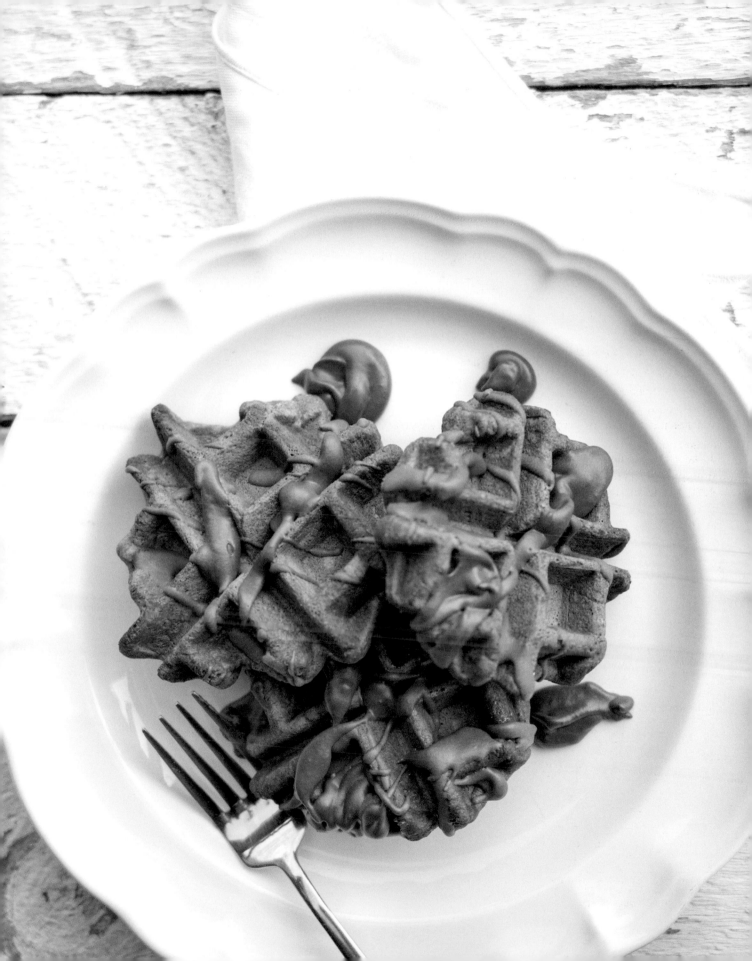

# lemon curd dutch baby

L M H KETO   option   prep time: 10 minutes (not including time to make the lemon curd)
cook time: 20 minutes • yield: 2 servings

2 tablespoons coconut oil

3 large eggs

¾ cup unsweetened (unflavored or vanilla-flavored) cashew milk, homemade (page 106) or store-bought, or almond milk (or hemp milk for nut-free)

¼ cup vanilla-flavored egg white protein powder

1 teaspoon baking powder

¼ cup Swerve confectioners'-style sweetener or equivalent amount of liquid or powdered sweetener (see page 81)

3 drops lemon oil or 2 teaspoons lemon extract

¼ teaspoon fine sea salt

¼ cup Lemon Curd (page 402), divided, for serving

Grated lemon zest, for garnish (optional)

1. Preheat the oven to 425°F.

2. In a medium cast-iron skillet over medium heat, melt the oil; set aside. In a blender, combine the eggs, cashew milk, protein powder, baking powder, sweetener, lemon oil, and salt. Blend for about 1 minute, until foamy.

3. Pour the batter into the skillet. Bake for 18 to 20 minutes, until the pancake is puffed and golden brown.

4. Meanwhile, make the lemon curd.

5. Remove the pancake from the oven, cut in half, and serve each portion with 2 tablespoons of the lemon curd. Garnish with lemon zest, if desired. Best served fresh.

busy family tip: *I make the pancake batter the night before and keep it in the fridge, ready to go for an easy breakfast the next morning.*

NUTRITIONAL INFO (per serving, with lemon curd)

| calories | fat | protein | carbs | fiber |
|---|---|---|---|---|
| 347 | 27g | 23g | 4g | 0g |
| | 70% | 26% | 4% | |

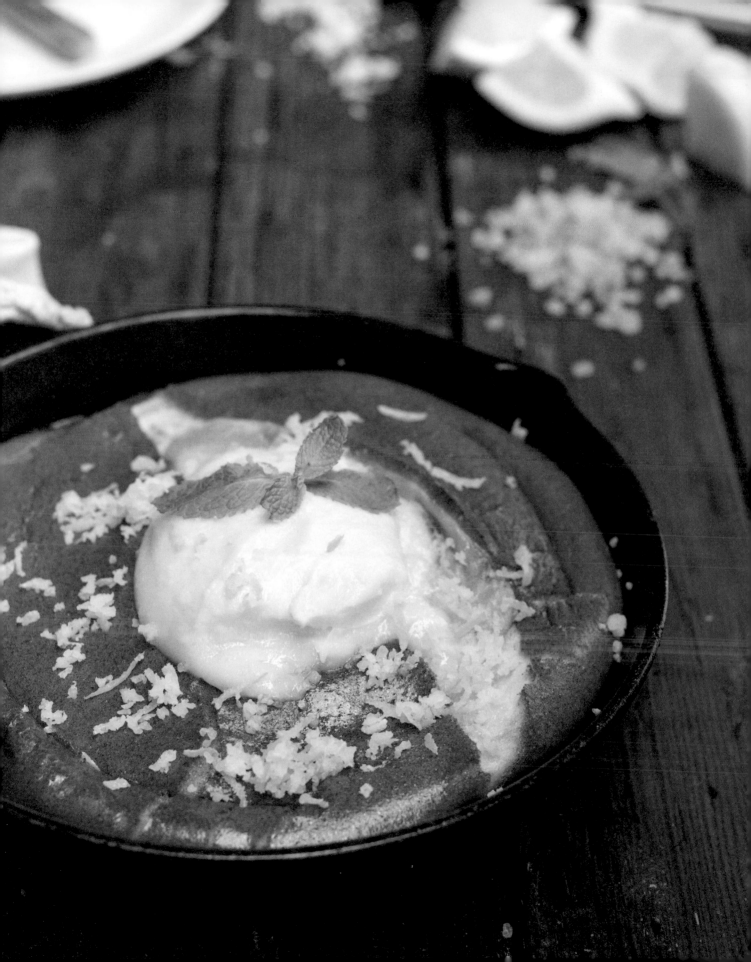

# chocolate pudding

L M H KETO

prep time: 5 minutes (not including time to hard-boil the eggs)
yield: 2½ cups (½ cup per serving)

I know this recipe sounds crazy, but you must try it! My son Kai hated eggs as a baby, so I devised this recipe to sneak some eggs into his breakfasts. He loves it!

10 hard-boiled eggs (see page 174), peeled (see note)

1 (13½-ounce) can full-fat coconut milk

½ cup Swerve confectioners'-style sweetener or equivalent amount of liquid or powdered sweetener (see page 81)

1 to 2 teaspoons stevia glycerite (or to desired sweetness)

¼ cup unsweetened cocoa powder

Seeds scraped from 2 vanilla beans or 2 teaspoons vanilla extract

1 teaspoon ground cinnamon

⅛ teaspoon fine sea salt

1. Place all the ingredients in a blender, starting with 1 teaspoon of stevia glycerite, and puree until *very* smooth. Add more sweetener and/or cocoa powder to taste.

2. Store in an airtight container in the fridge for up to 4 days.

note: *If you're making this dish for a child under the age of one, use only the egg yolks.*

NUTRITIONAL INFO (per serving)

| calories | fat | protein | carbs | fiber |
|---|---|---|---|---|
| 268 | 22g | 14g | 4g | 1g |
|  | 74% | 20% | 6% |  |

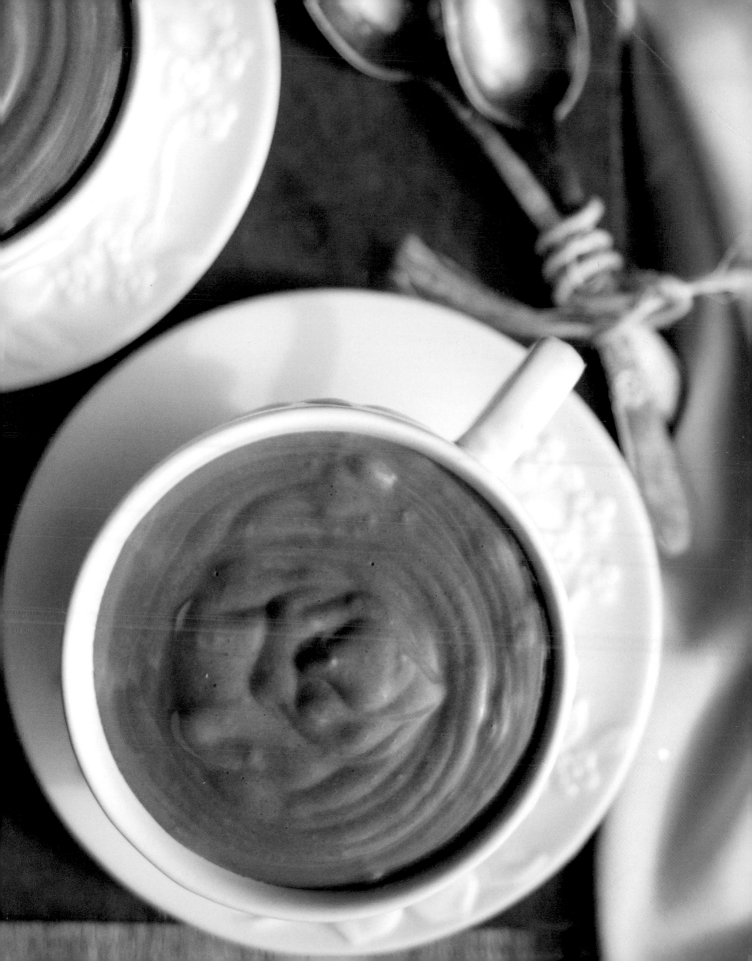

# keto english muffins

KETO · option · prep time: 2 minutes · cook time: 1 or 12 minutes, depending on cooking method · yield: 1 serving

This is an easy substitution for bagels or toast. Cut in half, a Keto English Muffin is the perfect vehicle for your favorite bagel spread or toppings. Try my Bacon Marmalade (page 122) or a lovely breakfast of Eggs Florentine (page 166)!

You can make these muffins in a microwave or a toaster oven. I love using my toaster oven for small jobs like this because it takes less time to preheat, plus it doesn't heat up the kitchen on hot summer days.

1 teaspoon coconut oil, for greasing the ramekin

1 large egg

2 teaspoons coconut flour

Pinch of baking soda

Pinch of fine sea salt

1. Grease a 4-ounce ramekin with the coconut oil. If using the toaster oven method, preheat the toaster oven to 400°F.

2. In a small mixing bowl, combine the egg and coconut flour with a fork until well combined, then add the rest of the ingredients and stir to combine.

3. Place the dough in the greased ramekin. *To cook in a microwave,* cook on high for 1 minute, until a toothpick inserted in the middle comes out clean. *To cook in a toaster oven,* bake for 12 minutes, until a toothpick inserted in the middle comes out clean.

4. Allow to cool in the ramekin for 5 minutes. Remove the muffin from the ramekin and allow to cool completely. Slice in half and serve.

note: *If you like your muffins with crispy edges, melt 2 teaspoons of coconut oil in a skillet over medium-high heat. When the oil is hot, place the muffin halves cut side down in the hot oil and fry until the edges are crispy.*

NUTRITIONAL INFO (per serving)

| calories | fat | protein | carbs | fiber |
|----------|-----|---------|-------|-------|
| 130 | 7g | 8.3g | 8.4g | 5g |
| | 48% | 26% | 26% | |

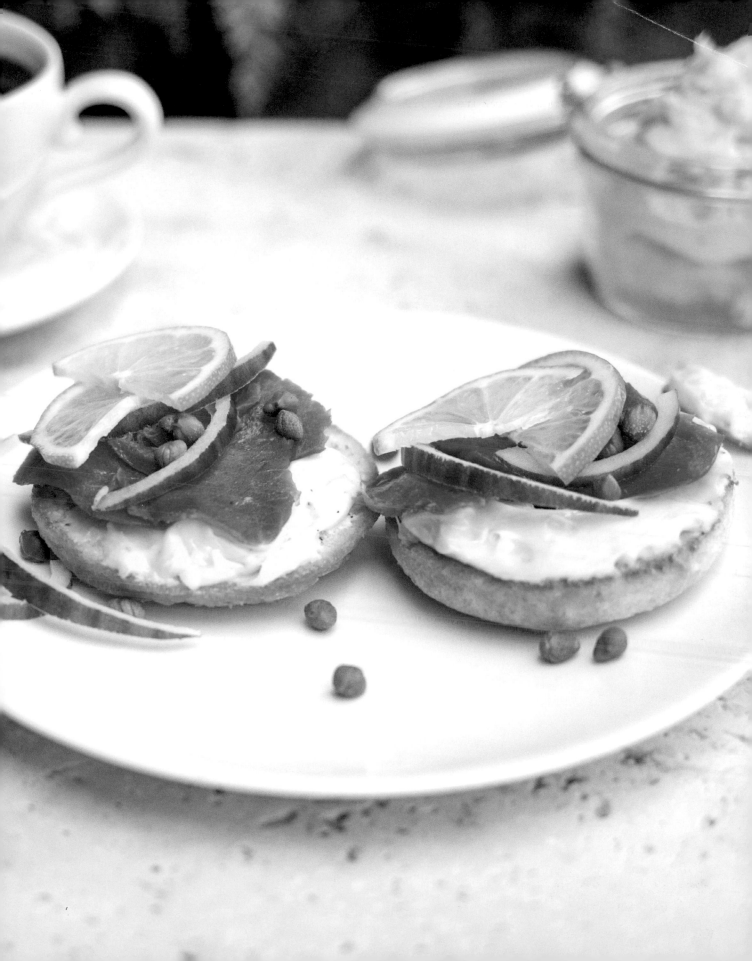

snacks
and appetizers

# bone broth fat bombs

L ⊤ H KETO  prep time: 5 minutes, plus 2 hours to chill • yield: 12 fat bombs (1 per serving)

These savory fat bombs are great for on-the-go energy. They remind me of a savory Jell-O bite. You can easily scale this recipe up or down; all you need to remember is to use 1 tablespoon of gelatin for every 2 cups of broth.

Besides eating these as a snack, you can also use them to intensify the flavor and up the healing properties of any stew or soup that calls for bone broth. Simply throw one or two fat bombs in and reduce the amount of broth called for in the recipe by that amount. The resulting dish with also have a thicker, more luxurious texture.

1 tablespoon grass-fed powdered gelatin

2 cups homemade bone broth, any type (page 108), warmed

**special equipment:**

Silicone mold with 12 (1⅞-ounce) cavities (see page 85)

1. Sprinkle the gelatin over the broth and whisk to combine.

2. Place the silicone mold on a rimmed sheet pan (for easy transport). Pour the broth into the mold. Place in the fridge or freezer until the gelatin is fully set, about 2 hours. To release the fat bombs from the mold, gently push on the mold to pop them out.

3. Store in an airtight container in the fridge for up to 5 days or in the freezer for several months.

NUTRITIONAL INFO (per serving)

| calories | fat | protein | carbs | fiber |
|---|---|---|---|---|
| 27 | 5.3g | 2g | 2.3g | 0g |
| | 60% | 19% | 21% | |

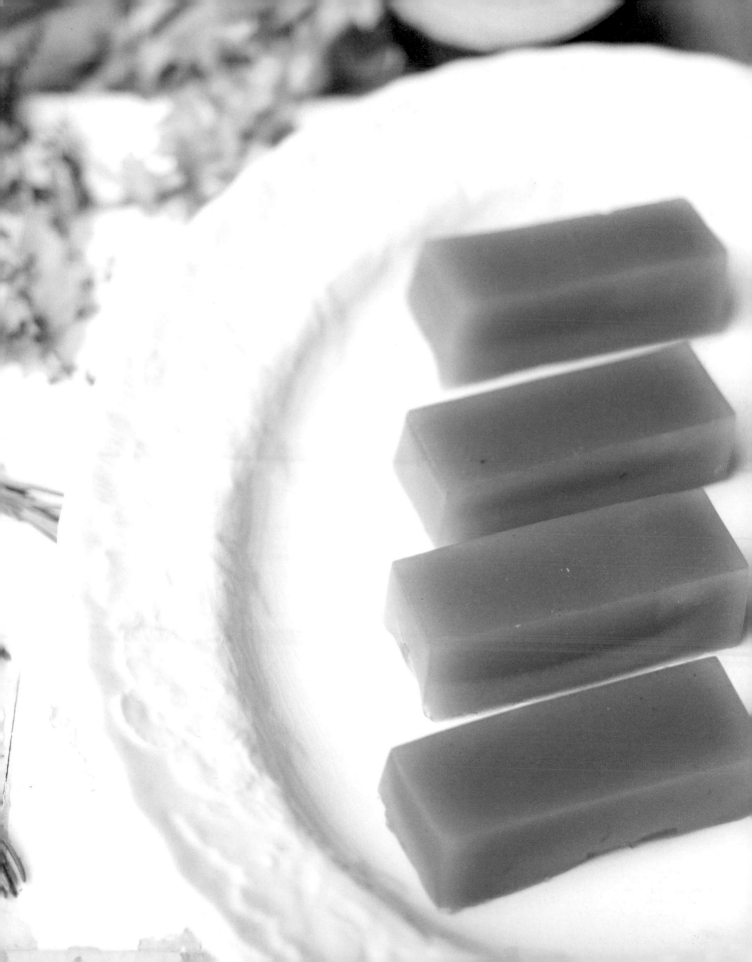

# paleo egg rolls

L M H KETO · prep time: 20 minutes • cook time: 10 minutes • yield: 10 egg rolls (1 per serving)

1 cup coconut oil, duck fat, or avocado oil, for frying (see note)

20 slices prosciutto

Sliced radishes, for serving (optional)

### filling:

1 pound ground pork

2 cups shredded cabbage

1 green onion, chopped

3 tablespoons coconut aminos

1 clove garlic, minced

1 teaspoon grated fresh ginger

½ teaspoon five-spice powder

½ teaspoon fine sea salt

### sweet 'n' sour sauce:

½ cup Swerve confectioners'-style sweetener or equivalent amount of liquid or powdered sweetener (see page 81)

½ cup coconut vinegar

2 tablespoons coconut aminos

1 tablespoon tomato paste

½ teaspoon minced garlic

1 teaspoon grated fresh ginger

¼ teaspoon guar gum (optional)

1. Heat the oil to 350°F in a deep-fryer or a 4-inch-deep (or deeper) cast-iron skillet over medium heat. The oil should be at least 3 inches deep; add more oil if needed.

2. While the oil is heating up, make the filling: In a large skillet over medium heat, brown the ground pork with the cabbage, green onion, coconut aminos, garlic, ginger, five-spice, and salt, stirring to break up the meat. Cook until the meat is cooked through and cabbage is tender, about 5 minutes. Remove the filling from pan and set aside until cool enough to handle.

3. Make the sauce: Heat the sauce ingredients, except the guar gum, in a small saucepan until simmering. Whisk until smooth. If you want a thicker sauce, sift the guar gum into the sauce; it will thicken in a few minutes.

4. To assemble the egg rolls: Lay one slice of prosciutto on a sushi mat or a sheet of parchment paper, with a short end facing you. Lay another slice of prosciutto on top of it, across the center at a right angle, forming a cross. Spoon 3 to 4 tablespoons of the filling into the center of the cross.

5. Fold the sides of the bottom slice up and over the filling to form the ends of the roll. Tightly roll up the long piece of prosciutto, starting at the edge closest to you, into a tight egg roll shape so that it overlaps by an inch or so. *Note:* If the prosciutto rips, it's okay. It will seal when you fry it. Repeat until all the prosciutto and filling are used.

6. Working in batches, fry the egg rolls by placing the tightly wrapped roll seam side down in the hot oil for about 2 minutes, until crisp on the outside. Remove from the oil and serve. Serve with sliced radishes, if desired.

7. Store extras in an airtight container for up to 3 days. To reheat, place in a skillet over medium heat and sauté for 3 minutes on all sides, or until warmed.

note: *Once cool, strain the used oil through cheesecloth and store it in mason jars in the fridge for future use.*

NUTRITIONAL INFO (per serving)

| calories | fat | protein | carbs | fiber |
|---|---|---|---|---|
| 190 | 13g | 15g | 3g | 2g |
| | 62% | 32% | 6% | |

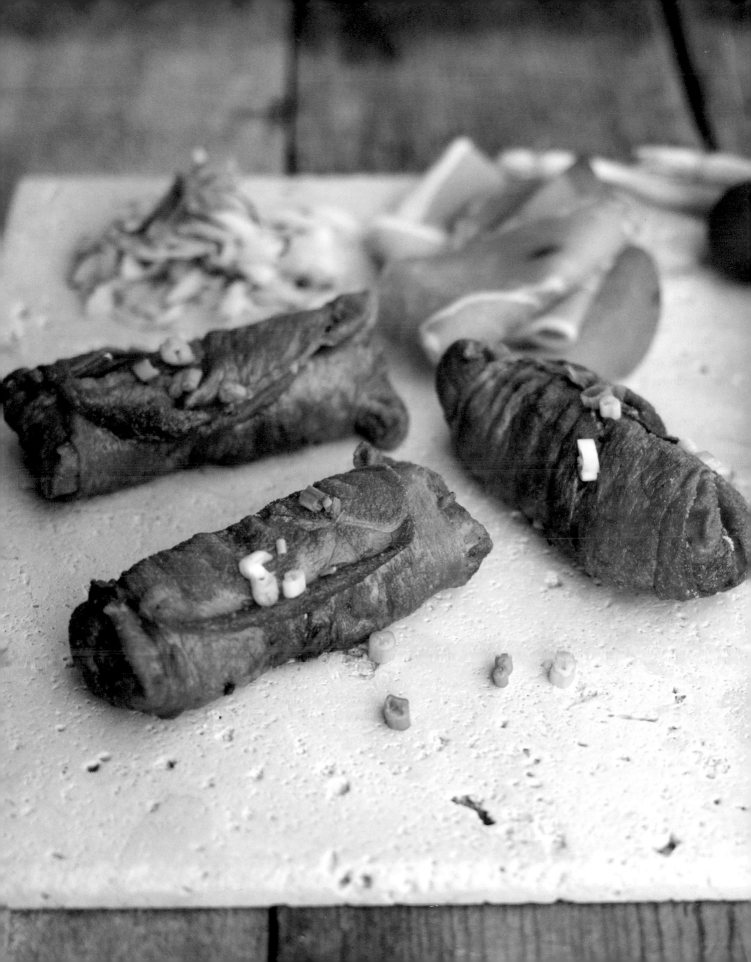

# scotch eggs

L M H / KETO  prep time: 10 minutes • cook time: 20 minutes • yield: 3 servings

The keys to making perfect Scotch eggs are to cook perfect soft-boiled eggs—not overcooked or rubbery ones—and to get the frying oil to the right temperature. Oil that's not hot enough creates soggy and oily fried foods, but if it's too hot, the exterior will burn before the interior—in this case the ground pork—has a chance to cook. The first time I made Scotch eggs, the oil was too hot. When I dropped my first egg in the pot, the oil boiled over and started a fire, and the prosciutto wrapper cooked so fast that the pork inside was still raw. Learn from my mistake and use a thermometer to check the oil temperature! The classic method for cooking Scotch eggs is to fry them, but I've also included an oven-cooked variation if you prefer to prepare them that way.

3 large eggs

1 cup coconut oil or other Paleo fat, such as lard, tallow, or duck fat, for frying

⅓ pound ground pork

¼ teaspoon fine sea salt

6 slices prosciutto

6 tablespoons whole-grain mustard, for garnish

1 tablespoon finely chopped fresh cilantro or other herb of choice, for garnish

**variation:** Baked Scotch Eggs.

*If you prefer to bake the eggs instead of frying them, preheat the oven to 425°F, place the eggs on a rimmed baking sheet, and bake for 20 minutes, or until the prosciutto is crisp and the pork is cooked through.*

1. To cook perfect soft-boiled eggs, fill a medium saucepan halfway with water and bring to a simmer, not quite a boil. Gently place the eggs in the simmering water and cook for 5 minutes, holding the water at a simmer, not a boil. Remove the eggs from the water and run under cool water. Once cool, carefully peel the eggs and set them aside.

2. Preheat the oil to 350°F in a deep-fryer or a 4-inch-deep (or deeper) cast-iron skillet over medium heat. The oil should be at least 3 inches deep; add more oil if needed. While the oil heats, assemble the eggs.

3. In a medium bowl, mix the ground pork with the salt until well combined. Place one-third of the pork on a piece of parchment paper, and, using your hands, flatten it out into as thin a circle as possible. Place a soft-boiled egg in the center of the meat and wrap the meat up and around the egg. Secure it closed by pressing the meat together, being careful not to break open the egg.

4. Lay out 2 pieces of prosciutto like an X on a sushi mat or a sheet of parchment paper. Place the pork-covered egg in the middle. Fold the prosciutto "arms" around the egg.

5. When the oil has reached 350°F (check it with a thermometer), fry the eggs: Gently drop one egg at a time into the hot oil. Fry for 5 to 6 minutes, until the prosciutto is crispy and the pork is cooked through. Remove from the oil and set aside on a paper towel to drain. Repeat with the remaining two eggs, frying them one at a time.

6. To serve, place six 1-tablespoon amounts of whole-grain mustard on a serving platter. Slice each fried egg in half with a very sharp serrated knife. Place the halves, cut side up, on top of the mustard (which keeps the eggs from sliding around on the platter). Garnish with the cilantro.

7. Reheat leftovers on a rimmed baking sheet in a 400°F oven for 7 minutes, or until heated through.

NUTRITIONAL INFO (per serving)

| calories | fat | protein | carbs | fiber |
|---|---|---|---|---|
| 430 | 33g | 33g | 1g | 0.2g |
|  | 69% | 30% | 1% |  |

**Notes on the Perfect Soft-Boiled Egg:**

*I grew up learning to make soft-boiled eggs with the "boil-and-rest" method: the eggs are put in a pot and covered with cold water, then brought to a boil, covered, and then removed from the heat to rest for 3½ minutes. Much to my mother's dismay, I found a better way to make perfect soft-boiled eggs, which is to place the eggs directly into simmering (not boiling!) water, as described in Step 1. When eggs are boiled, the whites coagulate and become rubbery. To make perfect ready-to-eat soft-boiled eggs, simmer the eggs for 6 minutes; in this recipe, the eggs are soft-boiled for just 5 minutes because they cook more when they're fried.*

# bacon cannoli

L M H KETO prep time: 10 minutes • cook time: 20 minutes • yield: 1 dozen cannoli (2 per serving)

This is a flexible recipe: once you get the method down, you can change up the savory filling to anything you like. This version is filled with egg salad. You might also try Doro Watt Chicken Salad Wraps (page 272), pureed or chopped Braunschweiger (page 214), or Simple Crab Salad (page 236).

12 slices bacon

**egg salad:**

8 large eggs

½ cup mayonnaise, homemade (page 124) or store-bought

2 tablespoons Dijon mustard

1 tablespoon chopped fresh dill or other herb of choice

1 teaspoon paprika

Fine sea salt and fresh ground black pepper, to taste

**for garnish:**

Chopped fresh dill, tarragon, or other herb of choice

Creamy Mexican Dressing (page 116) (optional)

**special equipment:**

12 cannoli tubes (1 inch around and 4 inches long)

1. Preheat the oven to 375°F. Line a rimmed baking sheet with parchment paper.

2. Wrap one slice of bacon around each cannoli tube. Wrap the bacon tightly, overlapping the edges so the bacon totally covers the tube.

3. Place the wrapped tubes on the prepared baking sheet and bake for 20 minutes, or until the bacon is crisp. Remove from the oven and allow to cool completely.

4. Meanwhile, make the egg salad filling: Place the eggs in a saucepan and cover with cold water. Bring the water to a boil, then cover, remove the pan from the heat, and let the eggs stand in the hot water for 10 to 12 minutes. Remove the eggs from the hot water and place them in a bowl of ice water to cool, then peel and chop them.

5. In a large bowl, combine the chopped eggs, mayonnaise, mustard, dill, paprika, and salt and pepper. Mash well with a fork or wooden spoon.

6. Use your hands to carefully wiggle the bacon to release it from the cannoli tubes while keeping its shape.

7. To assemble: When you're ready to fill the bacon tubes, place the filling in a pastry bag fitted with a tip or in a resealable plastic bag with one corner snipped off. Fill each cannoli, leaving some filling sticking out of each end. Garnish with fresh herbs and a drizzle of Dairy-Free Creamy Herb Dressing, if desired.

8. These are best served fresh. Store extra tubes and filling separately in airtight containers in the fridge for up to 3 days. To reheat, place the unfilled bacon tubes on a rimmed baking sheet and heat in a preheated 400°F oven for 4 minutes, or until the bacon is warmed and crispy. Fill with the egg salad or another savory filling of your choice.

NUTRITIONAL INFO
(per serving, without dressing)

| calories | fat | protein | carbs | fiber |
|----------|-----|---------|-------|-------|
| 199 | 18g | 9g | 0.3g | 0g |
| | 81% | 18% | 1% | |

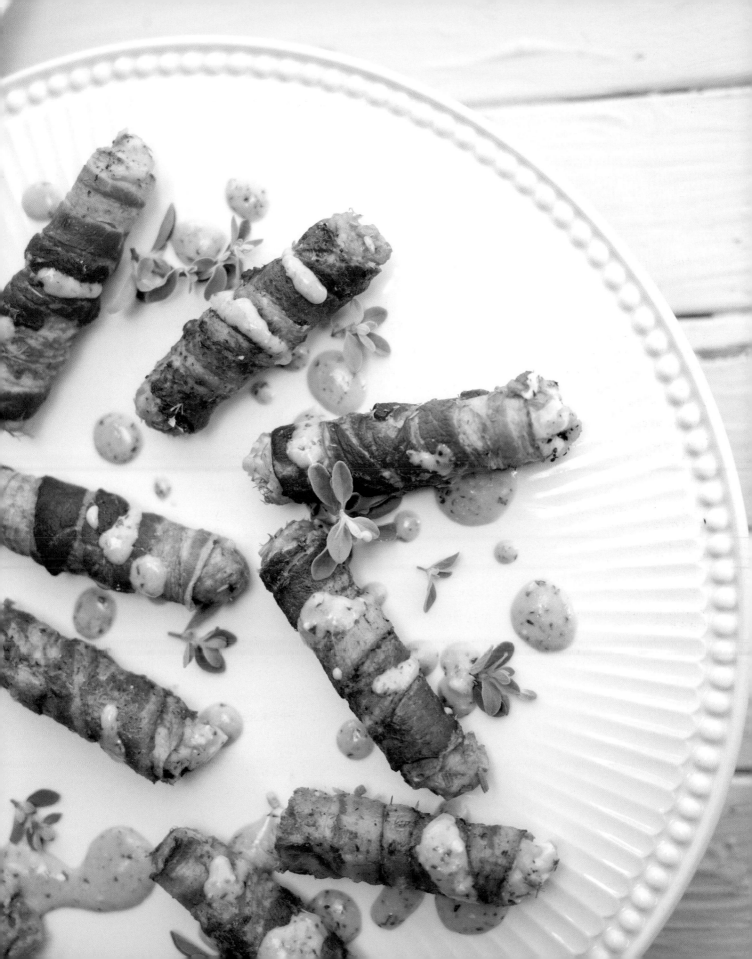

# chicken tinga wings

L→H M KETO ⬚ ⌀ ⌀  prep time: 10 minutes • cook time: 30 minutes • yield: 6 servings (2 wings per serving)

1 to 2 cups coconut oil, for frying

1 pound chicken wings (about 12 wings)

Fine sea salt and fresh ground black pepper

**tinga sauce:**

1 pound Mexican-style fresh (raw) chorizo

½ large white onion, chopped

1 clove garlic, minced

3 cups chopped tomatoes

1 cup chopped husked tomatillos

2 tablespoons pureed chipotles in adobo sauce

1½ teaspoons fine sea salt

1 teaspoon fresh ground black pepper

½ teaspoon dried oregano leaves

1 sprig fresh thyme

½ cup chicken bone broth, homemade (page 108) or store-bought

1. Preheat the oil to 350°F in a deep-fryer or a 4-inch-deep (or deeper) cast-iron skillet over medium heat. The oil should be at least 3 inches deep; add more oil if needed.

2. While the oil heats, make the sauce: Cook the chorizo, onion, and garlic in a large cast-iron skillet over medium heat until the meat is crumbled and cooked through, about 5 minutes. Add the tomatoes, tomatillos, chipotles, salt, pepper, and herbs and stir to combine. Continue cooking for 5 minutes. Add the chicken broth and cook for 5 more minutes. Remove the thyme sprig and set the sauce aside.

3. Fry about six wings at a time until golden brown on all sides and cooked through, about 8 minutes. Remove from the oil and sprinkle with salt and pepper. Repeat with the remaining wings.

4. Place the wings on a serving platter and serve with the sauce, or toss the wings in the sauce before serving. They are best served fresh. Store extra wings and sauce separately in airtight containers in the fridge for up to 3 days. To reheat, place the chicken wings on a rimmed baking sheet and heat in a preheated 400°F oven for 4 minutes, or until warmed. Heat the sauce in a saucepan over medium-low heat until warmed.

NUTRITIONAL INFO (per serving)

| calories | fat | protein | carbs | fiber |
|---|---|---|---|---|
| 247 | 17g | 19g | 5g | 2g |
|  | 62% | 31% | 7% |  |

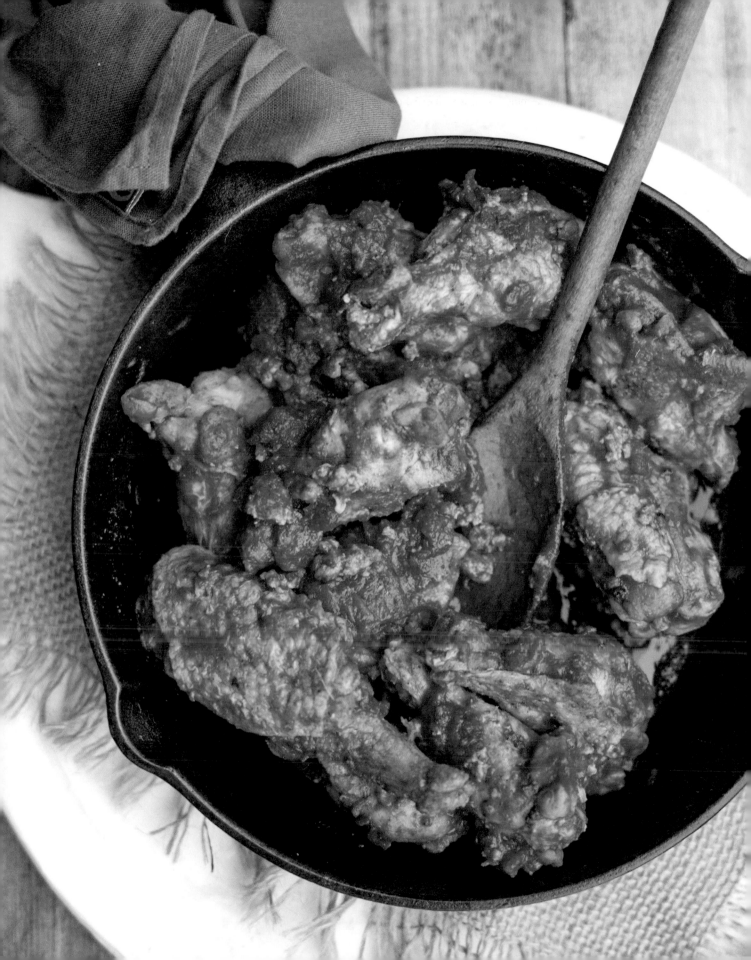

# lemon pepper wings

L⤳H KETO M  ▯ ⊘ ⊘ prep time: 5 minutes • cook time: 16 minutes • yield: 6 servings (2 wings per serving)

1 to 2 cups coconut oil or other Paleo fat, for frying

1 pound chicken wings (about 12 wings)

½ teaspoon fine sea salt, divided

1 teaspoon fresh ground black pepper, divided

## sauce:

¼ cup MCT oil or extra-virgin olive oil

Grated zest of 1 lemon

Juice of 1 lemon

1. Preheat the oil to 350°F in a deep-fryer or in a 4-inch-deep (or deeper) cast-iron skillet over medium heat. The oil should be at least 3 inches deep; add more oil if needed.

2. While the oil is heating, make the sauce: Place the MCT oil in a small dish. Add the lemon zest and juice and whisk to combine.

3. Fry the wings in the hot oil, about six at a time, until golden brown on all sides and cooked through, about 8 minutes. Remove the wings from the oil and sprinkle with half of the salt and pepper. Repeat with the remaining wings, salt, and pepper.

4. Place the wings on a serving platter and serve with the sauce. They are best served fresh. Store extra wings and sauce separately in airtight containers in the fridge for up to 3 days. To reheat, place the wings on a rimmed baking sheet and heat in a preheated 400°F oven for 4 minutes, or until the chicken is warm.

NUTRITIONAL INFO (per serving)

| calories | fat | protein | carbs | fiber |
|---|---|---|---|---|
| 286 | 24g | 16g | 1g | 0.5g |
|  | 76% | 23% | 1% |  |

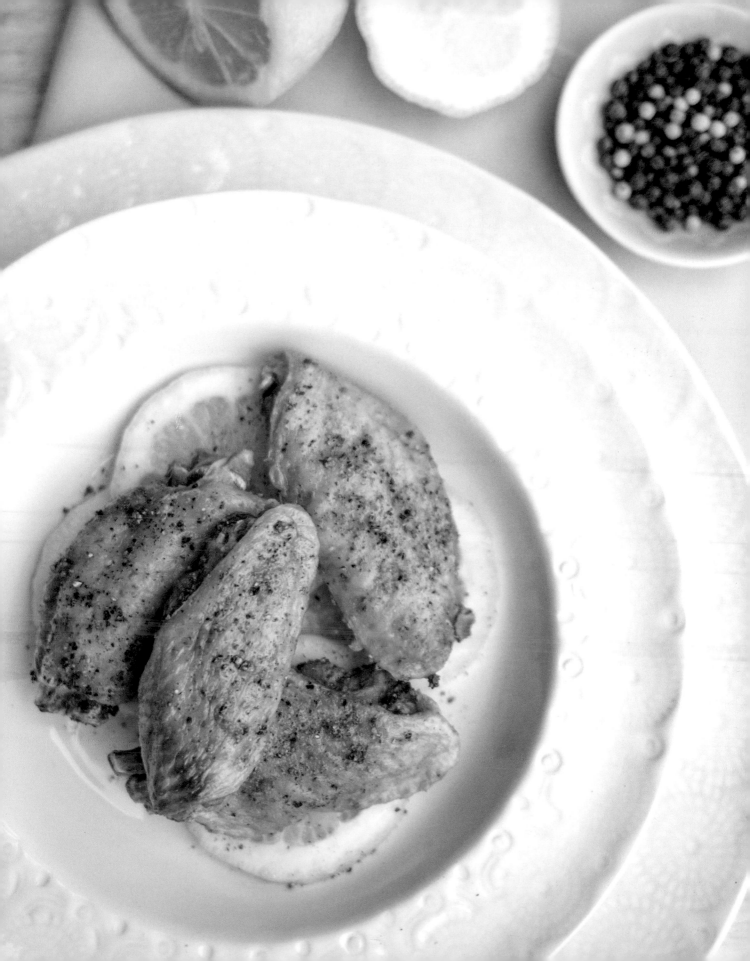

# fried prosciutto-wrapped deviled eggs

L M H KETO

prep time: 10 minutes • cook time: 10 minutes (not including time to hard-boil the eggs)
yield: 12 deviled eggs (2 per serving)

If you prefer to make these deviled eggs a little easier, you can skip the step of wrapping them in prosciutto and frying them.

1 cup coconut oil

6 slices prosciutto

6 hard-boiled eggs (see page 174), peeled

1 small red onion or 2 shallots, thinly sliced (optional)

½ cup mayonnaise, homemade (page 124) or store-bought

1 teaspoon prepared yellow mustard

½ teaspoon fine sea salt, divided

¾ teaspoon smoked paprika, for garnish

1. Preheat the oil to 350°F in a deep-fryer or a 4-inch-deep (or deeper) cast-iron skillet over medium heat. The oil should be at least 3 inches deep; add more oil if needed.

2. While the oil is heating, wrap 1 slice of prosciutto around each hard-boiled egg.

3. When the oil is hot, fry the wrapped eggs, three or four at a time, in the hot oil for about 2 minutes, or until crispy on the outside. Remove from the oil with a slotted spoon onto a paper towel.

4. Fry the onion, if using, in the hot oil until golden brown, about 1 minute. Remove from the oil with a slotted spoon, place on a paper towel, and dust lightly with salt while still hot. Go easy on the salt since prosciutto can be salty.

5. Slice the eggs in half and scoop the yolks into a small bowl. Set the whites aside on a serving platter.

6. Smash the yolks with the back of a fork until very crumbly. Add the mayonnaise, mustard, and salt and stir until smooth and creamy.

7. Spoon or pipe about 1 rounded tablespoon of the filling into each egg white half. If desired, top each deviled egg with some fried onion. Dust with smoked paprika.

8. These are best served immediately for maximum crispiness. Store extras in an airtight container for up to 3 days. Reheating is not recommended.

note: *If you are skipping the prosciutto wrapping and frying, you are welcome to cover and store the deviled eggs in the refrigerator until ready to serve. Top with the fried onion, if using, just before serving.*

NUTRITIONAL INFO (per serving)

| calories | fat | protein | carbs | fiber |
|----------|-----|---------|-------|-------|
| 232 | 21g | 10g | 1g | 0.1g |
| | 81% | 17% | 2% | |

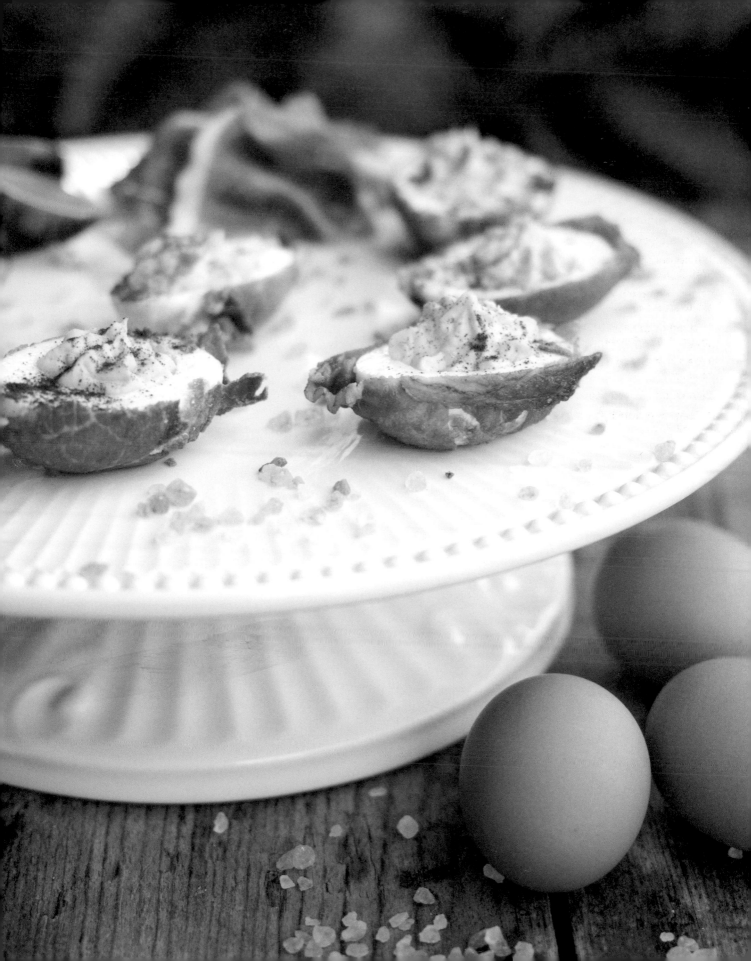

# chicharrón

L M H KETO · prep time: 5 minutes, plus 1 hour to 24 hours to cure
cook time: at least 2 hours • yield: 4 servings

2 teaspoons baking soda

1 teaspoon fine sea salt

1 pound fresh pork belly, skin on

Fine sea salt and fresh ground black pepper

Cajun Seasoning (page 112) or other spices of choice, such as ground cumin

1. Rub the baking soda and salt over the surface of the pork skin, taking care to distribute the powder evenly. Set the pork belly on a rack and place it, uncovered, in the refrigerator for at least an hour but preferably overnight and up to a full day.

2. Remove the pork belly from the refrigerator. Rinse well under running water and pat dry with paper towels.

3. Slice the pork belly into chip-sized pieces, about 2 inches square and ⅓ inch thick.

4. Place the pork chips in a pot and add enough water to cover all the pieces.

5. Heat on low for 2 hours, flipping the chips every 30 minutes, until the water has evaporated and the fat is rendered. Depending on how much moisture is in the pork belly, this process could take up to 3 hours.

6. When all the water has evaporated and there is liquid lard in the bottom of the pot, turn the heat to high to start the frying process—this happens quickly, so don't walk away from the pot!

7. Fry the chips in the rendered lard for 4 to 5 minutes, until they are golden brown. Using a slotted spoon, remove the chicharrónes to a plate lined with paper towels to drain. Sprinkle with salt and any other desired seasonings. (My favorite is my Cajun Seasoning, page 112.)

8. Store extras in an airtight container in the fridge for up to 1 week.

NUTRITIONAL INFO
(per serving)

| calories | fat | protein | carbs | fiber |
|---|---|---|---|---|
| 320 | 28g | 17g | 0g | 0g |
| | 79% | 21% | 0% | |

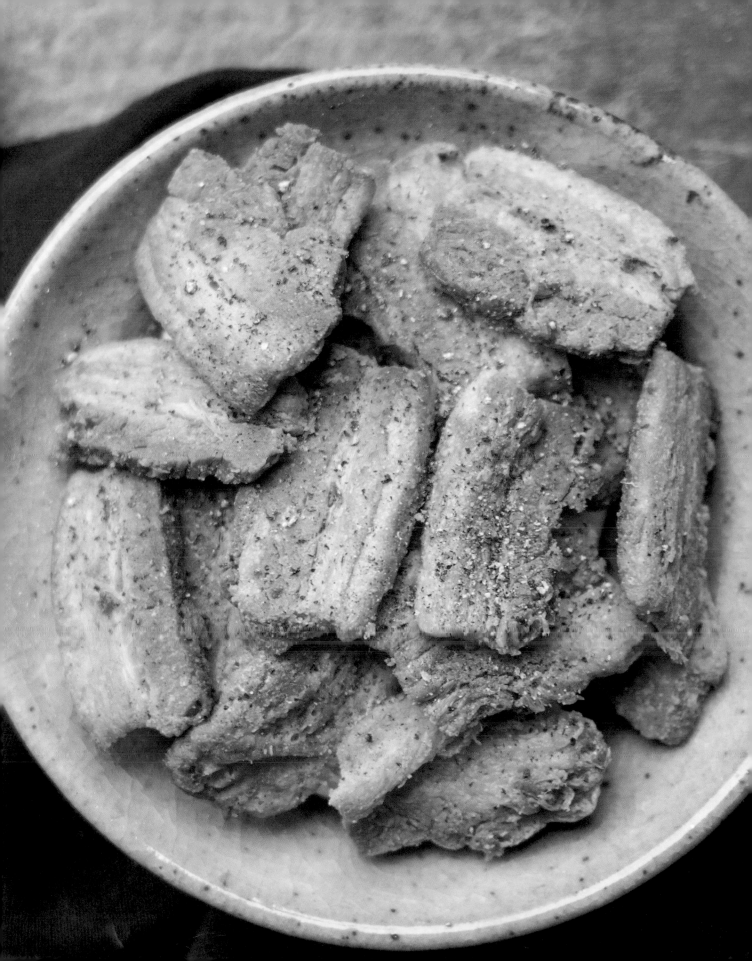

# italian marinated mushrooms

L M H KETO

prep time: 10 minutes, plus at least 24 hours to marinate
cook time: 3 minutes • yield: 8 servings

½ cup MCT oil or other liquid oil, such as extra-virgin olive oil

2 pounds button mushrooms, cleaned and halved or quartered, (very small mushrooms can be left whole)

¼ cup diced onions

¼ cup coconut vinegar or apple cider vinegar

2 cloves garlic, thinly sliced, or cloves from 1 head Garlic Confit (page 142)

Leaves from 1 bunch fresh basil

1 teaspoon Herbes de Florence (page 113)

1 teaspoon fine sea salt

½ teaspoon fresh ground black pepper

1. Heat the oil in a skillet over medium heat. Add the mushrooms and onions and sauté for 3 minutes.

2. Pour the mushroom mixture into a bowl. Add the vinegar, garlic, basil, Herbes de Florence, salt, and pepper and stir to combine. Transfer the mixture to a quart-sized mason jar, cover, and refrigerate for at least 24 hours before serving (marinate longer for a stronger flavor). Store in an airtight container in the fridge for up to 5 days.

note: *These mushrooms are delicious on their own, but I also love to serve them with my Pizza Meatballs in Red Gravy (page 330).*

| NUTRITIONAL INFO (per serving) | | | | |
|---|---|---|---|---|
| calories | fat | protein | carbs | fiber |
| 153 | 14g | 3g | 4g | 2g |
| | 82% | 8% | 10% | |

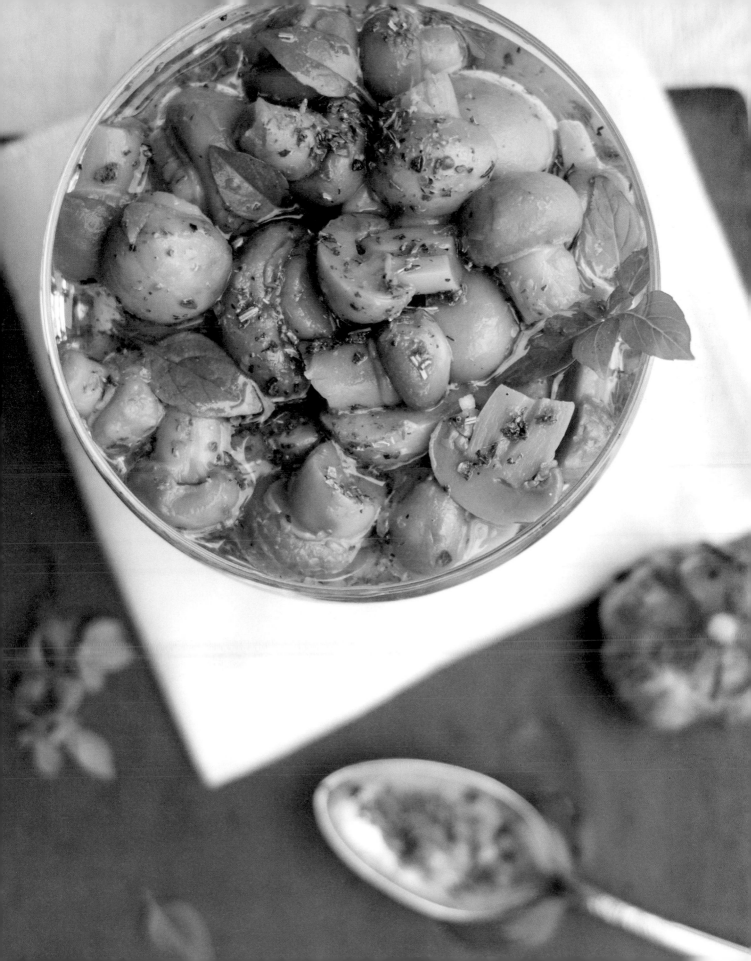

# chicken liver pâté

L →M→H KETO  prep time: 8 minutes (not including time to make the buns)
cook time: 15 minutes • yield: 4 servings

¼ cup chopped bacon (about 2 slices)

¼ cup diced onions

1 teaspoon minced garlic

3 tablespoons Paleo fat, such as duck fat or bacon fat, plus more, melted, for covering

½ pound chicken livers, white stringy parts removed

1 teaspoon chopped fresh thyme or other herb of choice

¼ teaspoon fine sea salt

⅛ teaspoon fresh ground black pepper

4 Keto Buns (page 256), sliced and pan-fried in fat, for serving

1. Cook the bacon in a cast-iron skillet over medium heat until crispy, about 4 minutes. Add the onions, garlic, and Paleo fat and sauté for 2 minutes. Add the chicken livers and cook for 8 minutes, or until the livers are cooked through (the exact time will depend on how thick the chicken livers are). Add the thyme to the pan.

2. Place the chicken liver mixture in a food processor and pulse until a smooth paste forms. Season with the salt and pepper and pulse to combine.

3. Divide evenly among four 4-ounce ramekins. Top with melted fat, which helps preserve the pâté.

4. Serve with toasted keto buns. Store extras in an airtight container in the fridge for up to 5 days.

NUTRITIONAL INFO (per serving)

| calories | fat | protein | carbs | fiber |
|---|---|---|---|---|
| 258 | 21g | 15g | 2g | 0.3g |
|  | 74% | 23% | 3% |  |

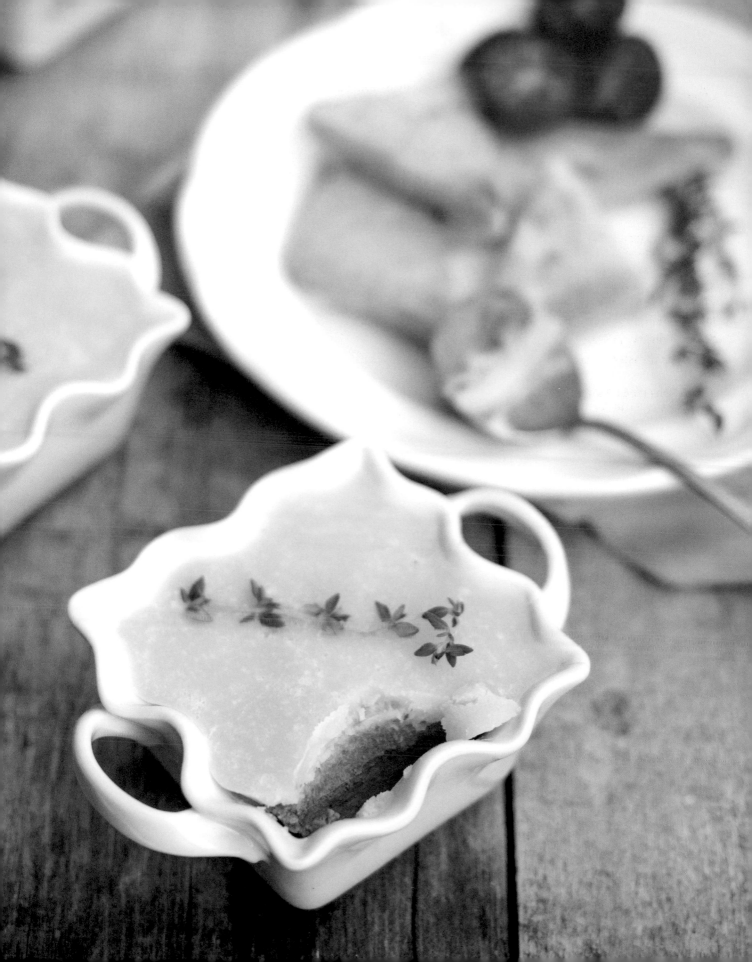

# pickled herring

L M H KETO · prep time: 4 minutes, plus 24 hours to brine and 5 days to pickle
cook time: 5 minutes • yield: 12 servings

It wouldn't be the holidays without my dad's pickled fish. He often goes ice fishing and pickles Northern Pike because it is hard to fillet all the bones out of that type of fish. When pickled, the bones get soft and disintegrate, so you can enjoy Northern Pike without crunching on the bones—and still get a ton of healthy calcium from the bones.

4 pounds herring or skinned Northern Pike fillets, cut into 2-inch pieces (see note)

## saltwater brine:

10 cups water

½ cup fine sea salt

## pickling brine:

½ cup thinly sliced red onions

Handful of fresh dill

2 cups water

2½ cups coconut vinegar

½ cup Swerve confectioners'-style sweetener or equivalent amount of liquid or powdered sweetener (see page 81)

2 teaspoons ground allspice

1 teaspoon dry mustard or mustard seeds

½ teaspoon grated fresh ginger

½ teaspoon prepared horseradish

½ teaspoon peppercorns

## for serving:

Hard-boiled eggs (see page 174), halved or quartered

Pickled ginger

Capers

Fermented pickles

Sliced red onions

Fresh dill sprigs

1. Place the fish in a large bowl with the 10 cups of water. Add the salt and stir. Cover and refrigerate for 24 hours, then drain the fish and rinse it well.

2. Place the drained and rinsed fish in a clean 2-liter glass jar, layering it with the sliced onions and dill.

3. In a large pot over medium heat, heat the 2 cups of water, coconut vinegar, sweetener, allspice, mustard, ginger, horseradish, and peppercorns. Once the sweetener has dissolved, about 5 minutes, allow the brine to cool a little, then pour over the fish packed in the jar. Cover and refrigerate overnight to allow the flavors to meld; the longer the better for stronger flavors. If you let it sit for 5 days, the bones will dissolve. The pickled fish will keep in an airtight container in the fridge for up to 1 month.

4. To serve, arrange the pickled fish on a platter with hard-boiled eggs, pickled ginger, capers, fermented pickles, sliced red onions, and fresh dill.

note: *If using Northern Pike fillets, ask your fishmonger to remove the skin for you. If the skin is left on, the pickled fish will be slimy.*

busy family tip: *If you do not fish or prefer not to prep the fish yourself, ask your local fishmonger to cut the fish into 2-inch pieces.*

NUTRITIONAL INFO (per serving)

| calories | fat | protein | carbs | fiber |
|---|---|---|---|---|
| 240 | 14g | 27g | 2g | 0.3g |
| | 52% | 45% | 3% | |

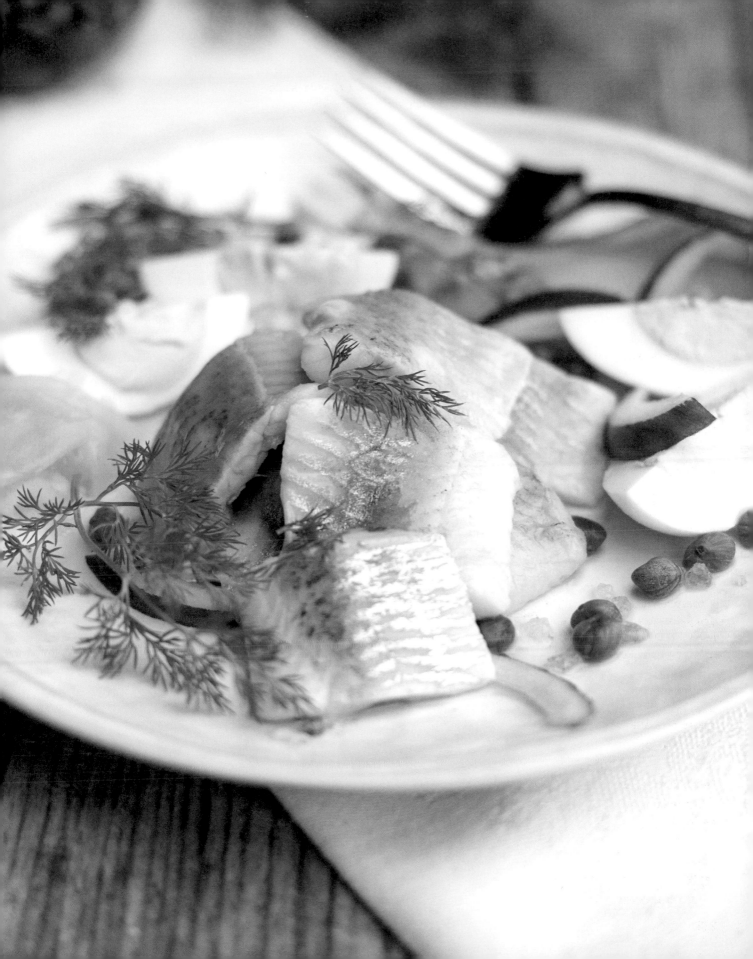

# braunschweiger

L M H KETO option  prep time: 10 minutes, plus 1 day to chill • cook time: 2 hours • yield: 16 servings

I grew up with Braunschweiger on the table whenever we had company. My dad adores it, but if you look at the ingredients on the package, most of them are unpronounceable, and it always contains corn syrup or some other form of sugar. If you prefer, you can leave the sweetener out of this recipe, but if you want Braunschweiger that tastes like the store-bought type, I suggest using it.

1¼ pounds pork liver or beef liver

½ pound pork shoulder or beef tongue

¾ pound pork fatback

½ cup diced yellow onions

1 tablespoon lard

1 tablespoon fine sea salt

1½ teaspoons Swerve confectioners'-style sweetener or equivalent amount of liquid or powdered sweetener (see page 81) (optional)

½ teaspoon ginger powder

¼ teaspoon ground cardamom

## serving suggestions:

Crudités, such as celery stalks, sliced cucumber, bell pepper strips,

Triangles of Keto Bread (page 256), toasted in fat

Chicharrón (page 206)

1. Cut the pork liver, pork shoulder, and fatback into cubes and freeze for an hour so that they can be ground without becoming mushy.

2. Meanwhile, sauté the onions in the lard until soft. Sprinkle with the salt, sweetener, and spices. Transfer to a food processor or blender.

3. Preheat the oven to 300°F and have a 9 by 5-inch loaf pan on hand.

4. Add the frozen liver, pork shoulder, and fatback to the food processor and pulse until you have a smooth puree. Pack the puree into the loaf pan and cover tightly with foil. Set the pan inside a roasting pan with an inch of boiling water and bake for about 2 hours, or until the meat is cooked but not browned; the internal temperature should be 160°F when done.

5. Remove the loaf pan from the roasting pan and let the meat cool completely in the pan. Refrigerate for 1 to 2 days before using. Serve with dippers, such as crudités, toasted Keto Bread slices, and/or chicharrón. Store in an airtight container in the fridge for up to 1 week.

NUTRITIONAL INFO (per serving)

| calories | fat | protein | carbs | fiber |
|---|---|---|---|---|
| 272 | 22g | 17g | 2g | 0.1g |
|  | 73% | 25% | 2% |  |

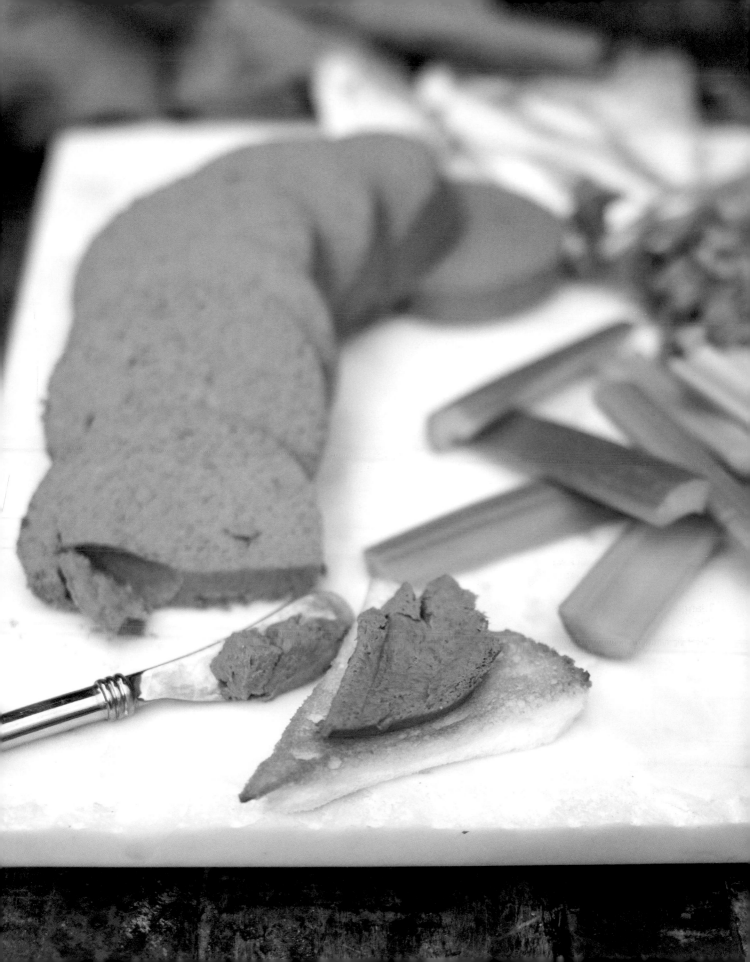

# oscar deviled eggs

12 large eggs

4 asparagus spears

½ cup mayonnaise, homemade (page 124) or store-bought

1 teaspoon prepared yellow mustard

½ teaspoon fine sea salt

¼ cup canned crabmeat (2 ounces)

Fresh basil leaves, thinly sliced, for garnish (optional)

¾ cup Easy Dairy-Free Hollandaise (page 136), for garnish (optional)

Cayenne pepper, for garnish

1. Place the eggs in a large saucepan and cover with cold water. Bring the water to a boil, then immediately cover the pan and remove it from the heat. Allow the eggs to cook in the hot water for 11 minutes.

2. Meanwhile, prepare the asparagus: Remove and discard the tough ends. Cut off the top 3 inches of each spear, and cut the rest on the diagonal into ¾-inch pieces. Place the asparagus in boiling water for 2 minutes, then quickly remove from the pan and rinse in cold water to maintain a bright green color. (*Note:* A skillet is best for this task, as the spears will fit easily and water boils faster with a larger bottom touching the heat source.)

3. After the 11 minutes are up, drain the eggs and rinse them with very cold water for a minute or two to stop the cooking process. Peel the eggs and cut them in half lengthwise. Remove the yolks and place them in a bowl (or a food processor); set the whites aside.

4. Mash or blend the egg yolks with a fork (or a food processor) until they are the texture of very fine crumbles. Add the mayonnaise, mustard, and salt and stir to combine. Fill the egg white halves with the yolk mixture.

5. Place an asparagus spear top and four deviled eggs on each serving plate. Garnish each deviled egg with a few pieces of canned crabmeat, a few pieces of asparagus, and some sliced basil, if desired. To up the keto level, drizzle each egg with 1½ teaspoons of hollandaise, if desired. Finish with a sprinkling of cayenne pepper.

6. Store leftover deviled eggs in an airtight container in the fridge for up to 5 days.

busy family tip: *I keep a dozen hard-boiled eggs in my fridge at all times. My boys, who are five and six, love to help me in the kitchen, and peeling eggs is one of the things they can do without my constant attention so I can prepare other food.*

NUTRITIONAL INFO
(per serving, with hollandaise)

| calories | fat | protein | carbs | fiber |
|---|---|---|---|---|
| 380 | 35g | 15g | 1g | 0.4g |
| | 83% | 16% | 1% | |

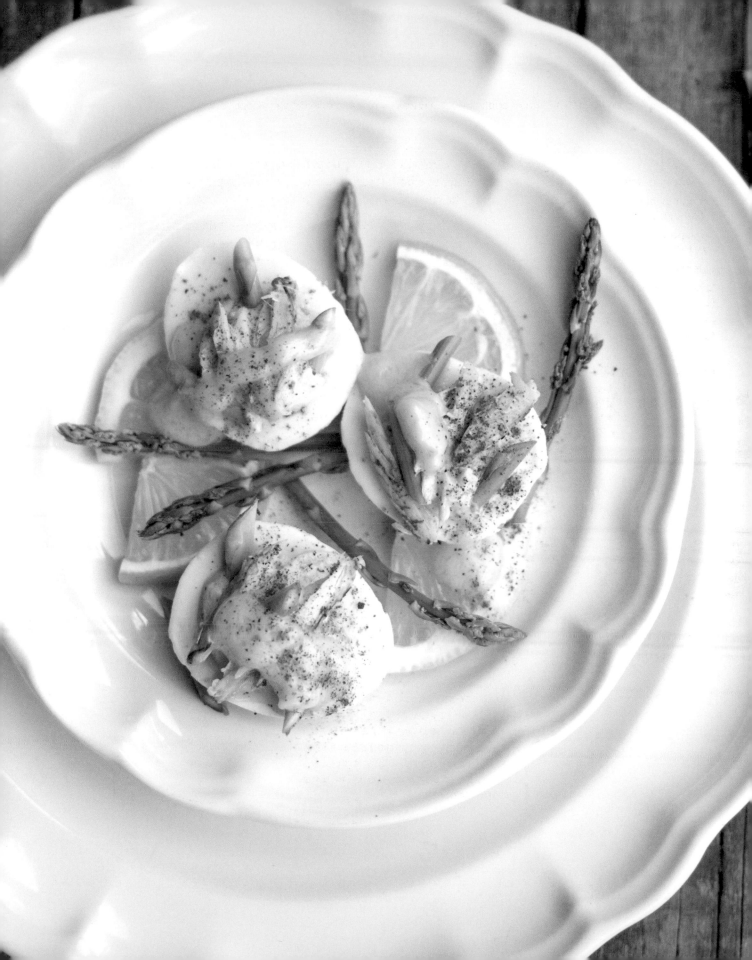

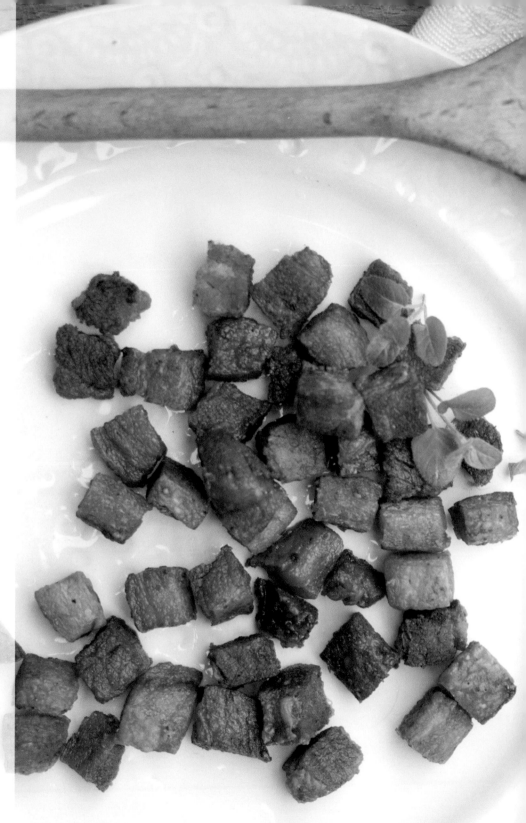

salads, soups,
and sides

# herbaceous salad

L M H KETO · prep time: 10 minutes • yield: 8 servings

### dressing:

¼ cup coconut vinegar or white wine vinegar

2 teaspoons Swerve confectioners'-style sweetener or equivalent amount of liquid or powdered sweetener (see page 81)

2 teaspoons Dijon mustard

½ teaspoon fine sea salt

½ teaspoon fresh ground black pepper

½ cup MCT oil or extra-virgin olive oil

### salad:

3 cups fresh basil leaves (preferably purple basil)

3 cups fresh flat-leaf parsley leaves

2 cups arugula leaves

½ cup fresh tarragon leaves

½ cup chopped fresh chives

1. To make the dressing: Place the vinegar, sweetener, mustard, salt, and pepper in a small food processor or blender and pulse until blended. With the machine running, slowly add the oil until the mixture is well combined and velvety. Set aside.

2. In a large bowl, combine the basil, parsley, arugula, tarragon, and chives. Add the dressing and toss to coat. Best served fresh.

NUTRITIONAL INFO (per serving)

| calories | fat | protein | carbs | fiber |
|---|---|---|---|---|
| 147 | 14g | 2g | 3g | 1g |
| | 86% | 6% | 8% | |

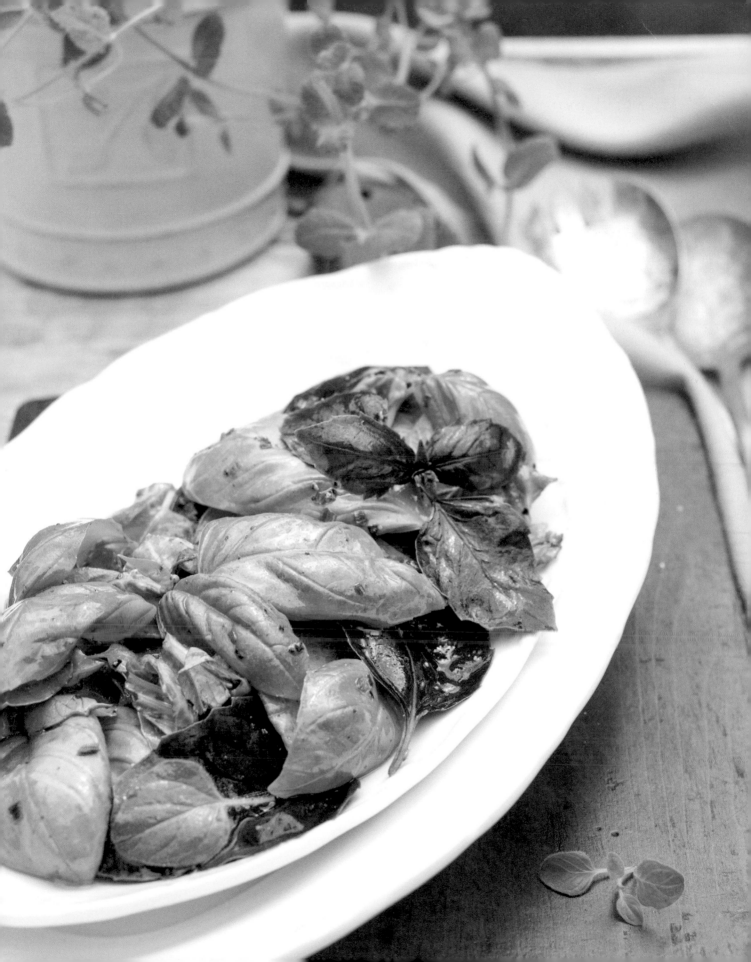

# asian chicken salad

L M H KETO / option / prep time: 5 minutes (not including time to cook the chicken) • yield: 2 servings

When I was first dating my now-husband, we enjoyed going to the Medford Café. They served a humongous Asian chicken salad that I loved. It was surrounded by mandarin oranges and crunchy rice noodles and smothered in a sweet Asian dressing. Here is my ketogenic version!

## dressing:

⅓ cup coconut vinegar or unseasoned rice vinegar

¼ cup coconut aminos or wheat-free tamari

3 tablespoons Swerve confectioners'-style sweetener or equivalent amount of liquid or powdered sweetener (see page 81)

3 tablespoons MCT oil

1 tablespoon grated fresh ginger

1 teaspoon untoasted, cold-pressed sesame oil

2 to 4 drops of orange oil or 1 teaspoon orange extract

## salad:

1 cup chopped romaine lettuce

½ cup chopped napa cabbage

½ cup coarsely chopped cooked chicken (see note, page 268)

## for garnish:

1 tablespoon thinly sliced green onions

1 tablespoon finely chopped purple cabbage

¼ cup finely diced cucumbers

2 tablespoons slivered almonds (omit for nut-free)

1. To make the dressing: Place all the dressing ingredients in a jar with a lid. Cover and shake well to combine. Add more salt, sweetener, or orange oil if desired.

2. Place the lettuce and cabbage on a serving platter and top with the chicken. Garnish the salad with green onions, purple cabbage, cucumbers, and slivered almonds, if using. Serve with the dressing.

busy family tip: *The dressing can be made up to 5 days ahead and stored in an airtight container in the fridge.*

NUTRITIONAL INFO (per serving)

| calories | fat | protein | carbs | fiber |
|----------|-----|---------|-------|-------|
| 402 | 35g | 12g | 10g | 7g |
| | 78% | 12% | 10% | |

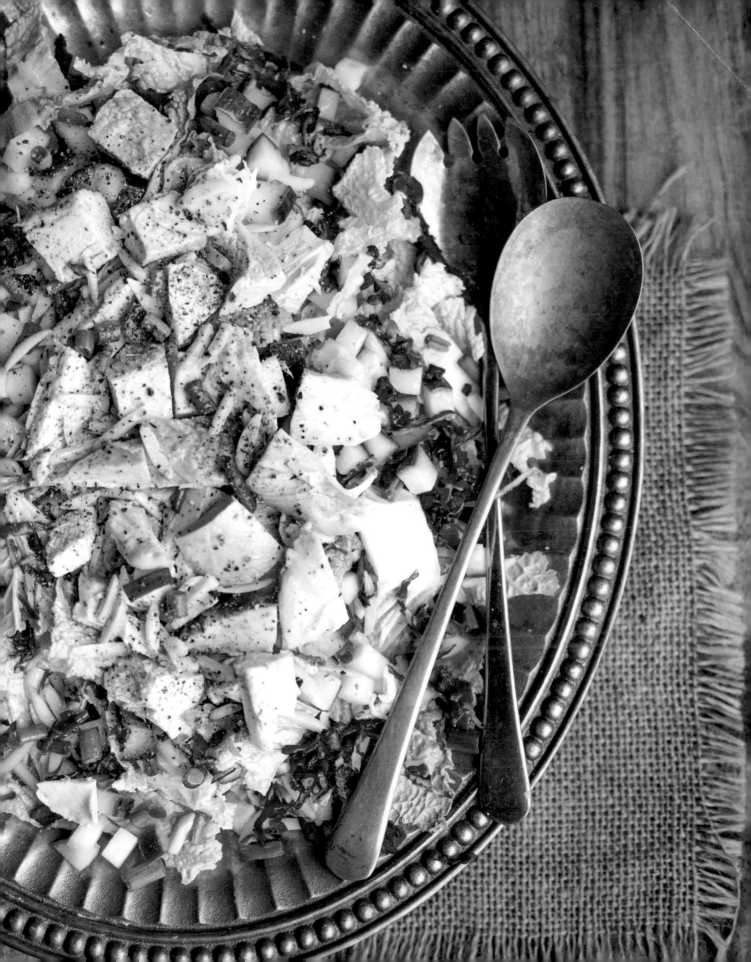

# keto "fruit" salad

L→M→H KETO · prep time: 7 minutes • yield: 4 servings

I often get asked if I ever eat fruit, and I giggle and say, "Of course! I eat cucumbers, olives, avocados, eggplant . . . those are all fruits!"

2 cucumbers

**dressing:**

¼ cup MCT oil or extra-virgin olive oil

1 teaspoon grated lime zest

3 tablespoons lime juice

1 tablespoon chopped fresh mint

½ teaspoon chopped fresh chives

½ teaspoon fine sea salt

½ teaspoon fresh ground black pepper

1. Using a julienne peeler or vegetable peeler, thinly slice the cucumbers lengthwise into wafer-thin ribbons and place them in a large bowl.

2. Place the ingredients for the dressing in a jar with a lid. Cover and shake well to combine. Pour the dressing into the bowl with the "fruit" and toss well to combine.

note: *If not eating right away, store the cucumber ribbons and dressing separately in airtight containers in the fridge for up to 3 days; dress the "fruit" right before serving.*

busy family tip: *The dressing can be made up to 1 week ahead and stored in an airtight container in the fridge.*

NUTRITIONAL INFO (per serving)

| calories | fat | protein | carbs | fiber |
|----------|-----|---------|-------|-------|
| 146 | 14g | 1g | 4g | 1g |
| | 86% | 3% | 11% | |

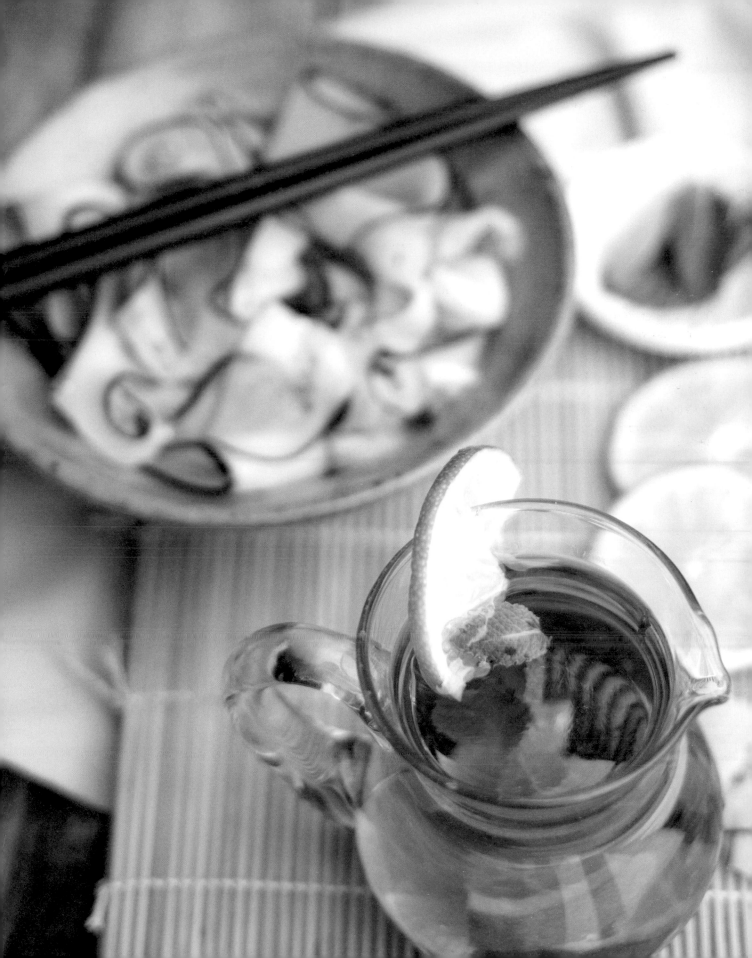

# warm spring salad
# with basil chimichurri and soft-boiled eggs

prep time: 10 minutes • cook time: 10 minutes • yield: 4 servings

I adore anything that includes a soft-boiled egg. This salad will surely impress any guest at your table. It looks lovely and tastes incredible!

¼ cup Paleo fat, such as lard, tallow, or coconut oil

1 pound portobello mushrooms, quartered

½ pound fresh asparagus, tough bottom ends trimmed, cut into 2-inch pieces

1 teaspoon fine sea salt

¼ teaspoon fresh ground black pepper

4 large eggs (omit for egg-free)

### basil chimichurri:

½ cup fresh basil leaves, plus more for garnish (optional)

¼ cup MCT oil or extra-virgin olive oil

2 tablespoons chopped fresh chives

2 tablespoons coconut vinegar or apple cider vinegar

½ teaspoon fine sea salt

¼ teaspoon fresh ground black pepper

1. Heat the Paleo fat in a large sauté pan. Add the mushrooms and asparagus pieces and sauté for 10 minutes, or until the mushrooms are golden brown and cooked through. Season with the 1 teaspoon of salt and ¼ teaspoon of pepper.

2. Meanwhile, make the soft-boiled eggs: Fill a medium saucepan halfway with water and bring to a simmer, not quite a boil. Gently place the eggs in the simmering water and cook for 6 minutes, holding the water at a simmer, not a boil. Remove the eggs from the water and run under cool water. Once cool, carefully peel the eggs and set them aside.

3. Make the chimichurri: Place the ingredients in a food processor and puree until smooth.

4. Place the mushroom and asparagus mixture on a serving platter. Slice the eggs in half and arrange them yolk side up on top of the mushroom mixture. Drizzle the chimichurri over the salad. Garnish with fresh basil leaves, if desired.

5. Store extras in an airtight container in the fridge for up to 4 days. This salad is best served fresh but will keep, undressed, in the fridge for a day. Drizzle leftover salad with chimichurri just before serving.

NUTRITIONAL INFO (per serving)

| calories | fat | protein | carbs | fiber |
|---|---|---|---|---|
| 380 | 34g | 12g | 7g | 3g |
| | 80% | 13% | 7% | |

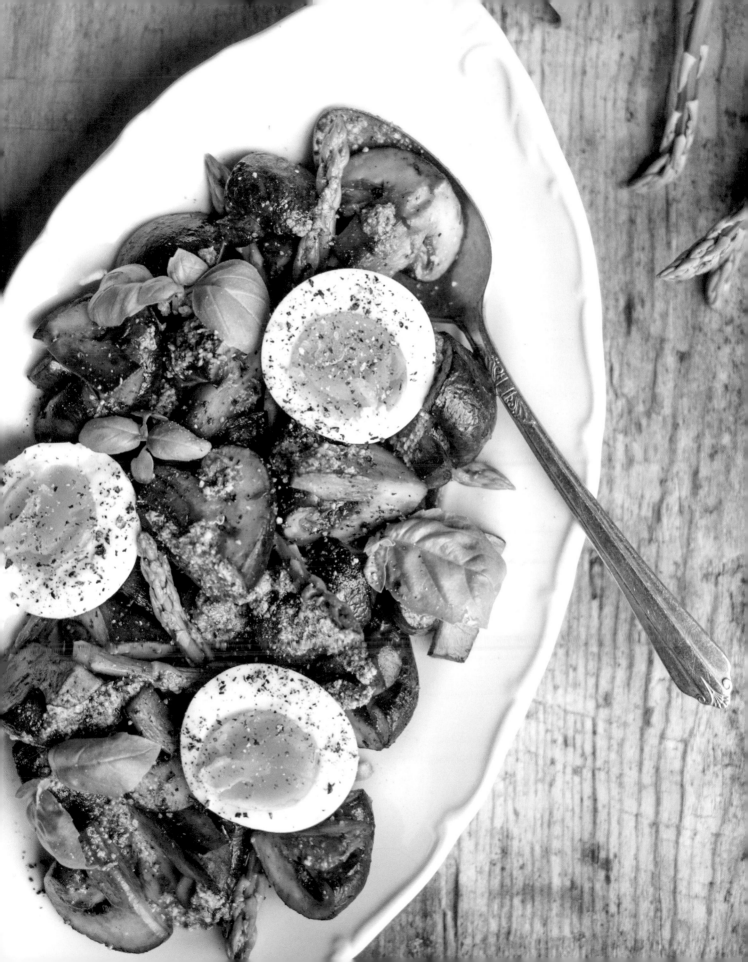

# 7-layer salad

prep time: 12 minutes, plus overnight to chill (not including time to hard-boil the eggs)
yield: 12 servings

6 cups chopped romaine lettuce, divided

½ teaspoon fine sea salt, divided

½ teaspoon fresh ground black pepper, divided

6 hard-boiled eggs (see page 174), sliced or coarsely chopped, divided (omit for egg-free)

2 cups chopped purple cabbage, divided

2 cups sliced black olives, divided

1 pound ham, diced, or bacon, diced and cooked, divided

¼ cup chopped red onions, divided

**dressing:**

1 cup Copycat Baconnaise or mayonnaise, homemade (page 124) or store-bought (or Egg-Free Keto Mayo, page 125, for egg-free)

¼ cup chicken or beef bone broth, homemade (page 108) or store-bought

2 tablespoons Swerve confectioners'-style sweetener or equivalent amount of liquid or powdered sweetener (see page 81)

**for garnish:**

¼ cup thinly sliced green onions

Diced avocado

Smoked paprika

1. Place half of the romaine lettuce in a large serving bowl and season it with half of the salt and pepper. Place half of the sliced or chopped hard-boiled eggs over the lettuce and sprinkle with more salt and pepper. Top the eggs with half of the chopped purple cabbage, half of the sliced olives, half of the ham, and half of the chopped red onions. Repeat with the rest of the ingredients, ending with the remaining red onions.

2. To make the dressing: In a small bowl, combine the mayonnaise, broth, and sweetener until very smooth. Pour the dressing evenly over the entire salad. Cover and chill overnight or for up to 24 hours. Just before serving, sprinkle with green onions, diced avocado, and smoked paprika.

NUTRITIONAL INFO (per serving)

| calories | fat | protein | carbs | fiber |
|----------|-----|---------|-------|-------|
| 312 | 27g | 12g | 5g | 1g |
| | 78% | 16% | 6% | |

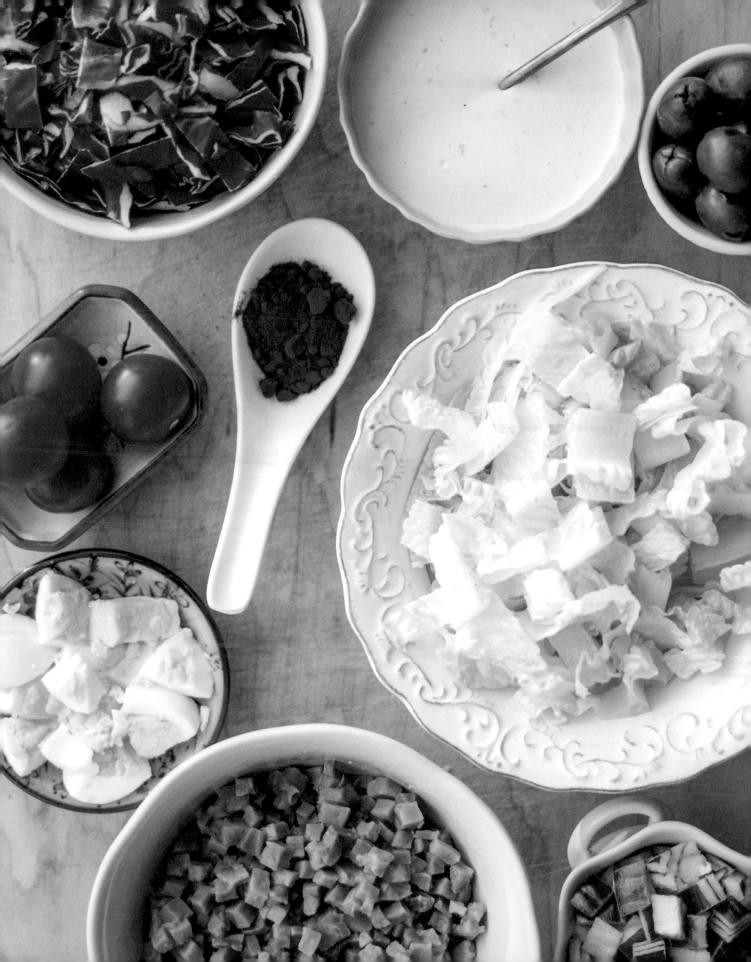

# chopped salad

L M H KETO   prep time: 10 minutes (not including time to make the dressing) • yield: 4 servings

4 cups chopped romaine lettuce

1 avocado, diced

1 cup diced cucumber

1 cup diced ham

1 cup pitted black olives, sliced

½ cup chopped purple cabbage

½ cup Dairy-Free Ranch Dressing (page 115) (or Egg-Free Keto Mayo, page 125, for egg-free)

Divide the romaine lettuce among four salad bowls. Top each bowl with a row each of avocado, cucumber, ham, olives, and cabbage. Drizzle each salad with 2 tablespoons of the ranch dressing.

NUTRITIONAL INFO (per serving)

| calories | fat | protein | carbs | fiber |
|----------|-----|---------|-------|-------|
| 388 | 33g | 15g | 8g | 4g |
| | 77% | 15% | 8% | |

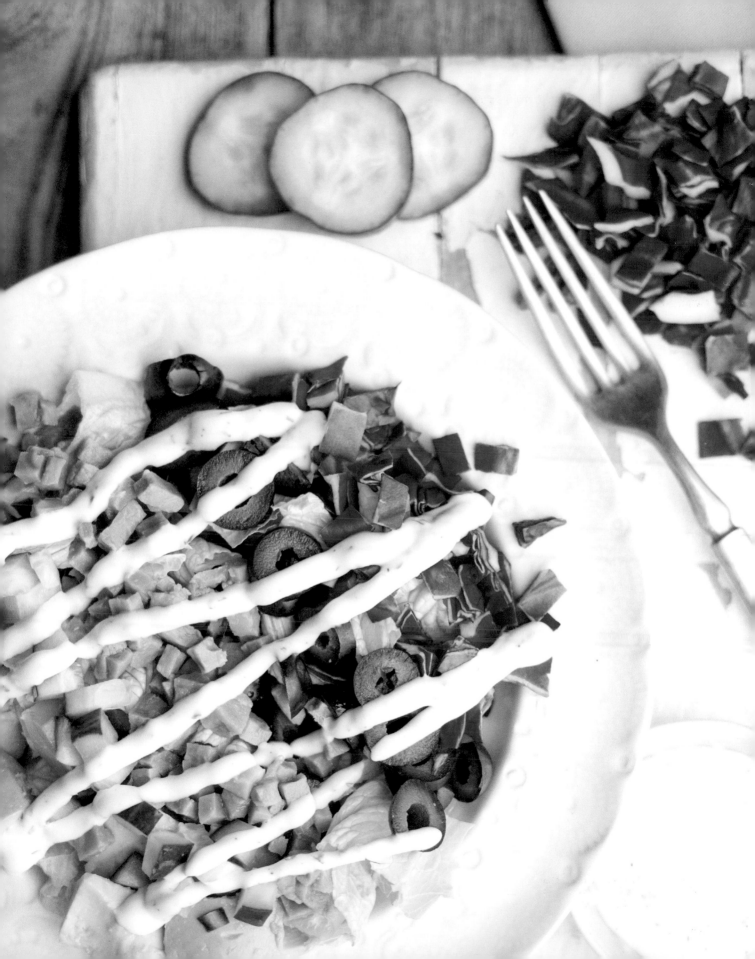

# mixed green salad with BLT deviled eggs and bacon vinaigrette

 KETO ∅ ∅ prep time: 15 minutes • cook time: 15 minutes • yield: 6 servings

12 large eggs

4 slices bacon, cut into ¼-inch dice

2 tablespoons diced onions

3 tablespoons plus 2 teaspoons coconut vinegar or red wine vinegar, divided

1 teaspoon Dijon mustard

3 tablespoons MCT oil or extra-virgin olive oil

½ cup mayonnaise, homemade (page 124) or store-bought

2 teaspoons prepared yellow mustard

½ teaspoon fine sea salt

6 cherry tomatoes, quartered

6 cups mixed greens, plus a few tablespoons finely chopped greens for garnish

Sliced fresh chives, for garnish

1. Place the eggs in a large saucepan and cover with cold water. Bring to a boil, then immediately cover the pan and remove it from the heat. Allow the eggs to cook in the hot water for 11 minutes.

2. Meanwhile, make the bacon vinaigrette: Cook the diced bacon in a skillet over medium heat until crispy, about 5 minutes. Remove the bacon from the pan, leaving the drippings in the skillet. Add the onions, 3 tablespoons of the vinegar, and the Dijon mustard. Cook over medium heat until the onions soften, about 2 minutes. While stirring with a whisk, slowly add the oil to the pan. Whisk well to combine. Set aside.

3. To make the deviled eggs: After the eggs cook for 11 minutes, drain the hot water and rinse the eggs with very cold water for a minute or two to stop the cooking process. Peel the eggs and cut them in half lengthwise. Remove the yolks and place them in a bowl (or food processor). Mash the yolks with a fork (or in a food processor) until they are the texture of very fine crumbles. Add the mayonnaise, remaining 2 teaspoons of vinegar, yellow mustard, and salt. Fill the egg white halves with the yolk mixture. Top each deviled egg with a cherry tomato quarter and sprinkle with the crispy bacon, chopped lettuce, and sliced chives.

4. Dress the rest of the lettuce with the bacon vinaigrette, divide among six plates, and place four deviled eggs on each plate.

5. If not serving immediately, do not dress the lettuce with the vinaigrette until just before serving. Store the vinaigrette in an airtight jar in the fridge for up to 5 days. Keep leftover deviled eggs in an airtight container in the fridge for up to 3 days.

busy family tip: *I keep a dozen hard-boiled eggs in my fridge at all times. My boys, who are four and six, love to help me in the kitchen, and peeling eggs is one of the things they can do without my constant attention so I can prepare other food.*

| NUTRITIONAL INFO | | | | |
|---|---|---|---|---|
| calories | fat | protein | carbs | fiber |
| 418 | 37g | 17g | 4g | 1g |
| | 80% | 16% | 4% | |

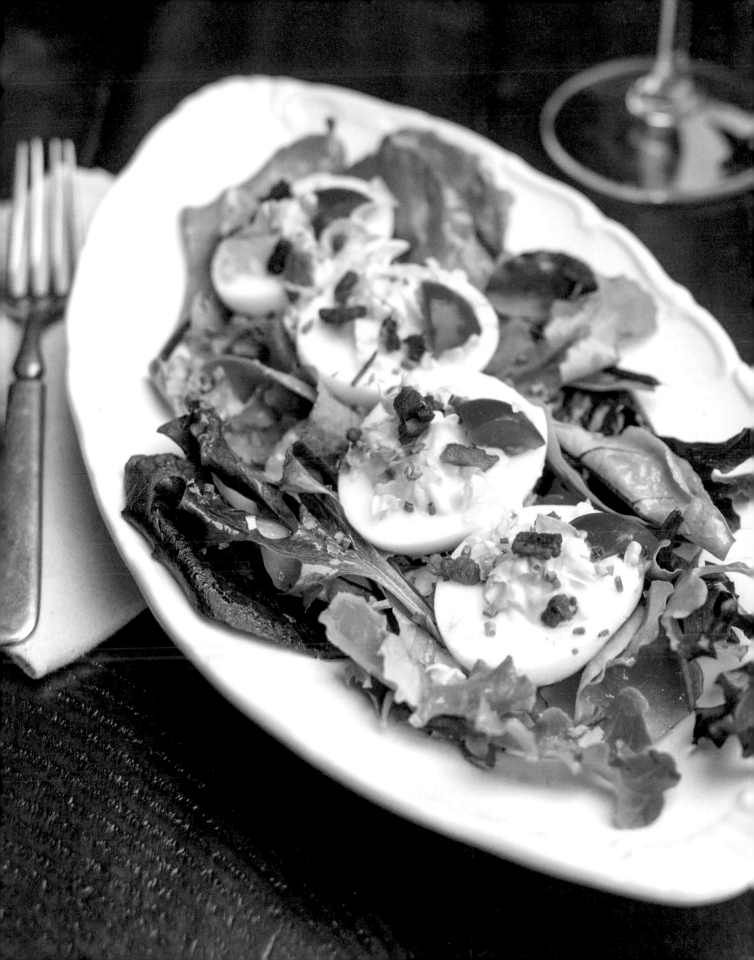

# panzanella salad

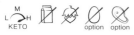

prep time: 10 minutes (not including time to make the croutons)
yield: 5 servings

Once the croutons are made, this lovely and tasty salad comes together very quickly. I've included a few different crouton options in this book, so take your pick. You could also use a different salad dressing than the one here, such as the Fat-Burning Herbes de Florence (page 121). The fish sauce is optional, but it adds a nice hit of umami; the sardines provide a healthy dose of omega-3s and calcium.

**dressing:**

½ cup MCT oil

¼ cup coconut vinegar or apple cider vinegar

1 teaspoon fine sea salt

½ teaspoon fresh ground black pepper

½ teaspoon fish sauce (optional) (omit for vegetarian)

1 (3¾-ounce) tin sardines, chopped fine (optional) (omit for vegetarian)

4 cups mixed greens

1 cup mixed cherry tomatoes and/or baby heirloom tomatoes, halved

1 recipe Crispy Keto Bread Croutons (page 256) or Crispy Pork Belly Croutons (page 260), or ½ recipe Crispy Chicken Skin Croutons (page 258)

1. To make the dressing: Place all the ingredients in a jar with a lid. Cover and shake vigorously.

2. Place the greens and tomatoes on a serving platter. Top with the croutons. Drizzle with the salad dressing and serve.

note: *This salad is best served fresh, but the salad ingredients will keep, undressed, in the fridge for up to 3 days. Store the croutons and vegetables separately in airtight containers; right before serving, assemble the salad and drizzle with the dressing.*

busy family tip: *The dressing can be made up to 2 weeks ahead and stored in an airtight container in the fridge.*

| NUTRITIONAL INFO | | | | |
|---|---|---|---|---|
| calories | fat | protein | carbs | fiber |
| 480 | 43g | 20g | 4g | 1g |
| | 80% | 17% | 3% | |

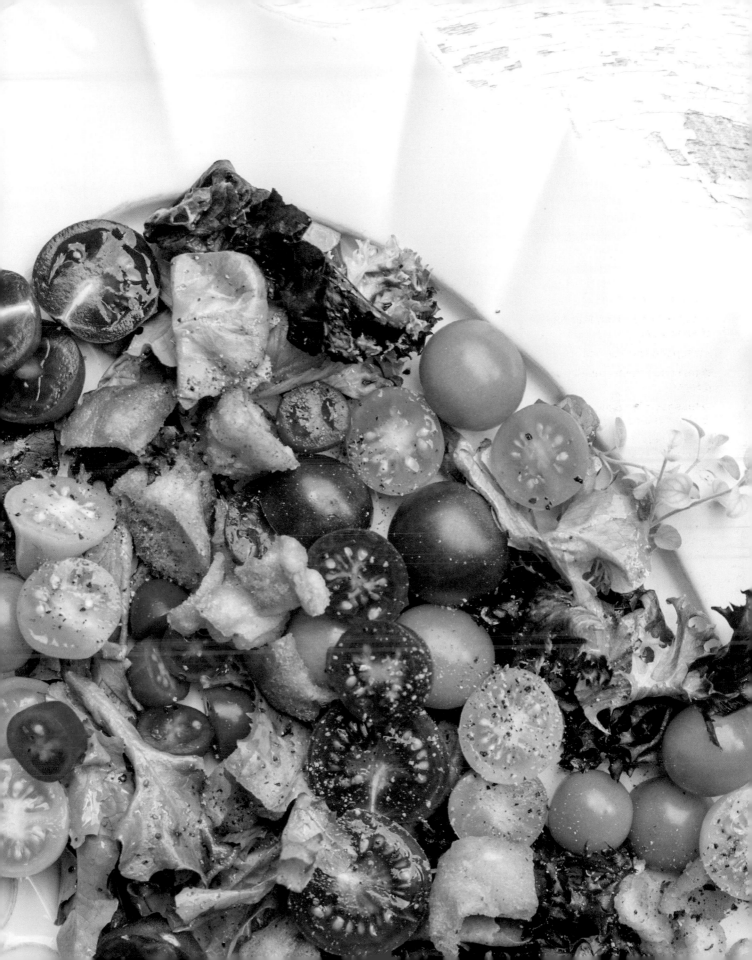

# simple crab salad

L M H KETO option  prep time: 5 minutes • yield: 2 servings

⅓ cup mayonnaise, homemade (page 124) or store-bought (or Egg-Free Keto Mayo, page 125, for egg-free)

1 teaspoon lemon juice

½ teaspoon Dijon mustard

1 teaspoon minced fresh tarragon leaves

½ teaspoon fine sea salt

2 (6-ounce) cans lump crabmeat, drained

½ cup diced celery

¼ cup diced red onions

## for serving:

1 cup coarsely chopped romaine lettuce

Fresh ground black pepper (optional)

1. Place the mayo, lemon juice, mustard, tarragon, and salt in a bowl. Stir well to combine. Add the crabmeat, celery, and onions. Gently fold the ingredients together until well combined.

2. If not using right away, cover the crab salad and store in the fridge for up to 4 days. Do not dress the lettuce with the crab salad until serving.

3. Just before serving, place the crab salad on a bed of romaine lettuce and sprinkle with fresh ground pepper, if desired.

| NUTRITIONAL INFO | | | | |
|---|---|---|---|---|
| calories | fat | protein | carbs | fiber |
| 382 | 27g | 31g | 4g | 1g |
| | 64% | 32% | 4% | |

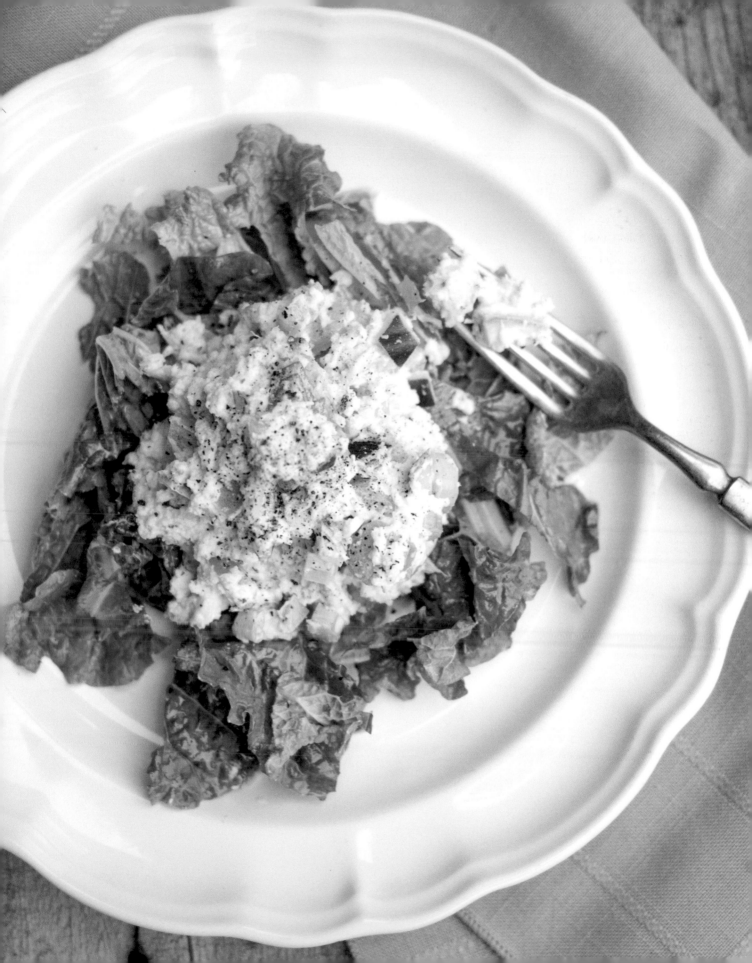

# chopped salad in jars

 L M H KETO  option   prep time: 8 minutes (not including time to cook the eggs and bacon or make the dressing)
yield: 4 servings

Packing salads in jars is a great way to make portable salads for lunches at work, or anywhere else you want to take them. And they're easily customizable: in addition to what's listed here, I sometimes throw in diced bell peppers or zucchini.

½ cup Dairy-Free Ranch Dressing (page 115) (or Egg-Free Keto Mayo, page 125, for egg-free)

1 cup diced tomatoes

1 cup diced cucumber

1 cup coarsely chopped radicchio or romaine lettuce

1 cup diced celery

4 hard-boiled eggs (see page 174), chopped (omit for egg-free)

4 slices bacon, diced and cooked until crispy

Have on hand four pint-sized mason jars. Place 2 tablespoons of ranch dressing in the bottom of each jar. Top with a quarter of the diced tomatoes. Then add the rest of the salad ingredients to the jars in the order listed, dividing the ingredients equally among the jars.

| NUTRITIONAL INFO | | | | |
|---|---|---|---|---|
| calories | fat | protein | carbs | fiber |
| 382 | 31g | 18g | 8g | 3g |
|  | 73% | 19% | 8% | |

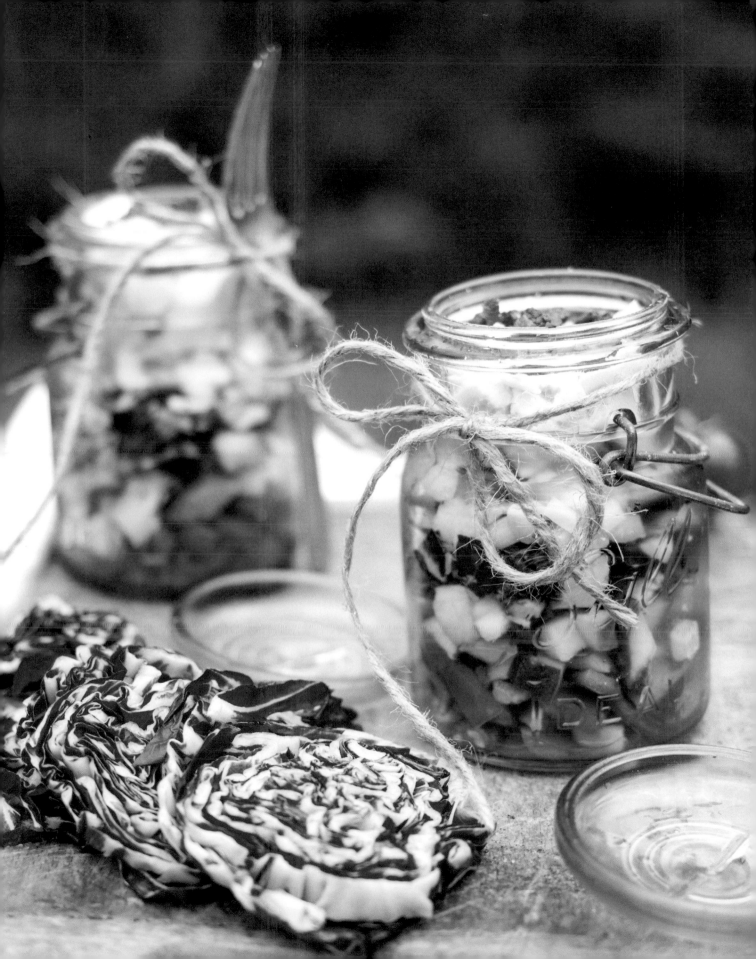

# cleansing ginger soup

L M H KETO 🗹 🚫 ∅   prep time: 8 minutes • cook time: 35 minutes • yield: 4 servings

1 tablespoon coconut oil

¼ cup diced onions

1 (1-inch) piece fresh ginger (about ½ ounce), scrubbed and cut into ½-inch-thick slices (leave peel on)

2 cloves garlic, crushed to a paste

4 bone-in, skin-on chicken thighs

8 cups filtered water

Fine sea salt and fresh ground black pepper

Fresh thyme leaves or other herb such as parsley or cilantro, for garnish

1. Heat the coconut oil in a large pot over medium heat. Add the onions, ginger, and garlic and sauté for 5 minutes, or until the onion is translucent. Add the chicken thighs and water to the pot and boil for 30 minutes, or until the chicken is cooked through and no longer pink inside.

2. Remove the ginger and discard it. Remove the chicken and, once cool enough to handle, remove the chicken skin (discard the skin or reserve it for making Crispy Chicken Skin Croutons, page 258, or cracklings, page 286). Shred the meat with two forks; discard the bones. Return the chicken to the soup and season the soup with salt and pepper to taste.

3. Divide the soup among four bowls and garnish with fresh herbs.

4. Store extras in airtight containers in the fridge for up to 4 days or in the freezer for up to a month.

NUTRITIONAL INFO

| calories | fat | protein | carbs | fiber |
|----------|-----|---------|-------|-------|
| 161 | 10g | 16g | 2g | 0.2g |
| | 56% | 40% | 4% | |

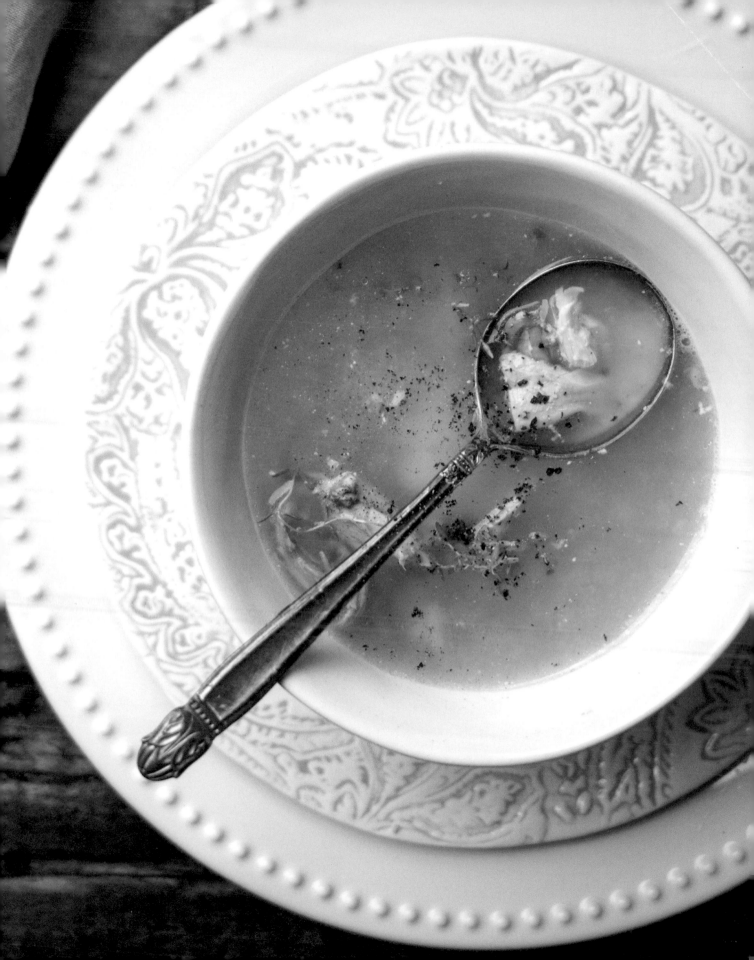

# bone marrow chili con keto

prep time: 12 minutes • cook time: 2 hours • yield: 12 servings

Bone marrow is a wonderful high-fat, moderate-protein food for a keto-adapted lifestyle. It is incredibly nutritious (see page 154) and delicious, yet I realize that not everyone is keen on eating it straight up, like I am. So I've come up with several ingenious ways to hide it in meals, like this chili. You can also try adding it to ground meat for extra moisture or to scrambled eggs for a keto jump on the day (see page 154).

4 slices bacon, diced

1 pound 80% lean ground beef

1 pound Mexican-style fresh (raw) chorizo, removed from casings

1 (26½-ounce) box diced tomatoes with juices

1 cup tomato sauce

¼ cup chopped onions

1 red bell pepper, chopped

2 green chiles, chopped

½ cup beef bone broth, home-made (page 108) or store-bought

2 tablespoons chili powder

2 teaspoons minced garlic

2 teaspoons dried oregano leaves

1 teaspoon ground cumin

½ teaspoon cayenne pepper

½ teaspoon paprika

½ teaspoon fine sea salt

½ teaspoon fresh ground black pepper

2 bay leaves

**bone marrow:**

8 (2-inch) cross-cut beef or veal marrow bones, split lengthwise

1 teaspoon fine sea salt

½ teaspoon fresh ground black pepper

**for garnish:**

Chopped fresh cilantro

1. In a large stockpot over medium-high heat, fry the bacon until crisp, then remove it from the pan and set aside, leaving the fat in the pot. Crumble the ground beef and chorizo into the hot fat and cook over medium-high heat until evenly browned, about 5 minutes.

2. Pour in the diced tomatoes and tomato sauce. Add the onions, bell pepper, chiles, beef broth, and half of the cooked bacon. Season with the chili powder, garlic, oregano, cumin, cayenne, paprika, salt, and pepper. Add the bay leaves and stir to combine. Cover and simmer over low heat for at least 2 hours, stirring occasionally.

3. After 2 hours, taste the chili and add more salt, pepper, or chili pow-der, if desired. The longer the chili simmers, the better it will taste. Remove the bay leaves before serving.

4. While the chili is simmering, make the bone marrow. Preheat the oven to 450°F. Rinse and drain the bones and pat dry, then season them with the salt and pepper.

5. Place the bones cut side up in a roasting pan. Roast for 15 to 25 min-utes, until the marrow in the center has puffed slightly and is warm. (The exact timing will depend on the diameter of the bones; if they are 2 inches in diameter, it will take closer to 15 minutes.)

6. To test for doneness, insert a metal skewer into the center of the bone. There should be no resistance when it is inserted, and some of the marrow will have started to leak from the bones. Using a small spoon, scoop the marrow out of the bones into each bowl of chili. Garnish with chopped cilantro before serving.

| NUTRITIONAL INFO | | | | |
|---|---|---|---|---|
| calories | fat | protein | carbs | fiber |
| 366 | 32g | 13g | 6g | 2g |
| | 79% | 14% | 7% | |

note:

*This recipe is featured in week 4 of the 30-day meal plan. It makes four more servings than you will need if you're feeding two people, but it's one of those dishes that is so worthwhile to make in a large batch. I recommend that you make the full recipe and freeze the leftovers in individual portions for easy meals after you've completed the meal plan.*

# chilled creamy cucumber soup

L M H KETO  option  ⌗⌀⌀  prep time: 8 minutes • yield: 6 servings

In the past, I always bought frozen avocados at Trader Joe's to store in my freezer. I was in a panic one day because I could no longer find them, and when I asked a stockperson, he said, "Why don't you just buy fresh ones and freeze those yourself?" I felt pretty silly, but I've done that ever since! It's a great way to keep avocados on hand for easy soup recipes like this. (See the tip on freezing avocados on page 176.) If you're a visual learner, check out the video that I made for this recipe on my website, MariaMindBodyHealth.com/videos/. Notice that the avocado I used in the video came right out of my freezer, and as you can see, it was perfect, creamy and green!

1 large cucumber, peeled, seeded, and coarsely chopped

1 avocado, peeled, halved, and pitted

2 tablespoons lime juice or lemon juice

¼ cup fresh cilantro leaves

2 tablespoons chopped leeks or green onions

1 cup sour cream or Dairy-Free Yogurt (page 178)

1 cup chicken bone broth, homemade (page 108) or store-bought (or vegetable broth for vegetarian)

1 teaspoon fine sea salt

### for garnish:

Extra-virgin olive oil, for drizzling

Diced cucumber

Fresh ground black pepper

Place all the ingredients in a blender and puree until smooth. Divide the soup among six bowls. Garnish each bowl with a drizzle of extra-virgin olive oil, diced cucumber, and a sprinkle of fresh ground pepper. Store leftover soup in an airtight container in the fridge for up to 3 days.

| NUTRITIONAL INFO | | | | |
|---|---|---|---|---|
| calories | fat | protein | carbs | fiber |
| 157 | 14g | 3g | 5g | 2g |
| | 80% | 8% | 12% | |

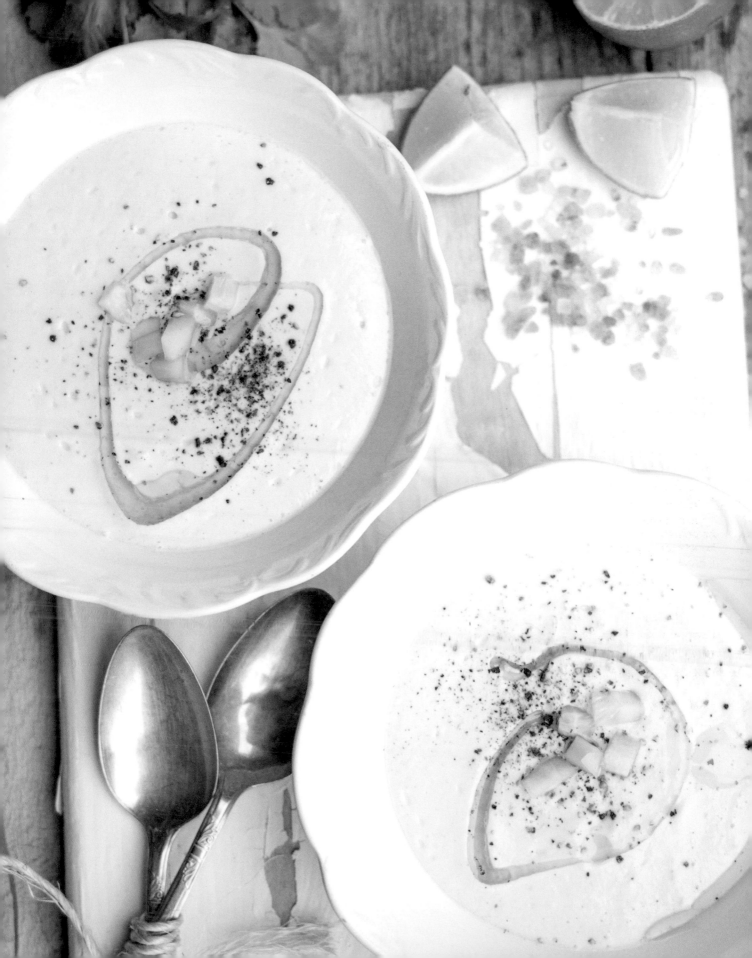

# creamy mushroom soup

L M H · KETO · prep time: 10 minutes • cook time: 30 minutes • yield: 4 servings

Using egg yolks to thicken soups is a great way to create a creamy soup without the cream! The only trick is to temper the egg yolks properly. It's easy—all you have to remember is to go slow.

2 slices bacon, cut into ¼-inch dice

2 tablespoons minced shallots or onions

1 teaspoon minced garlic or cloves from 1 head Garlic Confit (page 142)

1 pound button mushrooms, cleaned and quartered or sliced

1 teaspoon dried thyme leaves

2 cups chicken bone broth, homemade (page 108) or store-bought (see note)

1 teaspoon fine sea salt

½ teaspoon fresh ground black pepper

2 large eggs

2 tablespoons lemon juice

### for garnish:

Fresh thyme leaves

MCT oil or extra-virgin olive oil, for drizzling

1. Place the diced bacon in a stockpot and sauté over medium heat until crispy, about 3 minutes. Remove the bacon from the pan, but leave the drippings. Add the shallots and garlic to the pan with the drippings and sauté over medium heat for about 3 minutes, until softened and aromatic.

2. Add the mushrooms and dried thyme and sauté over medium heat until the mushrooms are golden brown, about 10 minutes. Add the broth, salt, and pepper and bring to boil.

3. Whisk the eggs and lemon juice in a medium bowl. While whisking, very slowly pour in ½ cup of the hot soup (if you add the hot soup too quickly, the eggs will curdle). Slowly whisk another cup of the hot soup into the egg mixture.

4. Pour the hot egg mixture into the pot while stirring. Add the cooked bacon, then reduce the heat and simmer for 10 minutes, stirring constantly. The soup will thicken slightly as it cooks. Remove from the heat. Garnish with fresh thyme and drizzle with MCT oil before serving.

5. This soup is best served fresh but can be stored in an airtight container in the fridge for up to 3 days. To reheat, place in a saucepan over medium-low heat until warmed, stirring constantly to keep the eggs from curdling.

note: *Using homemade broth will create a thicker soup, but boxed broth will work.*

| NUTRITIONAL INFO | | | | |
|---|---|---|---|---|
| calories | fat | protein | carbs | fiber |
| 185 | 13g | 11g | 6g | 2g |
| | 63% | 24% | 13% | |

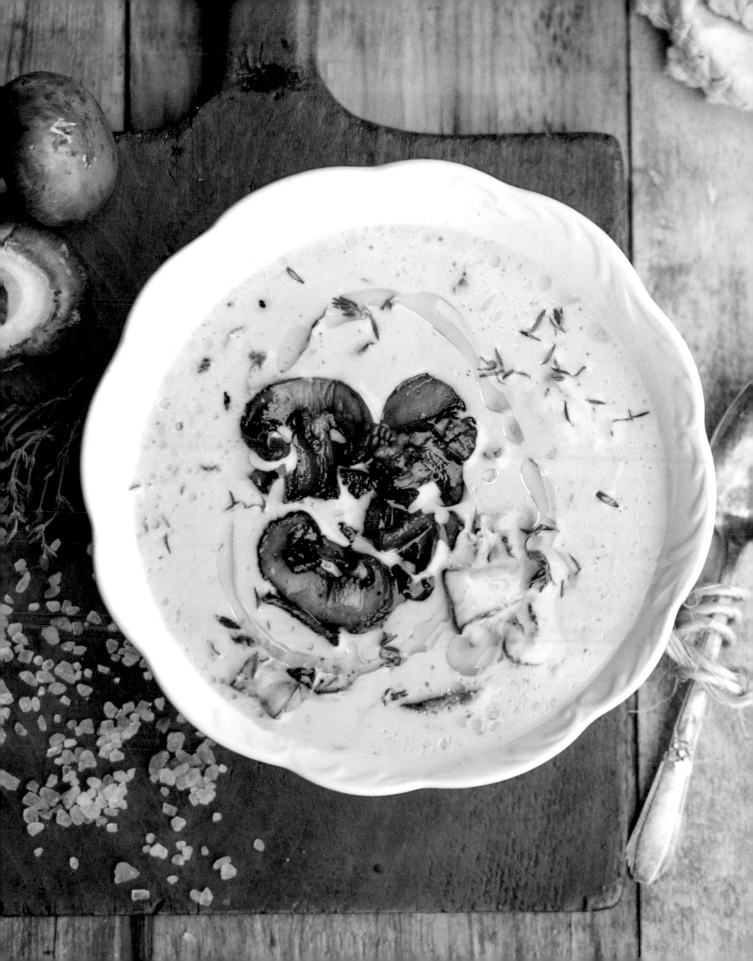

# hot-and-sour soup with pork meatballs

L M H KETO · prep time: 10 minutes · cook time: 15 minutes · yield: 4 servings

Traditionally, hot-and-sour soup is thickened with cornstarch. Instead, I use an egg yolk whisked into a cup of the cooled broth. Then I slowly whisk the mixture into the hot soup—the process is somewhat like thickening hollandaise, only in reverse.

## meatballs:

½ pound ground pork

1 tablespoon coconut aminos or wheat-free tamari

¼ teaspoon minced garlic

¼ teaspoon grated fresh ginger

¼ teaspoon fine sea salt

Pinch of fresh ground black pepper

## soup:

2 tablespoons coconut oil

1 pound shiitake or button mushrooms, sliced

1 tablespoon red chili paste

1 teaspoon grated fresh ginger

¼ cup coconut aminos or wheat-free tamari

¼ cup unseasoned rice vinegar

½ teaspoon fine sea salt

½ teaspoon fresh ground black pepper

5 cups chilled or room-temperature chicken bone broth, homemade (page 108) or store-bought, divided

1 large egg yolk

1 large whole egg

½ cup sliced green onions, for garnish

¼ cup fresh cilantro leaves, for garnish

1. To make the meatballs: Mix all the ingredients for the meatballs until well combined. Form into ¾-inch balls.

2. To make the soup: Heat the oil in a large soup pot over medium heat. Place the meatballs in the oil and sauté on all sides until they are cooked through, 5 to 7 minutes. Remove the meatballs from the pot and set aside. Add the mushrooms and sauté on both sides until golden brown, about 4 minutes. Add the chili paste and ginger and sauté for another minute. Season with the coconut aminos, rice vinegar, salt, and pepper.

3. Place 1 cup of the chicken broth in a small bowl. Whisk in the egg yolk (to act as a thickener). Add the remaining 4 cups of broth to the pot and bring to a simmer over medium heat. Slowly whisk in the 1 cup chicken broth with the yolk.

4. Beat the whole egg in a small bowl. Gently stir the egg into the hot soup to create strings of cooked egg. Return the meatballs to the soup and simmer gently for a couple minutes to heat through. Garnish each bowl of soup with green onions and cilantro leaves.

NUTRITIONAL INFO (per serving)

| calories | fat | protein | carbs | fiber |
|---|---|---|---|---|
| 388 | 30g | 21g | 9g | 4g |
| | 70% | 21% | 9% | |

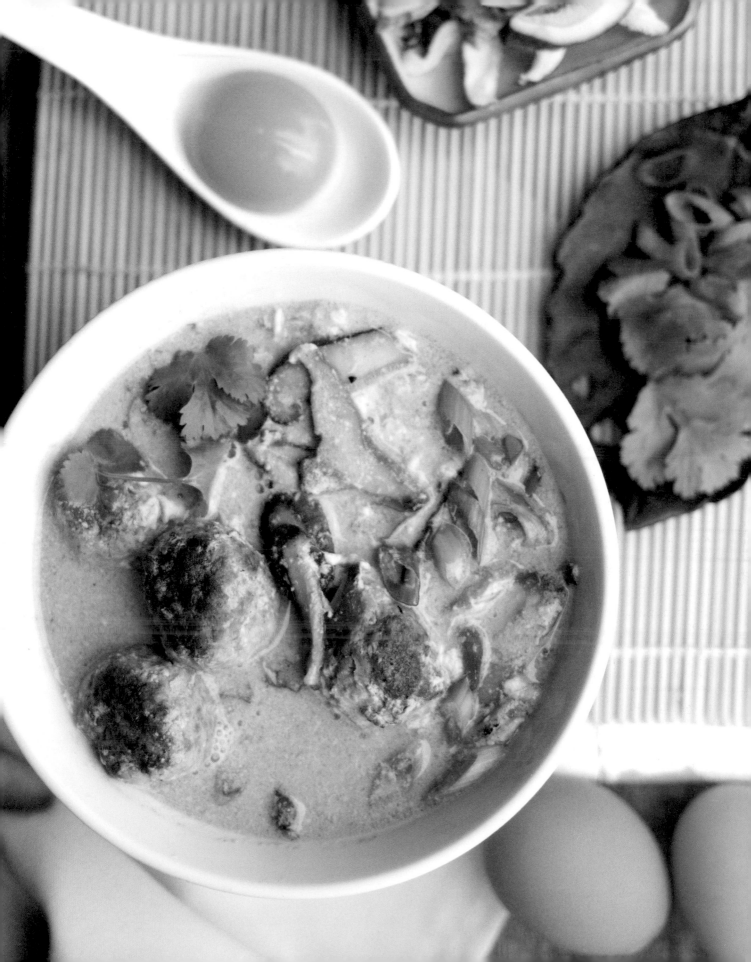

# bok choy and mushrooms with ginger dressing

LᴹTH KETO · prep time: 5 minutes • cook time: 10 minutes • yield: 4 servings

## ginger dressing:

¼ cup coconut aminos or wheat-free tamari

2 tablespoons beef bone broth, homemade (page 108) or store-bought (or vegetable broth for vegetarian)

2 tablespoons MCT oil or untoasted, cold-pressed sesame oil

1 tablespoon coconut vinegar or unseasoned rice vinegar

1 tablespoon lime juice

½ tablespoon grated fresh ginger

1 green onion, thinly sliced

2 tablespoons toasted sesame oil

1 pound mushrooms, sliced thin

4 heads baby bok choy (about 1 pound), sliced

Black sea salt or fine sea salt and fresh ground black pepper

1. Place the ingredients for the dressing in a jar with a lid. Cover and shake well to combine. Set aside.

2. Preheat a cast-iron skillet over medium heat, then add the toasted sesame oil. When the oil is hot, add the mushrooms and sauté until golden brown on both sides, about 4 minutes. Add the bok choy and sauté for about 5 minutes, until wilted. Season with salt and pepper to taste.

3. Place the bok choy and mushrooms on a platter and drizzle with the ginger dressing. Store extras in an airtight container in the fridge for up to 4 days.

busy family tip: *The dressing can be made up to 5 days ahead and stored in an airtight container in the fridge.*

| NUTRITIONAL INFO | | | | |
|---|---|---|---|---|
| calories | fat | protein | carbs | fiber |
| 173 | 15g | 4g | 8g | 4g |
| | 74% | 12% | 14% | |

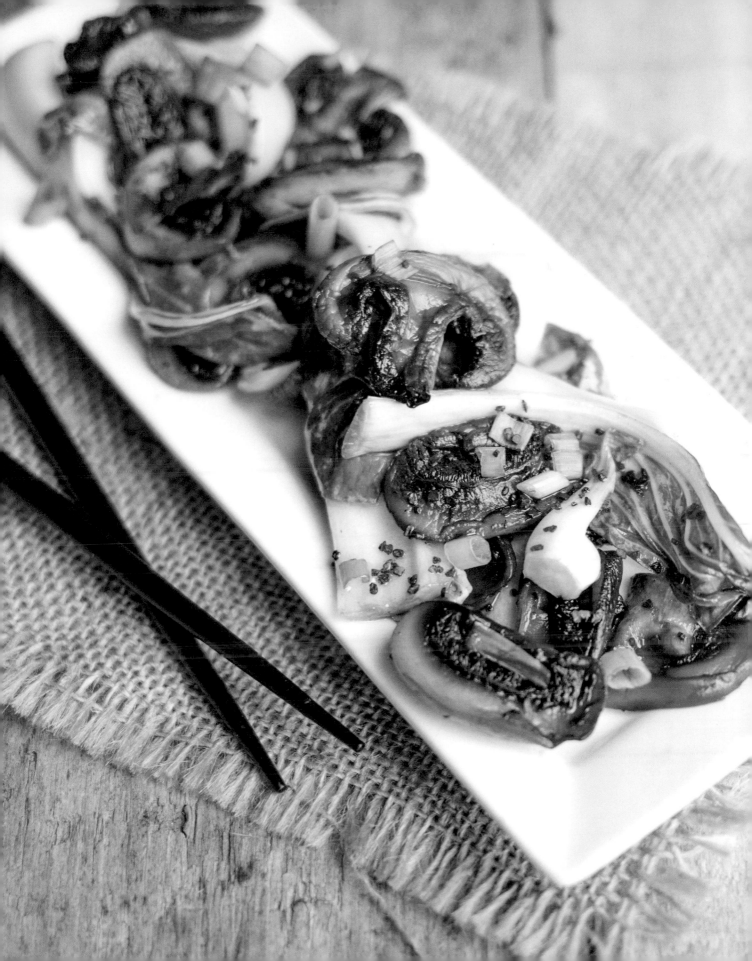

# green curry panna cotta

L M H
KETO · option · prep time: 10 minutes, plus 2 hours to chill · cook time: 5 minutes · yield: 6 servings

Collagen is a great prebiotic—food for those beneficial bacteria in the gut. So adding grass-fed gelatin, with its high amount of collagen, to foods like this panna cotta gives your digestive system a healthy dose of prebiotics without any carbs. (I like Great Lakes brand gelatin.)

2 teaspoons grass-fed powdered gelatin

¼ cup lime juice

1 cup unsweetened, unflavored cashew milk, homemade (page 106) or store-bought, or almond milk (or hemp milk for nut-free)

1 cup full-fat coconut milk

2 teaspoons green curry paste

1 stalk lemongrass, tough outer leaves removed and bottom half sliced (optional)

¼ teaspoon fish sauce (optional)

½ teaspoon fine sea salt (use ¾ teaspoon if omitting fish sauce)

### for garnish (optional):

Fresh cilantro leaves

Sliced green onions

1. In a small bowl, sprinkle the gelatin over the lime juice; allow to sit for 3 minutes to soften.

2. Meanwhile, combine the cashew milk, coconut milk, curry paste, lemongrass (if using), fish sauce (if using), and salt in a pot and heat gently over medium heat, stirring often. Remove the lemongrass.

3. Add the softened gelatin to the hot milk mixture and stir well to dissolve.

4. Pour the mixture into six 4-ounce ramekins and place them in the fridge to set for at least 2 hours or up to 4 hours. Garnish with cilantro and green onions, if desired, before serving.

note: *Cooks at Thai restaurants usually add sweetener to their curries. If you would like this recipe to taste more like the traditional curries you're used to eating at restaurants, add 2 tablespoons of Swerve confectioners'-style sweetener or the equivalent amount of liquid or powdered sweetener (see page 81). If you have been keto-adapted for a while and your sweet tooth has diminished, you likely will not miss the sweetness.*

gelatin tip: *Using gelatin is an easy way to make tasty treats, but foods made with gelatin can easily get too rubbery if they sit in the fridge overnight. If you plan on making this recipe ahead of time, use ¼ teaspoon less gelatin than called for; this quantity will create a perfect creamy texture even after a day or two of resting in the fridge.*

busy family tip: *Can be made up to 3 days ahead (with caveat—see gelatin tip).*

| NUTRITIONAL INFO | | | | |
|---|---|---|---|---|
| calories | fat | protein | carbs | fiber |
| 79 | 7g | 2g | 2g | 0.5g |
| | 80% | 10% | 10% | |

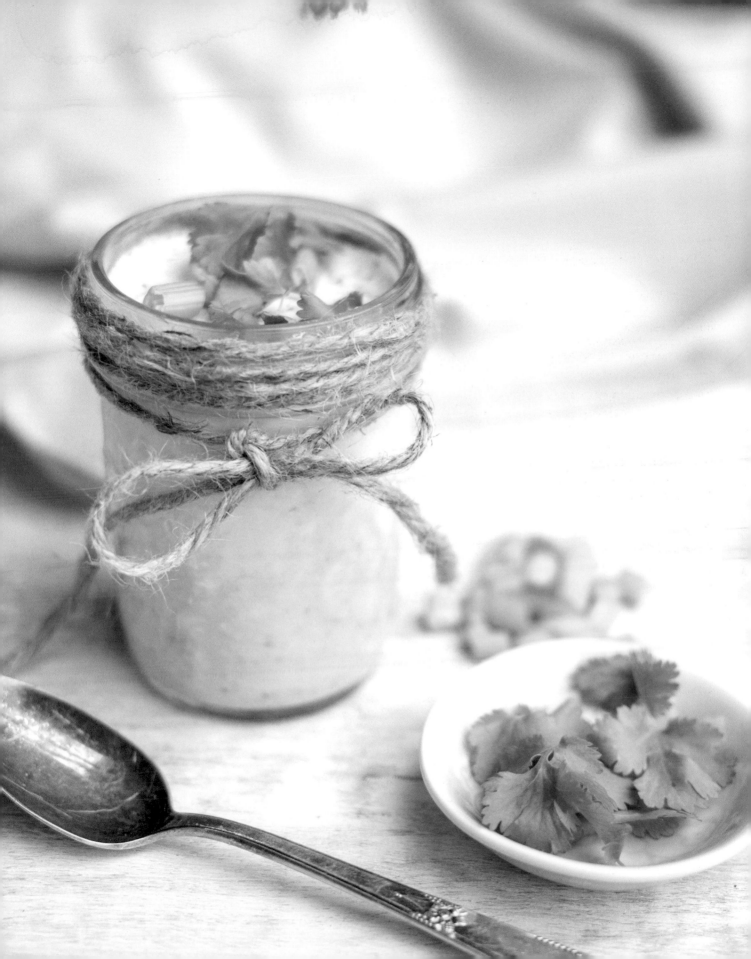

# wraps

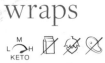

prep time: 4 minutes (not including time to hard-boil the eggs)
cook time: 8 minutes • yield: 2 wraps (1 per serving)

You'll have the most success with these wraps if you make them in a nonstick pan, but please do not use a Teflon pan! See page 84 for my recommendations for nonstick pans.

2 large eggs

2 hard-boiled eggs (see page 174), peeled

2 tablespoons chopped fresh cilantro or other fresh herbs of choice or green onions

½ teaspoon fine sea salt

1½ teaspoons coconut oil

1. Place the raw eggs, peeled hard-boiled eggs, herbs, and salt in a blender and combine until very smooth, without lumps.

2. Heat an 8-inch crepe pan or nonstick pan over medium-low heat, then add the oil. When the oil is hot, pour half of the egg mixture into the pan and tilt the pan to spread the eggs into a very large, thin wrap. Let the eggs set for 3 to 4 minutes, until cooked through. (Do not flip the wrap.) Slide the wrap onto a plate to cool. Repeat with the remaining half of the egg mixture.

3. Once cool, drizzle the wraps with the keto dressing of your choice (drizzling is easier than spreading, which often breaks the wrap) and fill with lettuce and other fillings of your choice. Wrap up like a burrito and enjoy! Store extras in an airtight container in the fridge for up to 3 days.

NUTRITIONAL INFO

| calories | fat | protein | carbs | fiber |
|----------|-----|---------|-------|-------|
| 172 | 13g | 13g | 1g | 0.5g |
| | 68% | 30% | 2% | |

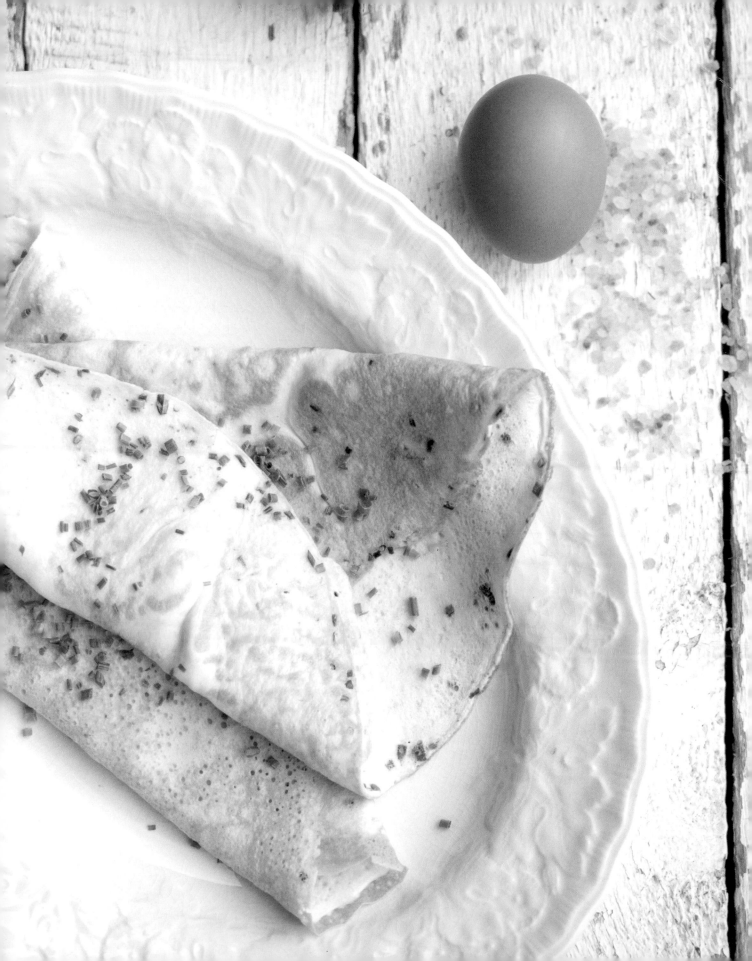

# keto bread

prep time: 10 minutes • cook time: 45 minutes
yield: one 9 by 5-inch loaf (14 slices, 2 per serving)

This recipe produces a light, fluffy bread with a texture that's often compared to that of Wonder Bread. If you whip the whites until very stiff, you won't end up something that's more like an eggy soufflé than bread—it will be light and airy. However, meringues and humidity do not mix. If your kitchen is very humid, you will not end up with airy bread. Please do not use egg whites in a carton, either; if you do, you won't end up with airy bread. It's best to use real eggs and separate the yolks from the whites.

6 large egg whites

¼ cup unflavored egg white protein powder

½ teaspoon onion powder or other seasonings/spices of choice (optional)

3 large egg yolks

1. Preheat the oven to 325°F. Grease a 9 by 5-inch loaf pan.

2. Using a stand mixer with the whisk attachment (or a mixing bowl and electric hand-held beaters), whip the egg whites until very stiff and the peaks hold their shape, about 10 minutes. (To test whether the whites are ready, turn the whisk upside down; if the peaks fold down on themselves, keep whipping.) Using a rubber spatula, slowly fold in the protein powder and any desired seasonings.

3. In a small bowl, beat the egg yolks, then gently fold the yolks into the whites (making sure that the whites don't fall).

4. Fill the prepared pan with the "dough." Bake for 40 to 45 minutes, until golden brown. Let completely cool before cutting or the bread will fall. Cut into 14 slices. Store in an airtight container in the fridge for up to 6 days or in the freezer for up to 1 month.

## variations:

**Garlic Keto Bread.** *Preheat the oven to 400°F. Brush slices of keto bread with MCT oil and rub on roasted garlic or Garlic Confit (page 142). Toast in the oven for 3 to 6 minutes, until golden brown.*

**Keto Buns.** *To make buns instead of a loaf, line two baking sheets with parchment paper and grease the paper.*

*To form hamburger buns, use a spatula to gently scoop up about ⅓ cup of the dough and place it on one of the prepared baking sheets. Using a spatula, form into a round bun, about 3½ inches in diameter. Repeat with the rest of the dough, placing seven buns on each baking sheet.*

*To form hot dog or hoagie buns, use a spatula to gently scoop up about ⅓ cup of the dough and place it on one of the prepared baking sheets. Using a spatula, form into an oblong shape, about 6 inches long and 2 inches wide. Repeat with the rest of the dough, placing seven buns on each baking sheet.*

*Bake the buns for 15 to 20 minutes, until golden brown. Let completely cool on the baking sheets before removing or cutting. Store in an airtight container in the fridge for up to 5 days or in the freezer for up to 2 months. Makes about 14 buns.*

**Crispy Keto Bread Croutons.** *Preheat the oven to 350°F. Cut a loaf of keto bread into cubes. Heat ¼ cup of bacon fat or MCT oil in a large sauté pan over medium heat, then add 1 to 2 teaspoons of minced garlic and the bread cubes and toss to coat. Place the croutons on a rimmed baking sheet and bake for 15 minutes, or until crispy. Let cool before using. Leftovers will keep in an airtight container in the fridge for up to 2 days. Makes 5 cups.*

busy family tip: *I often keep keto bread in my fridge or freezer for easy additions to meals.*

| NUTRITIONAL INFO (per serving) | | | | |
|---|---|---|---|---|
| calories | fat | protein | carbs | fiber |
| 70 | 4.3g | 7.5g | 0.4g | 0g |
| | 55% | 43% | 2% | |

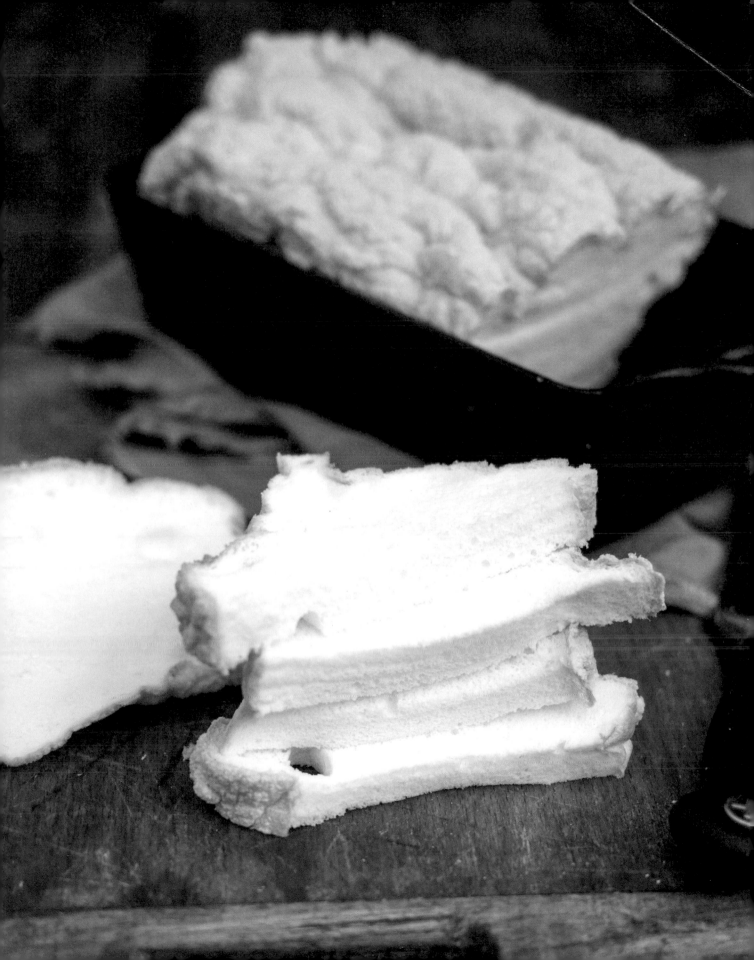

# crispy chicken skin croutons

L M H KETO  prep time: 5 minutes • cook time: 45 minutes • yield: 12 servings

1 pound chicken skin and fat

¼ cup diced onions

Minced garlic (optional)

Chopped fresh basil or other herbs of choice (optional)

Fine sea salt and fresh ground black pepper

1. Rinse the chicken skin and fat, pat dry, then cut it into ¼-inch pieces. Place the pieces in a large greased skillet set over low heat. Cover the skillet and cook for about 15 minutes. Liquid fat will start to accumulate at the bottom of the pan. Uncover and raise the heat to medium-low. Cook for another 15 to 20 minutes, breaking the pieces apart with a spatula and stirring until the skin starts to brown and curl at the edges. Remove the pan from the heat.

2. Pour the rendered fat from the skillet into a container, using a fine-mesh sieve to catch any small pieces of skin. Reserve the fat for later use.

3. After collecting the liquid fat, return the cooked chicken skin and fat to the skillet. Add the onions, garlic (if using), and herbs (if using) to the skillet. Season to taste with salt and pepper.

4. Turn the heat to medium and sauté the mixture for 15 to 20 minutes while stirring, until the pieces are dark brown (not black!) and crispy. Remove from the skillet and drain on a paper towel. Season again with salt and pepper to taste. Store the croutons in an airtight container in the fridge for up to 3 days. Reheat in a preheated 400°F oven or toaster oven for 3 minutes.

NUTRITIONAL INFO

| calories | fat | protein | carbs | fiber |
|----------|-----|---------|-------|-------|
| 169 | 15g | 8g | 0.4g | 0.1g |
| | 80% | 19% | 1% | |

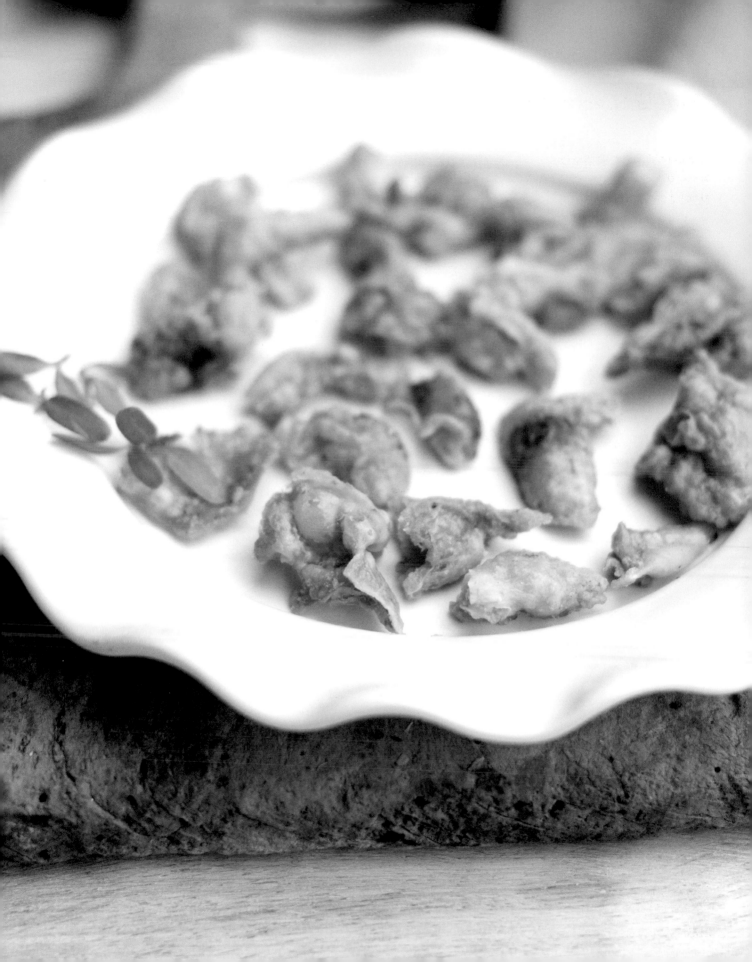

# crispy pork belly croutons

L →M H KETO  prep time: 5 minutes • cook time: 8 minutes • yield: 6 servings

1 (12-ounce) package fully cooked pork belly (see note)

1 tablespoon Paleo fat, such as coconut oil

1. Cut the pork belly into ¼-inch dice. Heat the oil in a cast-iron skillet over medium heat. Place the diced pork belly in the pan. Fry on all sides until crisp, about 8 minutes, stirring often. Remove from the skillet and serve on greens with keto dressing.

2. These croutons are best served fresh but can be stored in an airtight container in the fridge for up to 3 days. To reheat, place in 400°F oven or toaster oven for 3 minutes.

note: *Vacuum-sealed packages of fully cooked pork belly are available at Trader Joe's.*

| NUTRITIONAL INFO | | | | |
|---|---|---|---|---|
| calories | fat | protein | carbs | fiber |
| 236 | 21g | 12g | 0g | 0g |
| | 80% | 20% | 0% | |

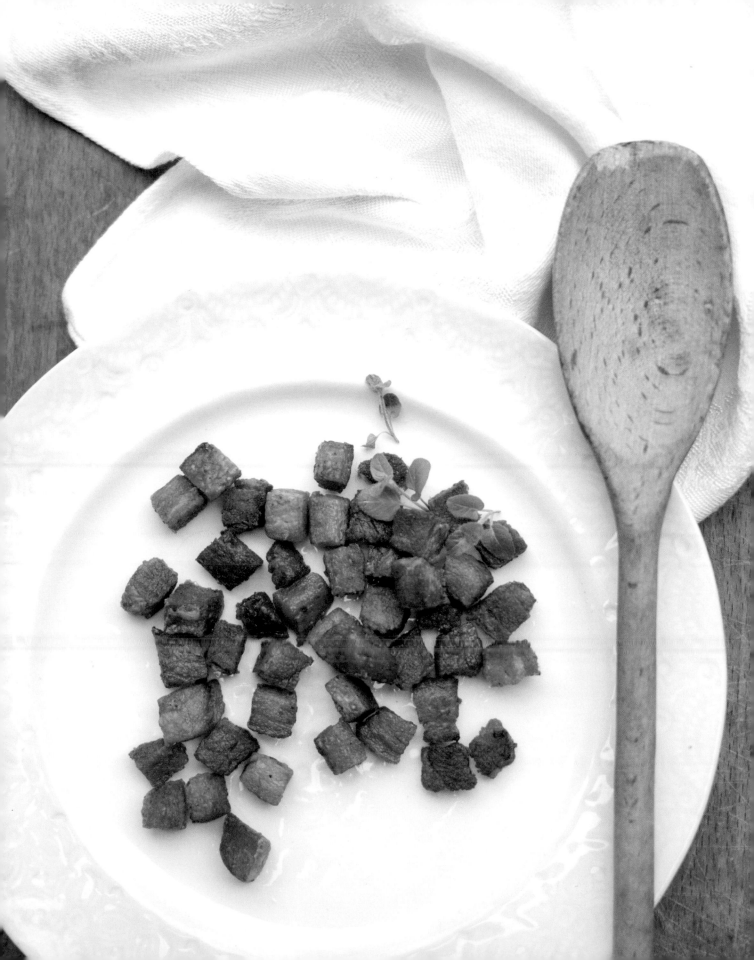

# zoodles

KETO · M L-H · prep time: 5 minutes • cook time: 20 minutes • yield: 4 cups (1 per serving)

"Zoodles" is a fun name for zucchini noodles! They are a wonderful replacement for traditional noodles (see the photo comparison on page 83). Zucchini is a wonderfully versatile and neutral vegetable that takes on other flavors easily, making it a perfect noodle substitute.

Here are my tricks for making the best zoodles:

1. Do not use zucchini that are too large and seedy. Find zucchini that are 10 to 12 inches long and 2 inches wide. Large seeds can ruin your spiral slicer.
2. Remove some of the excess moisture from the zoodles so you don't end up with a soggy bowl of pasta once you sauce them. My favorite way to do this is to dehydrate them in the oven (see method below). Though not quite as effective, you can also use this shortcut method: place the zoodles in a colander over the sink, sprinkle with a teaspoon of salt, and allow to drain for about 5 minutes, then gently press to wring out the excess water.

To increase the ketogenic level of this dish from medium to high, toss the noodles with a keto sauce, such as Creamy Mexican Dressing (page 116), Orange-Infused Dressing (page 119), or Keto Lemon Mostarda (page 138).

2 medium zucchini, not more than 12 inches long

**special equipment:**

Spiral slicer

busy family tip: *To enjoy zoodles throughout the week, prepare a double or triple batch of spiral-sliced zucchini by completing Steps 2 and 3. Store the raw noodles in an airtight container in the fridge for up to 5 days. Bake the amount of noodles you need, per Steps 1 and 4, just before serving.*

1. Preheat the oven to 250°F. Place a paper towel on a rimmed baking sheet.

2. Cut the ends off the zucchini to create nice even edges. If you desire white "noodles," peel the zucchini.

3. Using a spiral slicer, swirl the zucchini into long, thin, noodlelike strips, gently pressing down on the handle while turning it clockwise.

4. Spread out the zucchini noodles on the prepared baking sheet and bake for 20 minutes. Remove from the oven and serve immediately.

5. Zoodles are best consumed as soon as they're baked, so it's best to make the exact amount you need (but to save time, you can spiral-slice the zucchini in advance; see tip). If you have leftover zoodles, store them unsauced in an airtight container in the fridge for up to 5 days. Freezing is not recommended because the zoodles tend to get soggy.

NUTRITIONAL INFO (per serving)

| calories | fat | protein | carbs | fiber |
|---|---|---|---|---|
| 16 | .2g | 1g | 3g | 1g |
| | 11% | 25% | 64% | |

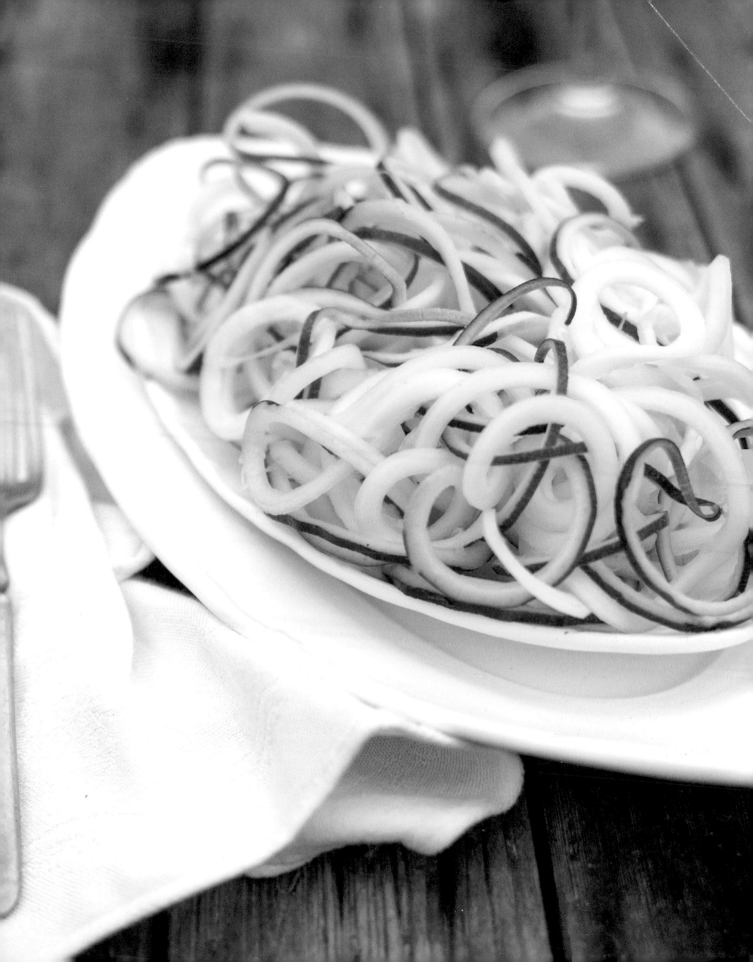

main dishes: chicken

# chiles rellenos

L M H KETO · prep time: 16 minutes · cook time: 30 minutes (not including time to cook the chicken)
yield: 2 servings (1 chile per serving)

This recipe takes a few extra steps—like roasting the peppers to remove the skins and give them a nice charred flavor. I find that coring and removing the seeds from the peppers is easier to do before roasting and keeps the peppers from tearing when you stuff in the chicken. If you aren't a fan of poultry, you could also fill the poblanos with shredded pork or beef.

2 medium poblano chiles (about 1 pound)

Fine sea salt and fresh ground black pepper

**filling:**

1 cup shredded leftover Simple Slow Cooker Chicken Thighs (page 290)

**fried coating:**

2 large eggs, separated, at room temperature

¼ teaspoon fine sea salt, plus more as needed

¼ cup coconut oil, for the pan

**for serving:**

½ cup salsa, pureed

2 tablespoons chopped fresh cilantro

1. Lay a chile on a cutting board so that it sits flat. Using a knife, make two cuts to form a T. First, cut down the middle of the chile lengthwise from stem to tip, then make a second cut perpendicular to the first, about ½ inch from the stem, slicing through only one side of the chile (be careful not to cut off the stem end completely).

2. Open the flaps of the pepper and use a paring knife to carefully cut out and remove the core and seeds. Then, using a small spoon, gently scrape the inside of the pepper to remove any remaining seeds, ribs, and core. Repeat with the second pepper. Close the flaps once all the seeds are removed.

3. The next step is to roast the peppers. Doing so over a gas flame is the best option because the shorter time over the heat helps keep the peppers' shape and texture intact during frying, but if you don't have a gas stove, you can use the broiler in your oven.

   *To roast over a gas flame,* turn two gas burners to medium-high heat. Place 1 chile directly on each burner and roast, turning occasionally with tongs, until blackened and blistered on all sides, 5 to 7 minutes. Remove to a large heatproof dish.

   *To roast under the broiler,* place an oven rack in the upper third of the oven and turn the broiler to high. Place the chiles directly on the rack and broil, turning occasionally with tongs, until blackened and blistered on all sides, 8 to 10 minutes. Remove to a large heatproof dish.

   Cover the dish tightly with plastic wrap or a baking sheet and let the chiles steam until cool enough to handle, about 15 minutes. Using a butter knife, scrape away and discard the chile skins, being careful not to tear the chiles; set the chiles aside.

4. Season the inside and outside of the chiles with salt and pepper.

5. Fill each chile with shredded chicken. If you used the broiler rather than a gas flame to roast the chiles, be extra careful when filling them to avoid tearing them.

6. Whip the egg whites in a bowl until soft peaks form. Beat the yolks together with the salt. Gently fold the yolks into the whites.

NUTRITIONAL INFO (per serving)

| calories | fat | protein | carbs | fiber |
|----------|-----|---------|-------|-------|
| 585 | 48g | 31g | 8g | 2g |
| | 74% | 21% | 5% | |

7. Pour the pureed salsa into a serving platter and set aside.

8. Heat the coconut oil in a cast-iron skillet over medium-high heat. When the oil is hot, dip each chile into the egg mixture to coat the whole chile. Fry the coated chiles on all sides until golden brown, 2 to 3 minutes per side. *Note:* If the coating doesn't stick, dollop about 3 tablespoons of the egg coating into the hot oil in the shape of the chile and fry until it is light golden brown, then place the chile on the egg mixture and dollop another 3 tablespoons of the egg coating over the top of the chile and smooth with a spoon to cover the entire chile. Flip the coated chile over to fry the other side until light golden brown.

9. Remove the fried chiles from the pan and place them on the serving platter over the salsa. Garnish with the cilantro.

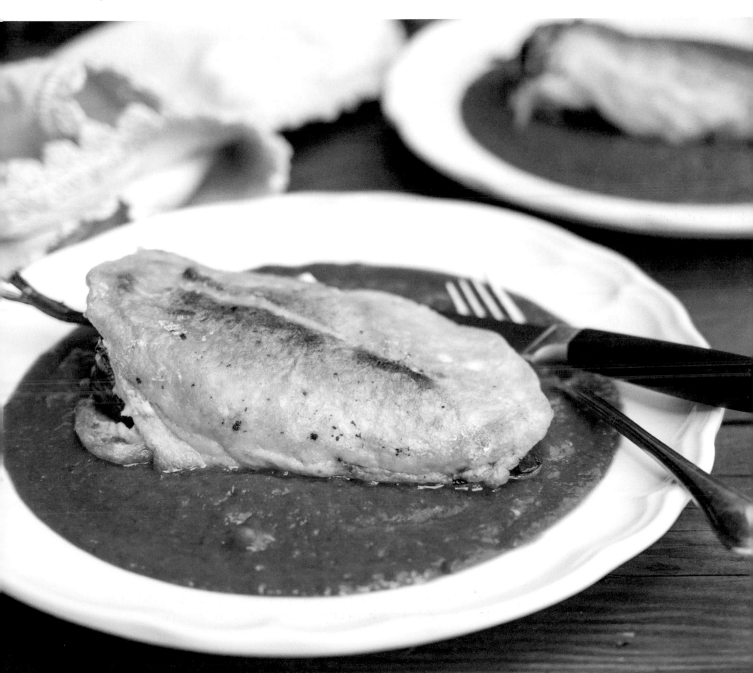

# deconstructed spicy chicken stack

L M H KETO

prep time: 5 minutes (not including time to make the guacamole or cook the chicken)
yield: 4 servings

## spicy mayo:

2 tablespoons mayonnaise, homemade (page 124) or store-bought

1 teaspoon medium-hot hot sauce, homemade (page 134) or store-bought (see notes)

## stack:

2 hard-boiled eggs (see page 174), diced

¼ cup mayonnaise, homemade (page 124) or store-bought

Fine sea salt and fresh ground black pepper

1 cup Guacamole (page 140)

1 cup diced cooked chicken (see notes)

1 cup chopped romaine lettuce

Snipped fresh chives, for garnish

1. To make the spicy mayo, combine the mayonnaise and hot sauce until well combined. Set aside.

2. In a medium bowl, combine the diced hard-boiled eggs, mayonnaise, and salt and pepper to taste.

3. To serve, place ¼ cup of the guacamole in the center of a small serving plate and spread into a thick 3- to 4-inch circle. Mound the guacamole with ¼ cup of the diced chicken, followed by ¼ cup of the chopped lettuce and one-quarter of the egg salad mixture. Repeat with the remaining ingredients to make a total of four salads. Serve with a drizzle of the spicy mayo and a sprinkling of fresh chives. Store extras in an airtight container in the fridge for up to 2 days.

notes: *If you're using a store-bought hot sauce, check the label to make sure that it's free of sugar.*

*If you don't have leftover cooked chicken on hand, you can use my easy recipe for Simple Slow Cooker Chicken Thighs on page 290. Or purchase an organic rotisserie chicken from your local market.*

NUTRITIONAL INFO (per serving)

| calories | fat | protein | carbs | fiber |
|---|---|---|---|---|
| 444 | 38g | 20g | 6g | 4g |
| | 77% | 18% | 5% | |

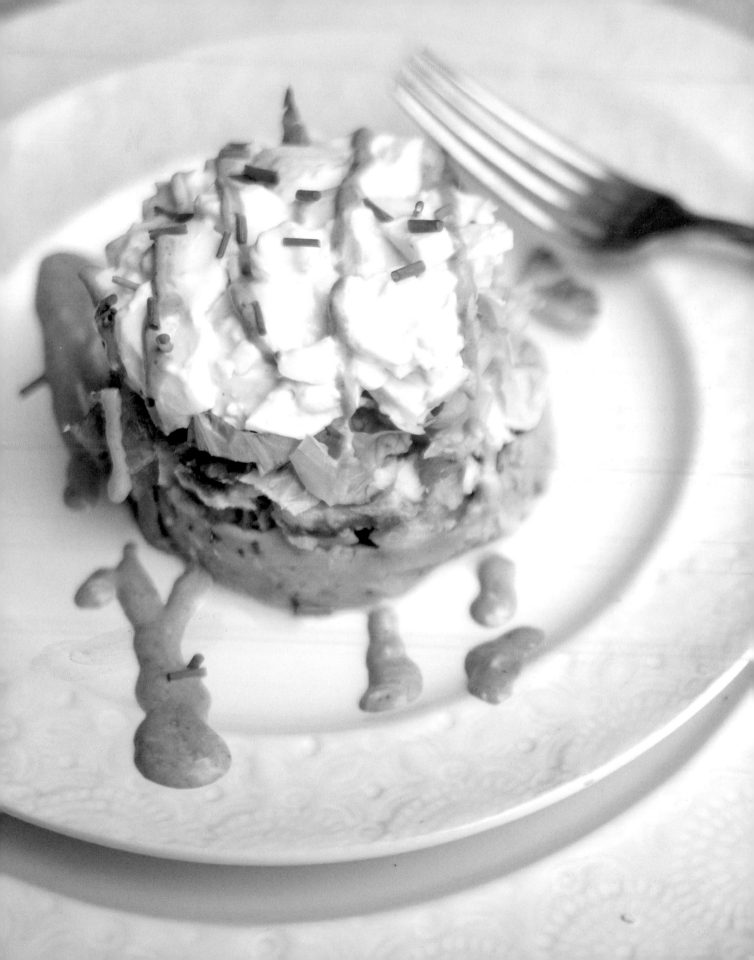

# easy egg foo young

L M H KETO ☒ ⊘ prep time: 10 minutes • cook time: 25 minutes (4 to 6 minutes per omelet) • yield: 4 servings

I adore ginger root, but I don't use it often. To avoid wasting it, I cut it into 1-inch sections and freeze it. I love having it on hand for an amazing flavor addition to meals.

1 tablespoon MCT oil or coconut oil, plus more as needed

6 large eggs

2 ounces deli chicken, turkey, ham, or roast beef, finely chopped

2 ounces button mushrooms, stemmed and thinly sliced

1 cup thinly sliced green or napa cabbage

½ cup thinly sliced green onions

1 tablespoon grated fresh ginger, divided

1 large clove garlic, crushed to a paste

1 teaspoon fine sea salt

½ teaspoon fresh ground black pepper

## sauce:

¾ cup chicken bone broth, homemade (page 108) or store-bought

¼ cup coconut oil

¼ cup coconut aminos or wheat-free tamari

½ teaspoon hot sauce, homemade (page 134) or store-bought (adjust amount for desired heat)

Reserved grated ginger (from above)

¼ to ½ teaspoon guar gum

¼ cup diced roasted red pepper, for garnish

1. Heat the MCT oil in a large skillet over medium heat.

2. While the oil is heating, whisk the eggs in a large mixing bowl. Stir in the deli meat, mushrooms, cabbage, green onions, ¾ tablespoon of the grated ginger, and the garlic. Season with the salt and pepper.

3. Using a measuring cup or large spoon, dollop ½ cup of the egg mixture into the skillet. Cook the omelet until golden, 2 to 3 minutes, then flip and cook for another 2 to 3 minutes. Remove from the pan and set aside. Repeat with the remaining egg mixture, adding more oil to the skillet if needed between batches.

4. Meanwhile, make the sauce: Combine the chicken broth, coconut oil, coconut aminos, hot sauce, and remaining ¼ tablespoon grated ginger in a small saucepan. Whisk in ¼ teaspoon of guar gum. Heat until the sauce is boiling and has reduced a bit, about 5 minutes. If you prefer a thicker sauce, add another ¼ teaspoon of guar gum, whisk until smooth, and boil until thickened, about another 5 minutes.

5. To serve, place 2 puffed omelets on each plate and top with 3 tablespoons of the sauce. Garnish with roasted red pepper. The omelets are best served fresh, but extras can be stored in an airtight container in the fridge for up to 2 days. To reheat, lightly grease a skillet with avocado oil or coconut oil and set over medium heat. Place the omelet in the skillet and heat for 2 minutes on each side, or until warm.

NUTRITIONAL INFO (per serving)

| calories | fat | protein | carbs | fiber |
|---|---|---|---|---|
| 452 | 38g | 18g | 9g | 6g |
| | 76% | 17% | 7% | |

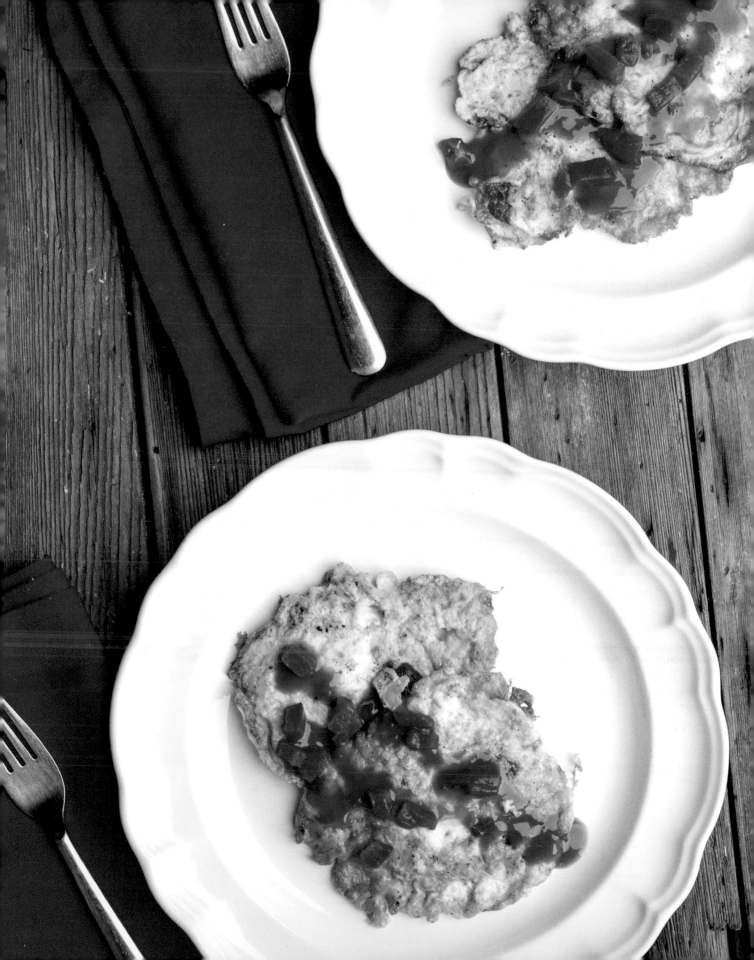

# doro watt chicken salad wraps

prep time: 8 minutes (not including time to cook the chicken, hard-boil the eggs, or make the mayo) • yield: 12 servings

Doro watt is a traditional dish that my husband and I enjoyed during our visits to Ethiopia to meet and then adopt our baby boys. I've added my twist on it here, turning it into a chicken salad and using my Berbere Mayo to give it an ethnic flair. If you want to make this recipe even easier, pick up an organic rotisserie chicken and use it to make the chicken salad.

1 recipe Simple Slow Cooker Chicken Thighs (page 290)

1 cup Berbere Mayo (page 126) (see note)

1 tablespoon lemon juice

1 head Boston leaf lettuce, for wrapping

**for garnish (optional):**

Chopped fresh cilantro or other herb of choice

Diced tomatoes or roasted red peppers

Sliced hard-boiled eggs (see page 174) (omit for egg-free)

1. Remove the meat from the slow-cooked chicken thighs and discard the bones. Shred the meat and place it in a large bowl. Add the Berbere Mayo and lemon juice and toss until the chicken is evenly coated.

2. To serve, place a large spoonful of the chicken salad in the center of a lettuce leaf. Garnish with cilantro, diced tomatoes, and/or sliced hard-boiled eggs, if desired. Roll the lettuce up and around the filling to make a wrap. Repeat to make additional wraps. Store extras in an airtight container in the fridge for up to 4 days.

note: *For an egg-free version, use my Egg-Free Keto Mayo (page 125) to make the Berbere Mayo.*

NUTRITIONAL INFO (per serving)

| calories | fat | protein | carbs | fiber |
|----------|------|---------|-------|-------|
| 334 | 28g | 20g | 1g | 0.3g |
| | 75% | 24% | 1% | |

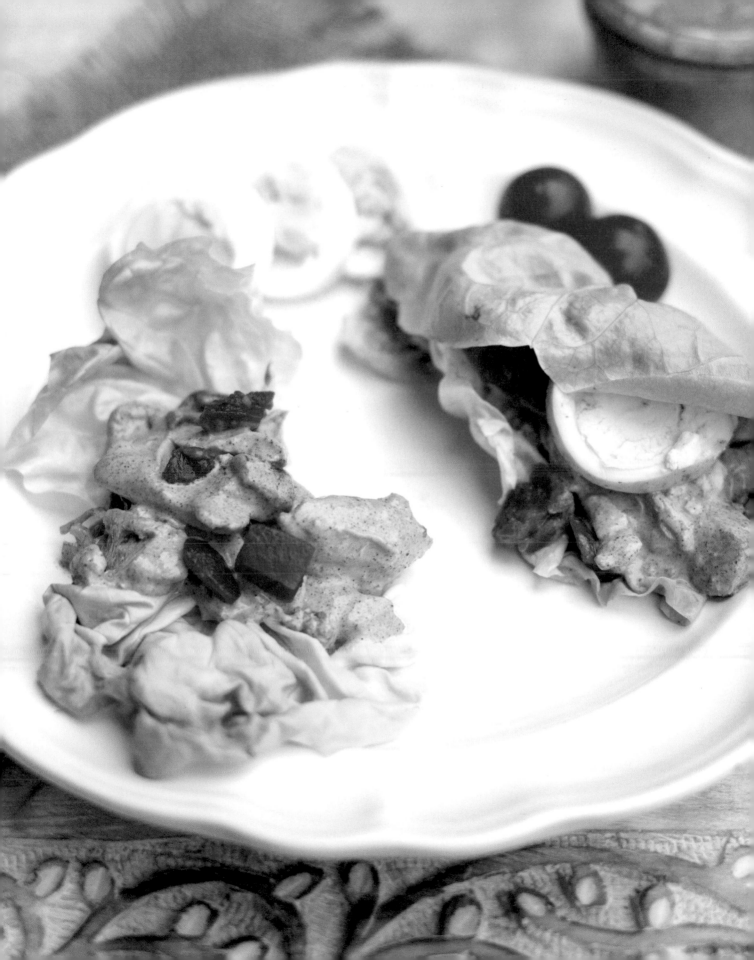

# slow cooker ethiopian spicy chicken stew

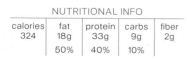 prep time: 10 minutes • cook time: 7 hours • yield: 8 servings

When we traveled to Ethiopia to adopt our boys, my mouth was introduced to some amazing new and exotic flavors! If you've ever been to Ethiopia, you know the word *berbere*. It is the main spice mix that Ethiopians use in their cooking. It is quite spicy, so you can add more or less to your liking. I've included a recipe for it on page 110, but if you don't want to make a batch yourself, you can find berbere in specialty spice stores as well as online.

Chicken thighs are more ketogenic and tastier than bland, skinless chicken breasts, and the skin helps make this dish more ketogenic by increasing the fat ratio. But I have to admit, I'm not a fan of soggy, chewy skin. In this recipe, I use the skin to make cracklings to add another layer of texture and flavor to this amazing stew.

2½ pounds bone-in, skin-on chicken thighs

4 cups chopped onions

2 cups chicken bone broth, homemade (page 108) or store-bought

1½ cups diced tomatoes with juices (about 2 tomatoes)

¼ cup Berbere Spice Mix (page 110)

2 tablespoons melted coconut oil

5 cloves garlic, minced

1 tablespoon minced fresh ginger

1 teaspoon fine sea salt

8 hard-boiled eggs (see page 174), peeled, for serving (optional)

1. Remove the skin from the chicken thighs and reserve for cracklings.

2. Place the onions, chicken broth, tomatoes, spice mix, coconut oil, garlic, ginger, and salt in a 4-quart (or larger) slow cooker. Stir well to combine. Place the chicken on top.

3. Cover and cook on low for 7 hours or until the chicken is fork-tender. Meanwhile, make the chicken cracklings by following the method in Step 2 on page 286.

4. When the chicken is done, remove the thighs from the slow cooker and place them in a bowl or casserole dish (to catch the juices as you work). Remove the meat from the bones, discard the bones, and shred the meat using two forks. Return the shredded chicken to the slow cooker along with any accumulated juices and stir to combine the shredded chicken into the stew.

5. Garnish with the cracklings and serve with hard-boiled eggs, if desired. Store extras in an airtight container in the fridge for up to 4 days.

**tip: slow cook your way to sanity**

*If you tend to get overwhelmed by the prospect of cooking homemade meals, or you know you have a busy day coming up, try this strategy: Have your spouse or other kitchen helper clean up the kitchen after dinner while you prepare dinner for the next night and fill your slow cooker. All you need to do is store the slow cooker insert in the fridge and then, the next morning, take it out of the fridge and let the slow cooker do the work of cooking the meal for you. Dinner is taken care of, as well as yummy leftovers for easy lunches. This is my go-to trick—it saves me from a lot of stress. (Note: There are ten slow cooker meals in this book. To quickly find them, see the index on page 418.)*

| NUTRITIONAL INFO | | | | |
|---|---|---|---|---|
| calories | fat | protein | carbs | fiber |
| 324 | 18g | 33g | 9g | 2g |
| | 50% | 40% | 10% | |

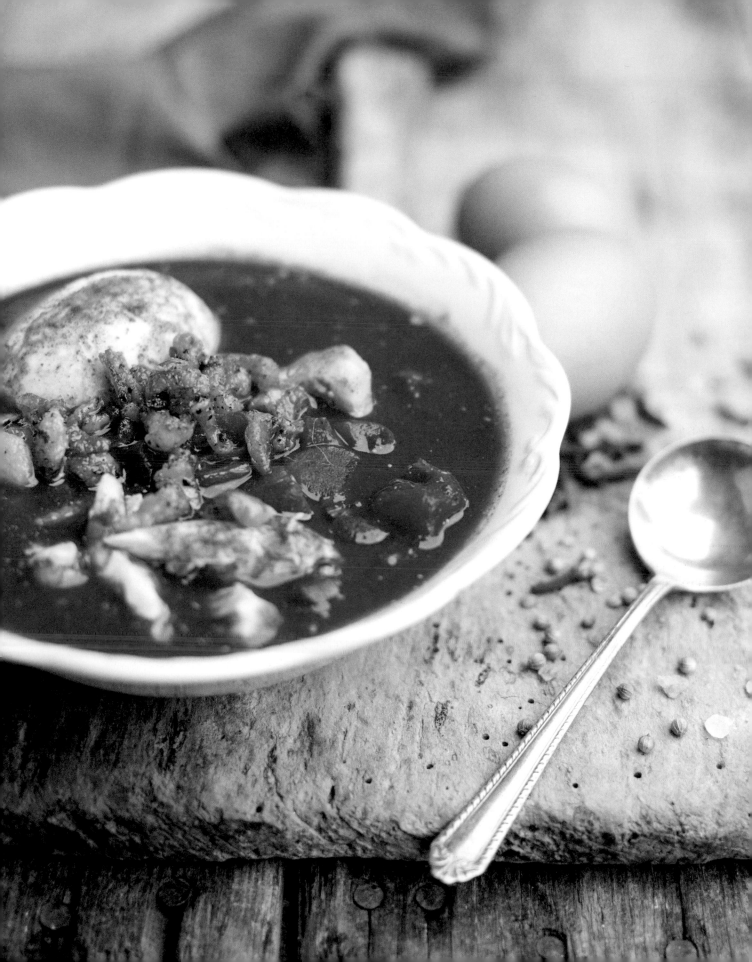

# california club wraps

L M→H KETO

prep time: 10 minutes • cook time: 3 minutes (not including time to cook the chicken, make the tortillas, or hard-boil the eggs) • yield: 4 wraps (1 per serving)

This is a great on-the-go sandwich option. You can assemble the wraps for two days of lunches, or prepare all the ingredients and store them in the fridge for up to five days, assembling the wraps as needed for a week of easy lunches. The latter is a great option for single-serving portions, too!

4 slices bacon

2 cups shredded cooked chicken (see notes)

½ cup mayonnaise, homemade (page 124) or store-bought

½ teaspoon fine sea salt, plus more for seasoning the avocado

½ teaspoon fresh ground black pepper, plus more for seasoning the avocado

1 small avocado (see notes)

4 Wraps (page 254) or large lettuce leaves

2 hard-boiled eggs (see page 174), sliced

2 cups shredded romaine lettuce

1 small tomato, diced

1. Heat a cast-iron skillet over medium-high heat and fry the bacon until crisp, about 3 minutes. Remove from the heat and set aside.

2. While the bacon is frying, place the shredded chicken in a medium bowl. Stir in the mayo, salt, and pepper.

3. Cut the avocado in half, then remove the pit. Slice the avocado into ¼-inch slices and, using a spoon, scoop the slices from the skin. Sprinkle the avocado with salt and pepper.

4. To assemble the wraps: Lay a wrap on a clean work surface and place one-quarter of the dressed chicken along the edge closest to you, leaving about a 1-inch border for easy rolling. Top the chicken with one-quarter of each of the remaining filling ingredients. Fold the ends of the wrap over the filling and roll it up. Repeat with the remaining three wraps and filling ingredients.

5. Slice the assembled wraps in half before serving. Store extras in an airtight container in the fridge for up to 2 days.

notes: *If you don't have leftover cooked chicken on hand, you can use my easy recipe for Simple Slow Cooker Chicken Thighs on page 290. Or purchase an organic rotisserie chicken from your local market.*

*If you do not plan to serve all the wraps immediately, slice just enough of the avocado needed for the number of wraps you're serving, then add the remaining avocado to the remaining wraps right before serving.*

busy family tip: *For a week of easy on-the-go lunches, prepare all the ingredients for the wraps, except the avocado, and store them separately in the fridge for up to 5 days. Prepare single-serving wraps as needed for easy meals, cutting avocado slices and adding them to the wraps just before serving.*

NUTRITIONAL INFO (per serving)

| calories | fat | protein | carbs | fiber |
|----------|-----|---------|-------|-------|
| 750 | 63g | 30g | 7g | 4g |
| | 78% | 18% | 4% | |

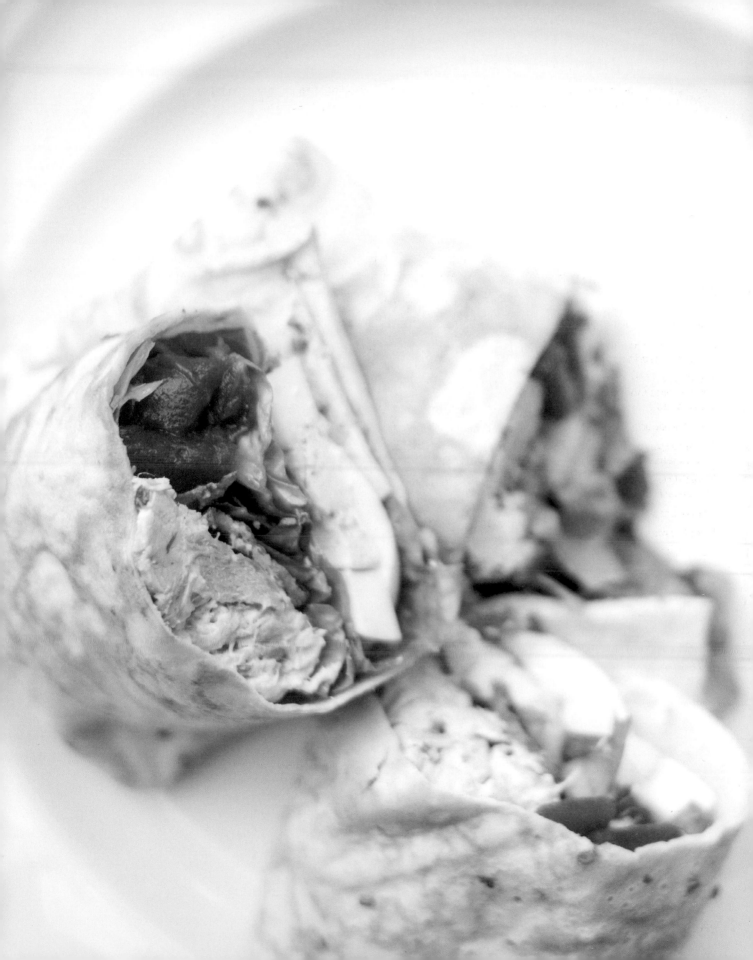

# chicken oscar

L M H KETO

prep time: 5 minutes • cook time: 20 minutes (not including time to make the hollandaise)
yield: 4 servings

1 pound medium-thick asparagus

1 tablespoon MCT oil or extra-virgin olive oil

1 teaspoon fine sea salt, divided

1 teaspoon fresh ground black pepper, divided

2 tablespoons Paleo fat, such as lard, tallow, or coconut oil

4 (3- to 4-ounce) boneless, skinless chicken thighs

½ cup Easy Dairy-Free Hollandaise (page 136), warm

8 ounces canned crab claw meat

Purple sea salt, for garnish

Chopped fresh flat-leaf parsley, for garnish

1. Preheat the oven to 450°F. Cut off the tough bottom ends of the asparagus and place the spears in a single layer on a rimmed baking sheet. Pour the MCT oil over the asparagus and roll them around to coat. Sprinkle with ¼ teaspoon of the salt and ¼ teaspoon of the pepper. Bake for 10 minutes, or until slightly brown.

2. To cook the chicken: Heat the Paleo fat in a cast-iron skillet over medium-high heat. Place the chicken thighs in a large resealable plastic bag and, using a rolling pin, pound the thighs until they're ¼ inch thick. Remove from the plastic bag and season both sides with the remaining ¾ teaspoon each of salt and pepper. Once the oil is hot, add the chicken to the skillet and cook until golden brown on both sides and cooked through, about 4 minutes per side. Remove to a cutting board and let rest for a minute or two, then slice.

3. To serve, divide the roasted asparagus among four plates. Top each with a sliced chicken thigh, one-quarter of the hollandaise, and one-quarter of the crabmeat. Garnish with purple salt and chopped parsley. Though best served fresh, leftovers will keep in an airtight container in the fridge for up to 2 days.

NUTRITIONAL INFO (per serving)

| calories | fat | protein | carbs | fiber |
|----------|-----|---------|-------|-------|
| 397 | 29g | 29g | 5g | 2g |
| | 66% | 29% | 5% | |

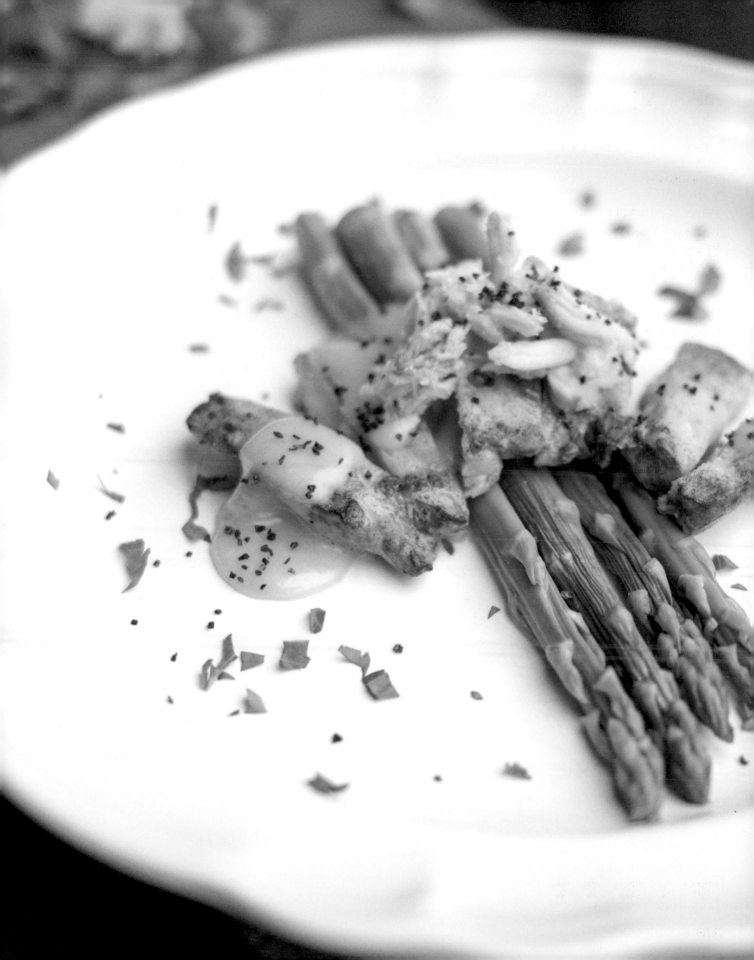

# chicken neapolitan

L ⫟ H
KETO

prep time: 5 minutes (not including time to make the garlic bread)
cook time: 20 minutes • yield: 8 servings

8 bone-in, skin-on chicken thighs

2 teaspoons fine sea salt

1 teaspoon fresh ground black pepper

3 tablespoons MCT oil

1 pound mushrooms, quartered

1 cup chopped onions

4 cloves garlic, minced

2 cups diced tomatoes with juices

1 cup pitted black olives, drained

1 cup fresh basil leaves

8 slices Garlic Keto Bread (page 256), for serving

1. Sprinkle the chicken with the salt and pepper. Heat the oil in a large skillet over medium-high heat. Once hot, add the chicken thighs to the pan and sear for 8 to 9 minutes, until the skin is golden brown. Flip the thighs over, then add the mushrooms, onions, and garlic. Cook for 8 minutes, or until a meat thermometer reaches 170°F when inserted into a chicken thigh.

2. Lower the heat to medium-low, then add the tomatoes, olives, and basil and cook just until warmed through. Serve with Keto Garlic Bread. Store extras in an airtight container in the fridge for up to 2 days. Reheat in a skillet over medium heat until warmed.

NUTRITIONAL INFO (per serving)

| calories | fat | protein | carbs | fiber |
|----------|-----|---------|-------|-------|
| 378 | 23g | 33g | 12g | 2g |
| | 60% | 29% | 11% | |

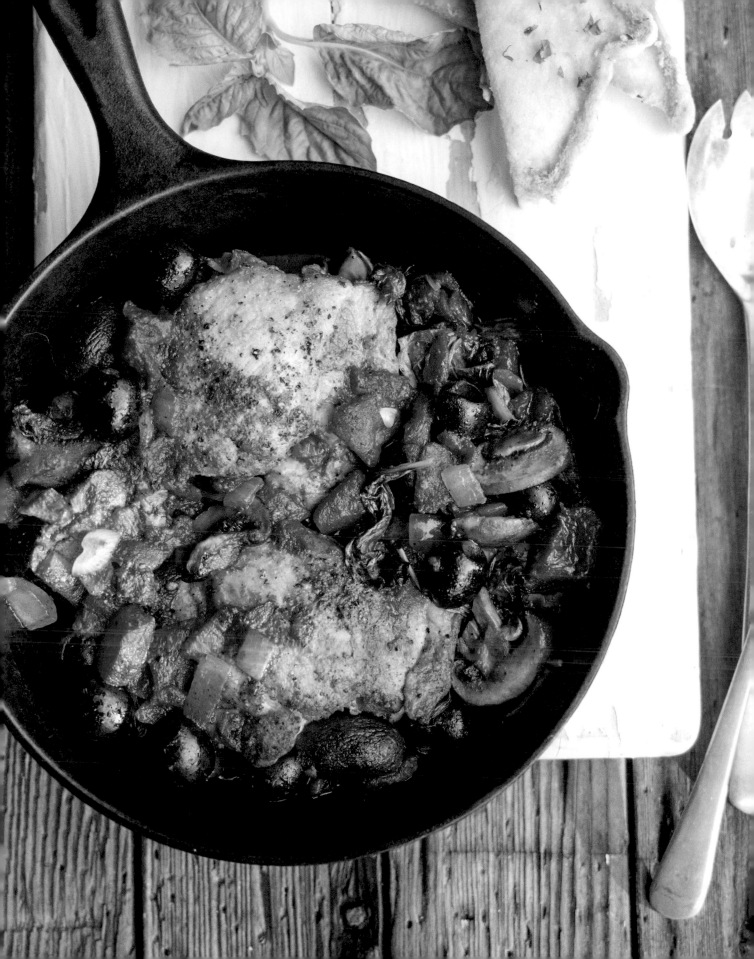

# lemon pepper chicken

4 boneless, skinless chicken thighs

½ teaspoon fine sea salt

1 teaspoon fresh ground black pepper

2 tablespoons coconut oil

Juice of 1 lemon

2 tablespoons capers

Chopped fresh flat-leaf parsley, for garnish

Lemon slices, for garnish

1. Pat the chicken thighs with a paper towel to remove the excess moisture. Using a heavy skillet, pound the thighs to an even thickness of about ½ inch, then season both sides well with the salt and pepper.

2. Heat the oil in a cast-iron skillet over medium-high heat. Sear the chicken thighs for 5 minutes per side, or until cooked through and no longer pink inside. Remove the pan from the heat. Place the chicken on a platter, leaving the drippings in the pan.

3. Add the lemon juice and capers to the skillet and use a whisk to scrape up the brown bits from the bottom of the pan. Pour the sauce over the chicken on the platter and garnish with chopped parsley and lemon slices.

4. Store extras in an airtight container in the fridge for up to 2 days. Reheat in a skillet over medium heat until warmed.

NUTRITIONAL INFO (per serving)

| calories | fat | protein | carbs | fiber |
|----------|-----|---------|-------|-------|
| 220 | 17g | 16g | 1g | 1g |
| | 69% | 29% | 2% | |

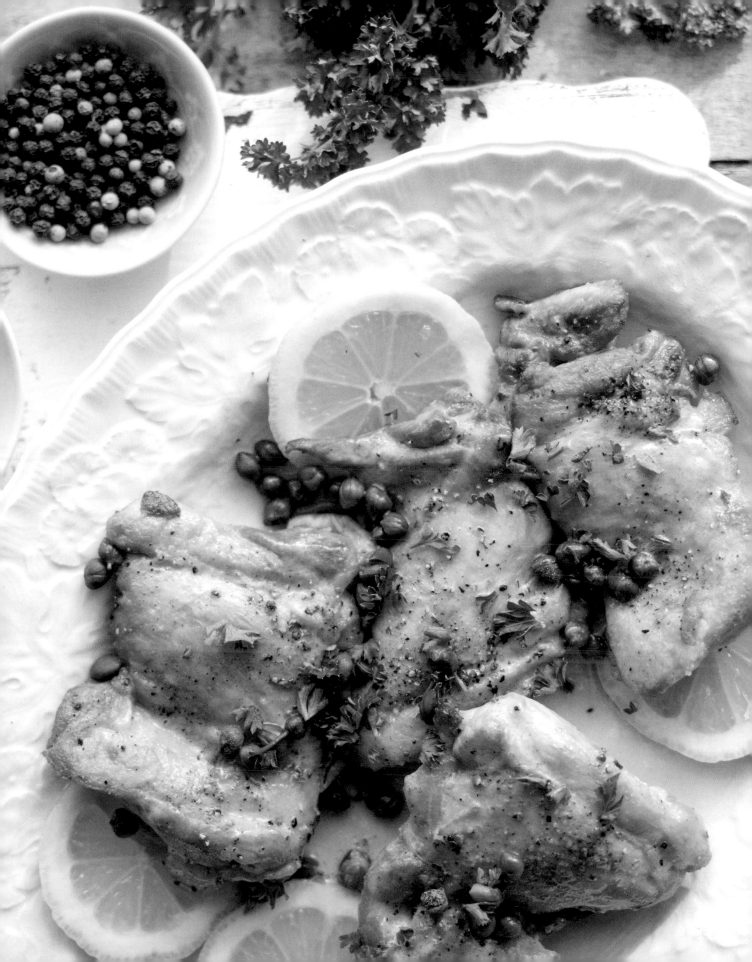

# tom ka gai (thai coconut chicken)

L M H KETO · prep time: 10 minutes · cook time: 30 to 50 minutes · yield: 4 servings

When you hear "tom ka gai," you may think soup, and it is, but here, I've turned it into a thicker and heartier option that is more of a main dish.

2 tablespoons MCT oil or extra-virgin olive oil, divided

1 cup thinly sliced napa cabbage

¼ teaspoon fine sea salt, plus more for the chicken

1 pound boneless, skinless chicken breasts, cut into 2-inch pieces

3 shallots, diced

1½ to 3 tablespoons red curry paste

1½ cups chicken bone broth, homemade (page 108) or store-bought

1 (13½-ounce) can full-fat coconut milk

¼ cup fresh cilantro leaves, chopped, plus more for garnish

2 green onions, cut into ½-inch pieces, plus more for garnish

Juice of 1 lime

1. Heat 1 tablespoon of the oil in a cast-iron skillet over medium heat. Add the thinly sliced cabbage and sauté until wilted, about 3 minutes. Season with the salt and set aside in a bowl.

2. Place the same skillet back over medium heat and add the remaining tablespoon of oil. Sprinkle salt all over the chicken pieces and sauté them in the skillet for 4 to 5 minutes, until seared on all sides. They do not need to be cooked through; they will finish cooking in the broth.

3. Add the shallots to the skillet and sauté until tender, about 2 minutes. Reduce the heat to low. Whisk in the curry paste, broth, and coconut milk. Simmer, uncovered, for 20 to 40 minutes, or until the broth has reduced a bit. The longer you simmer it, the thicker the sauce will be.

4. Once the chicken is cooked through, add the sautéed cabbage and cook for about a minute to heat through. Stir in the cilantro, green onions, and lime juice. Immediately remove from the heat and transfer to serving bowls. Garnish each bowl with additional sliced green onions and cilantro leaves.

5. Store extras in an airtight container in the fridge for up to 4 days or in the freezer for up to a month. Reheat in a skillet over medium heat until warmed.

NUTRITIONAL INFO (per serving)

| calories | fat | protein | carbs | fiber |
|---|---|---|---|---|
| 478 | 33g | 38g | 8g | 2g |
| | 62% | 32% | 6% | |

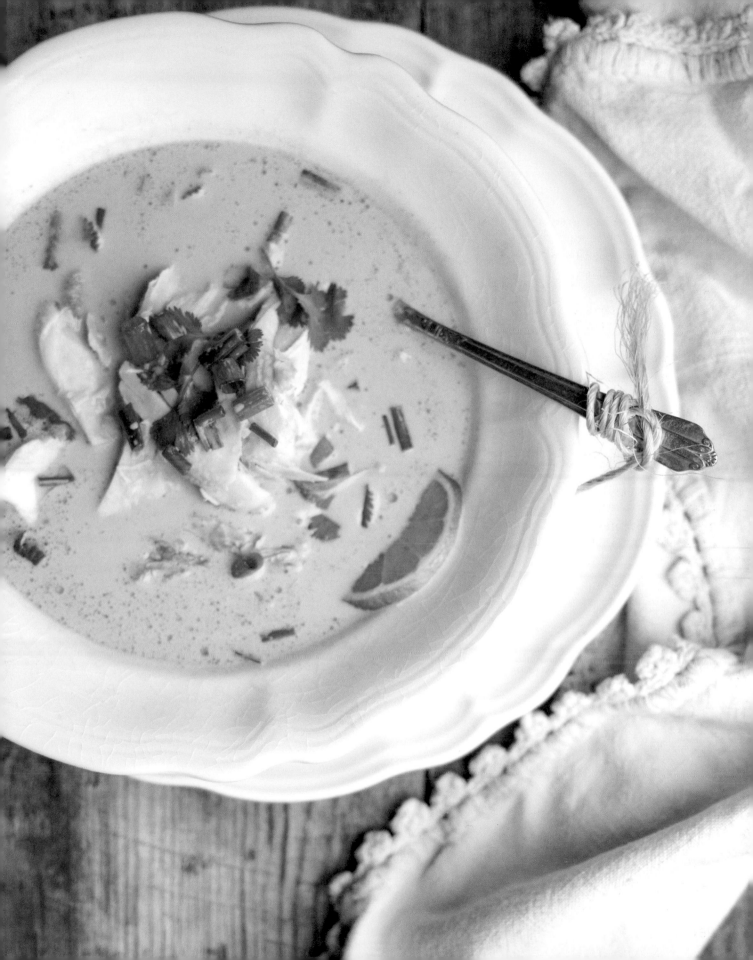

# keto greek avgolemono

Avgolemono is a traditional Greek soup, but in my version the chicken is left on the bone. Think of it as a main dish with a lot of sauce! That's how I roll—I love tasty sauces (particularly creamy sauces) with chicken and other meats. If you are missing the creamy mouthfeel that you get from dairy, look no further! This creamy bowl of saucy chicken will leave your body satisfied.

4 bone-in, skin-on chicken thighs

¼ cup diced onions

1 sprig fresh thyme

4 cups chicken bone broth, homemade (page 108) or store-bought, plus more if needed (see note)

Fine sea salt and fresh ground black pepper

2 large eggs

2 tablespoons lemon juice

4 tablespoons extra-virgin olive oil or MCT oil, for drizzling (optional)

## cracklings:

Chicken skin (from above)

½ teaspoon fine sea salt

½ teaspoon fresh ground black pepper

1½ teaspoons Paleo fat, such as lard, tallow, or avocado oil

1. Remove the skin from the chicken thighs and set aside (you will use it to make cracklings). Place the skinless chicken, diced onions, and thyme in a large pot and fill with broth so that the broth covers the thighs by 1 inch. Add a couple pinches each of salt and pepper. Bring to a boil and cook for 20 minutes, or until the chicken is tender and easily falls off the bone.

2. While the chicken is cooking, make the cracklings: Cut the chicken skin into ¼-inch pieces and season with the ½ teaspoon each of salt and pepper. Heat the Paleo fat in a skillet over medium-high heat, then add the chicken skin and fry until golden brown and crispy, about 8 minutes. Set the cracklings aside on a paper towel to drain.

3. When the chicken thighs are done, place them in individual serving bowls and set aside.

4. In a medium bowl, whisk the eggs and lemon juice. While whisking, very slowly pour in ½ cup of the hot broth (if you add the hot broth too quickly, the eggs will curdle). Slowly whisk another cup of hot soup into the egg mixture.

5. Pour the hot egg mixture into the pot while stirring to create a creamy soup without the cream. Reduce the heat and simmer for 10 minutes, stirring constantly. The soup will thicken slightly as it cooks.

6. Pour one-quarter (about 1 cup) of the creamy soup over each chicken thigh. Top with the cracklings. Drizzle each bowl with 1 tablespoon of olive oil, if desired.

7. This dish is best served fresh to avoid curdled eggs from reheating, but leftovers can be stored in an airtight container in the fridge for up to 2 days. Reheat in a saucepan over medium-low heat until warmed, stirring constantly to keep the eggs from curdling.

NUTRITIONAL INFO (per serving)

| calories | fat | protein | carbs | fiber |
|----------|-----|---------|-------|-------|
| 275 | 20g | 22g | 2g | 1g |
| | 65% | 32% | 3% | |

note: *Using homemade broth will create a thicker soup, but boxed broth will work.*

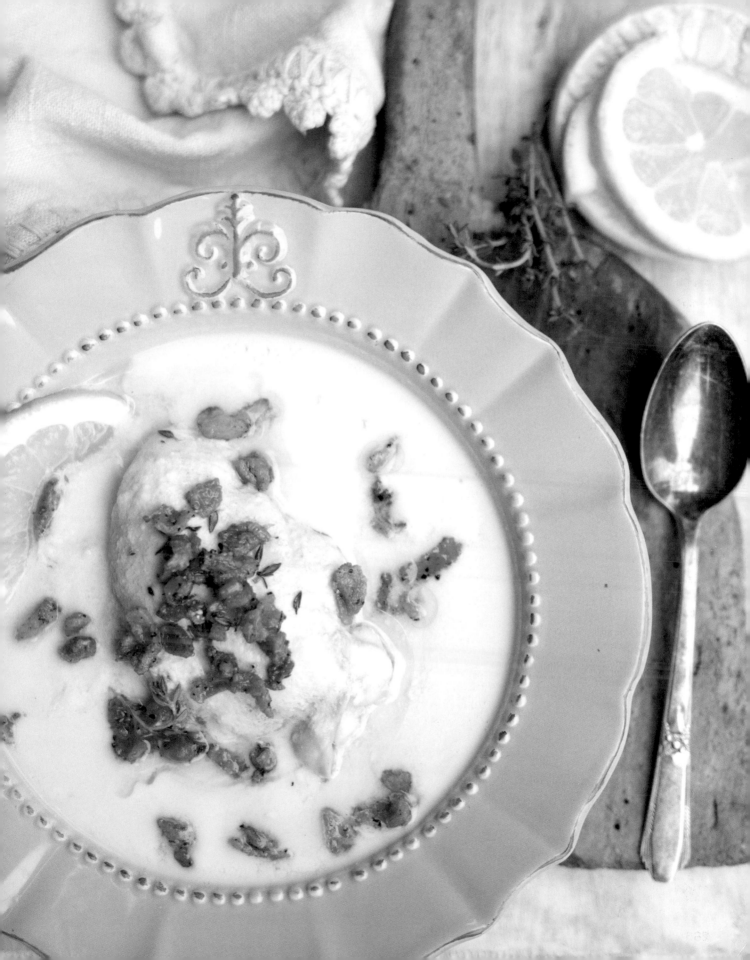

# stewed chicken and sausage

KETO · prep time: 10 minutes · cook time: 1 hour 10 minutes · yield: 8 servings

This hearty dish is so amazing. The three different textures from the chicken, sliced chorizo, and crumbled chorizo really add another level of enjoyment!

2 pounds Mexican-style fresh (raw) chorizo

1 tablespoon coconut oil

2 boneless, skinless chicken thighs, cut into ½-inch pieces

1 cup chopped onions

1½ (18-ounce) jars whole peeled tomatoes with juices

3 chipotle chiles in adobo sauce

3 tablespoons minced garlic

2 tablespoons smoked paprika

1 tablespoon ground cumin

1 tablespoon dried oregano leaves

2 teaspoons fine sea salt

1 teaspoon cayenne pepper

2 cups chicken bone broth, homemade (page 108) or store-bought

¼ cup lime juice

¼ cup chopped fresh cilantro

1. Slice 1 pound of the chorizo into rounds; crumble the remaining pound.

2. Heat the oil in large soup pot over medium-high heat. Add the sliced and crumbled chorizo, chicken, and onions and cook until the onions are soft and the chicken is cooked through, about 5 minutes, stirring to break up the crumbled chorizo.

3. Meanwhile, place the tomatoes and their juices and the chiles in a food processor. Puree until smooth; set aside.

4. Add the garlic, paprika, cumin, oregano, salt, and cayenne pepper to the soup pot and sauté for another minute while stirring.

5. Add the pureed tomato mixture and broth to the soup pot. Bring to a gentle boil, then reduce the heat to low and simmer for 1 hour to allow the flavors to open up. Just before serving, stir in the lime juice and cilantro.

6. Store extras in an airtight container in the fridge for up to 2 days. Reheat in a saucepan over medium heat until warmed.

NUTRITIONAL INFO (per serving)

| calories | fat | protein | carbs | fiber |
|----------|-----|---------|-------|-------|
| 415 | 33g | 20g | 10g | 2g |
| | 72% | 19% | 9% | |

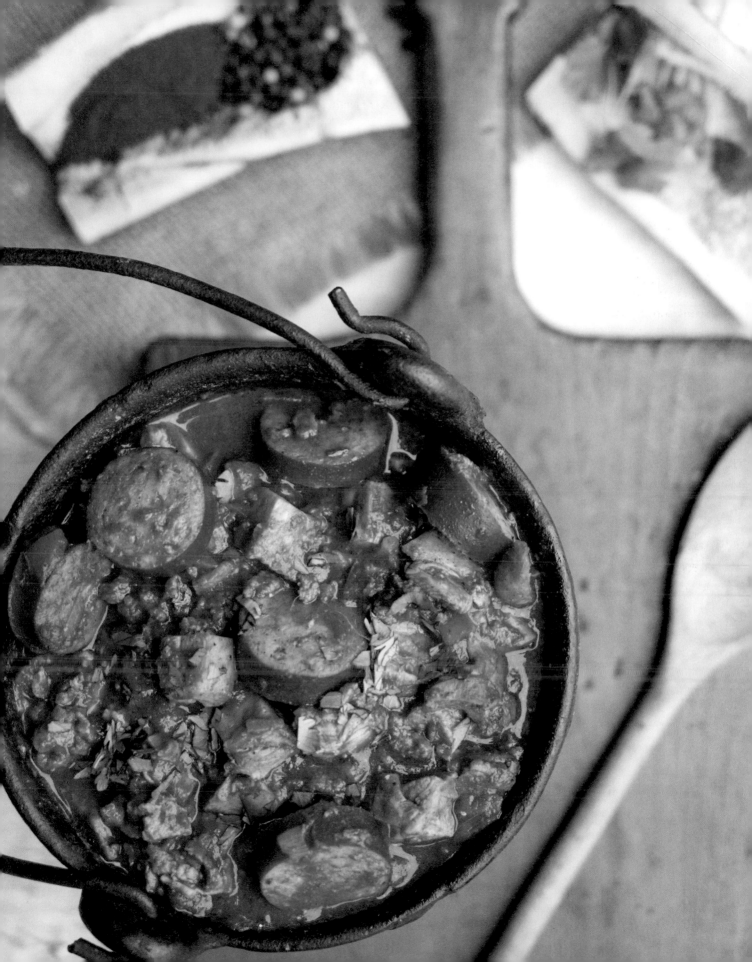

# simple slow cooker chicken thighs

L M H KETO 🗹 ⌀ ⌀  prep time: 10 minutes • cook time: 6 hours • yield: 3 cups shredded chicken (6 servings)

This is a great way to have shredded chicken ready for easy dinners, such as my California Club Wraps (page 276).

2 pounds bone-in, skin-on chicken thighs

2 cups chicken bone broth, homemade (page 108) or store-bought

¼ cup diced onions

2 teaspoons minced garlic

1 teaspoon fine sea salt

½ teaspoon fresh ground black pepper

Place all the ingredients in a 6-quart (or larger) slow cooker. Cover and cook on low until the chicken is fork-tender, about 6 hours. Remove the chicken from the slow cooker, then remove the skin (reserve the skin for making Crispy Chicken Skin Croutons, page 258, or cracklings, page 286). Remove the meat from the bones, discard the bones, and shred the meat using two forks. Store the chicken in an airtight container in the fridge for up to 5 days, or freeze for up to 1 month.

tip: *If you're not using the chicken right away, store it with some of the juices from the slow cooker. It will help keep the meat moist until you use it.*

NUTRITIONAL INFO (per serving)

| calories | fat | protein | carbs | fiber |
|----------|-----|---------|-------|-------|
| 389 | 25g | 39g | 2g | 0.3g |
| | 58% | 40% | 2% | |

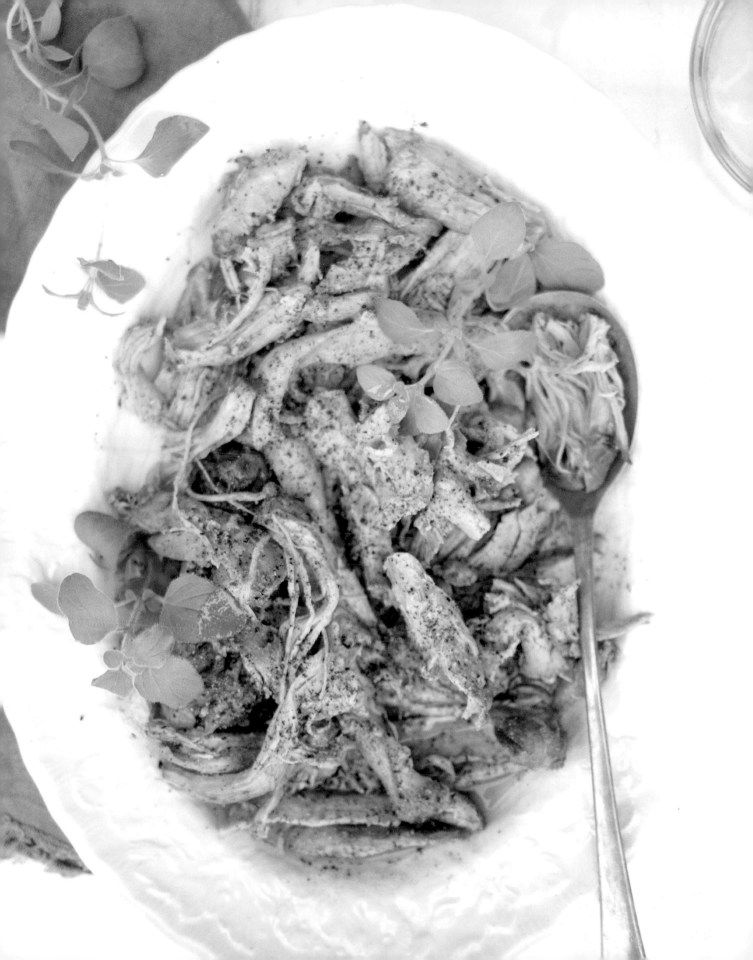

# main dishes: beef

# smothered bacon and mushroom burgers

KETO ⟶ option    prep time: 10 minutes • cook time: 15 minutes • yield: 4 servings

5 slices bacon, diced

1 tablespoon plus 1 teaspoon Paleo fat, such as lard, tallow, or coconut oil

1²/₃ pounds mushrooms, sliced

²/₃ cup thinly sliced onions

2 teaspoons fine sea salt, divided

1¼ heaping teaspoons fresh ground black pepper, divided

1¹/₃ pounds 80% lean ground beef

8 large lettuce leaves, for "buns"

Cherry tomatoes, cut in half, for garnish

### special sauce:

¼ cup plus 2 tablespoons mayonnaise, homemade (page 124) or store-bought (or Egg-Free Keto Mayo, page 125, for egg-free)

¼ cup tomato sauce

2 tablespoons plus 2 teaspoons Swerve confectioners'-style sweetener or equivalent amount of liquid or powdered sweetener (see page 81)

1½ scant teaspoons coconut vinegar or apple cider vinegar

½ rounded teaspoon fine sea salt

½ rounded teaspoon fresh ground black pepper

1. Heat a large cast-iron skillet over medium-high heat and sauté the bacon until crispy, about 3 minutes. Add the Paleo fat to the pan, along with the mushrooms and onions, and sauté until the mushrooms are cooked through, about 4 minutes. Season with ¾ teaspoon of the salt and ½ teaspoon of the pepper. Using a slotted spoon, remove the bacon, mushrooms, and onions from the pan and set aside. Leave the fat in the pan.

2. Using your hands, form the meat into four ¾-inch-thick patties. Season the outsides of the patties with the remaining salt and pepper. Fry the burgers in the skillet over medium-high heat on both sides until cooked to your desired doneness (see the chart below).

3. Meanwhile, make the sauce: Place all the ingredients in an 8-ounce jar with a lid. Cover and shake vigorously to combine.

4. To serve, place a burger on a lettuce leaf, then top it with one-fourth of the fried bacon, mushroom, and onion mixture, followed by 2 tablespoons of the sauce and another lettuce leaf (for a top "bun"). Repeat with the remaining burgers and toppings, and garnish each plate with cherry tomatoes.

note: *This is one of the recipes featured in week 3 of the 30-day meal plan. To help curb your sweet tooth during the cleanse, I suggest you reduce the amount of sweetener in the Special Sauce to 2 teaspoons.*

tip: *To keep the burgers moist inside and out, season only the outsides of the patties; don't mix salt into the meat. Salt removes water and dissolves some of the meat protein, causing the insoluble proteins to bind together. That's great for making sausage, where you want a springy texture, but not great for creating tender, juicy burgers.*

### BURGER DONENESS

| °F | |
|---|---|
| 170 | |
| 165 | |
| 160 | WELL DONE |
| 155 | |
| 150 | MEDIUM-WELL |
| 145 | |

### NUTRITIONAL INFO (per serving)

| calories | fat | protein | carbs | fiber |
|---|---|---|---|---|
| 570 | 45g | 25g | 6g | 2g |
| | 71% | 25% | 4% | |

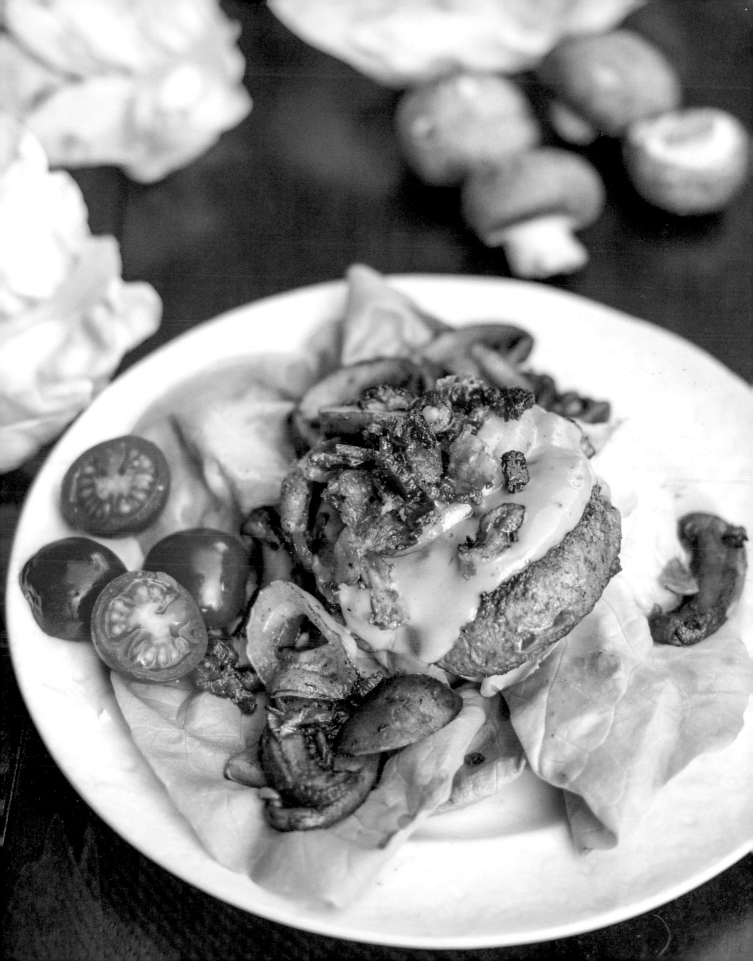

# umami burgers

prep time: 5 minutes (not including time to make the buns)
cook time: about 25 minutes • yield: 4 servings

I call these "umami burgers" because they are seasoned with a touch of fish sauce and topped with mushrooms—both wonderful sources of umami. Umami is the fifth taste, after sour, salty, bitter, and sweet. It is usually described as the "savory" taste. Umami's amazing savory taste is produced by ribonucleotides, molecules that help boost flavor naturally in many foods, including beef broth and aged cheeses. These burgers are topped with bone marrow, providing that creamy mouthfeel that we crave without dairy. The bone marrow also packs a huge nutritional punch!

## bone marrow:

5 (2-inch) cross-cut beef or veal marrow bones, split lengthwise

½ teaspoon fine sea salt

¼ teaspoon fresh ground black pepper

1 tablespoon plus 1 teaspoon Paleo fat, such as lard, tallow, or coconut oil

⅔ pound mushrooms, sliced

¾ cup sliced onions

2 teaspoons fine sea salt, divided

1¾ teaspoons fresh ground black pepper, divided

1⅓ pounds 80% lean ground beef

1½ scant teaspoons fish sauce

4 Keto Buns (page 256), for serving

Lettuce, for serving (optional)

Cornichons or other pickles, for garnish

1. Preheat the oven to 450°F.

2. Rinse, drain, and pat the bones dry. Season them with the ½ teaspoon of salt and ¼ teaspoon of pepper and place them cut side up in a roasting pan.

3. Roast the bones for 15 to 25 minutes (the exact timing will depend on the diameter of the bones; if they are 2 inches in diameter, it will take closer to 15 minutes), until the marrow in the center has puffed slightly and is warm. To test for doneness, insert a metal skewer into the center of the bone; there should be no resistance when it is inserted, and some of the marrow will have started to leak from the bones.

4. Meanwhile, heat the Paleo fat in a large cast-iron skillet over medium-high heat. Fry the mushrooms and onions in the skillet until the mushrooms are soft. Season with half of the salt and pepper, then remove from the pan.

5. Place the ground beef in a mixing bowl and sprinkle it with the fish sauce. Using your hands, mix the meat and fish sauce together to evenly distribute the sauce, then form the meat into four ¾-inch-thick patties. Season the outsides of the patties with the remaining salt and pepper.

6. When the marrow is nearly done, fry the burgers on both sides in the skillet over medium-high heat until cooked to your desired doneness (see the chart at left). Remove from the pan and set aside.

7. Split the buns in half and fry them in the leftover fat in the skillet until golden brown. Scoop the marrow from the marrow bones with a small spoon.

8. Serve the burgers on the fried buns with lettuce leaves, if desired, and topped with the marrow and fried mushrooms and onions. Garnish the plates with cornichons. These burgers are best served fresh.

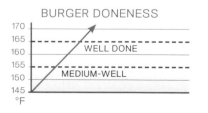

BURGER DONENESS

| °F | |
|---|---|
| 170 | |
| 165 | |
| 160 | WELL DONE |
| 155 | |
| 150 | MEDIUM-WELL |
| 145 | |

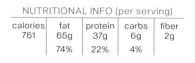

NUTRITIONAL INFO (per serving)

| calories | fat | protein | carbs | fiber |
|---|---|---|---|---|
| 761 | 65g | 37g | 6g | 2g |
| | 74% | 22% | 4% | |

# sloppy joes

1 pound 80% lean ground beef

2 tablespoons chopped onions

1 stalk celery, chopped

1 clove garlic, minced

¾ cup water or beef bone broth, homemade (page 108) or store-bought

¼ cup tomato paste

2 tablespoons Swerve confectioners'-style sweetener or equivalent amount of liquid or powdered sweetener (see page 81)

1½ teaspoons coconut vinegar

½ teaspoon prepared yellow mustard

½ teaspoon fine sea salt

⅛ teaspoon fresh ground black pepper

4 Keto Buns (page 256), split and fried in fat until golden brown, or lettuce leaves, for serving

1. In a large sauté pan, brown the ground beef with the onions, celery, and garlic for about 8 minutes; drain the fat. Stir in the remaining ingredients. Simmer on low heat for 20 minutes to allow the flavors to open up and the sauce to thicken.

2. Serve on keto buns or in lettuce wraps. Store extras in an airtight container in the fridge for up to 5 days, or freeze for up to a month.

note: *Because this recipe is slightly sweetened, it's best to avoid it while you're adapting to the keto lifestyle and trying to curb your sweet tooth.*

busy family tip: *I usually make a double batch of this recipe and store the second batch in the freezer with a batch of keto buns for easy weekday meals.*

NUTRITIONAL INFO (per serving)

| calories | fat | protein | carbs | fiber |
|---|---|---|---|---|
| 299 | 23g | 20g | 3g | 1g |
| | 69% | 27% | 4% | |

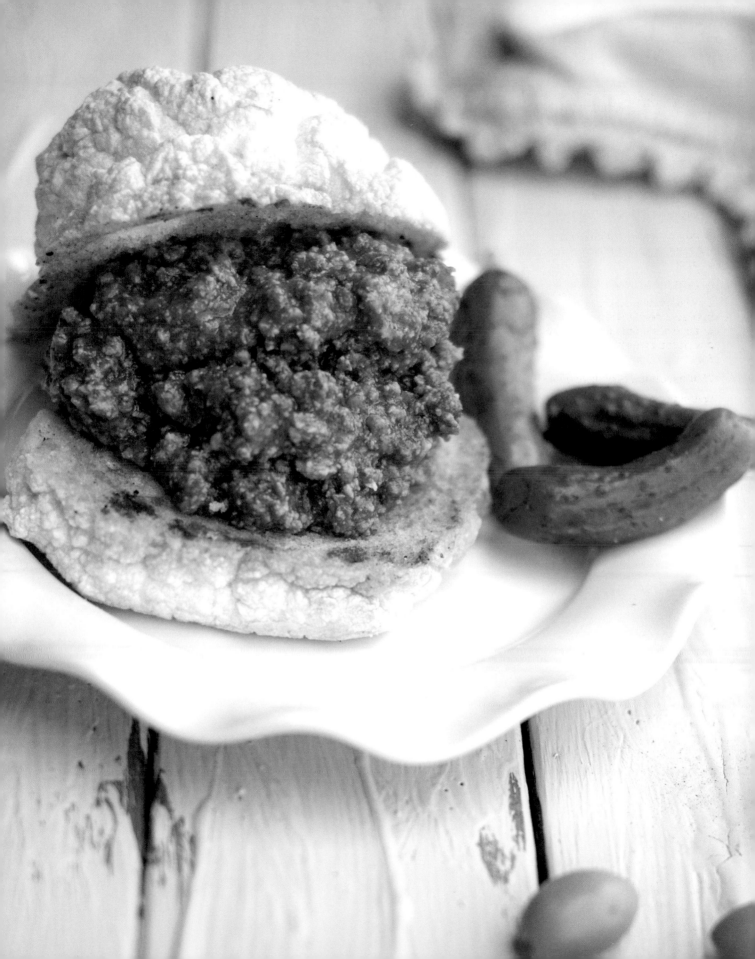

# reuben meatballs

L M H KETO · prep time: 10 minutes (not including time to make the dressing)
cook time: 35 minutes • yield: 8 servings

Using a very hot oven results in meatballs that are crispy outside and tender inside. Adding a little water or other liquid to the meatball mixture helps bind the fat to the meatballs when cooking, which creates a moist cooked meatball. Here I've used a couple tablespoons of sauerkraut juice to add both moisture and flavor.

1 tablespoon coconut oil

¼ cup chopped onions

1 clove garlic, minced

1 teaspoon fine sea salt

1 pound corned beef, finely diced

1 pound ground pork

1¼ cups sauerkraut, finely chopped and excess moisture squeezed out

2 tablespoons sauerkraut juice

1 teaspoon caraway seeds

1 large egg

Sauerkraut, warmed, for serving

Dairy-Free Thousand Island Dressing (page 118), for serving

Finely chopped purple cabbage, for garnish

1. Preheat the oven to 425°F.

2. Heat the oil in a skillet over medium heat. Add the onions and garlic and season them with the salt; cook until the onions are translucent, about 5 minutes. Transfer the onion mixture to a small bowl and set aside to cool.

3. Combine the corned beef, ground pork, sauerkraut, sauerkraut juice, caraway seeds, and egg in a large mixing bowl. When the onion mixture is no longer hot to the touch, add it to the bowl with the meat and work everything together with your hands.

4. Shape the meat mixture into 2-inch balls and place on a rimmed baking sheet. Bake for 30 minutes, or until cooked through.

5. Serve the meatballs on a bed of sauerkraut, drizzled with Thousand Island dressing and sprinkled with purple cabbage. This dish is best served fresh, but extras can be stored in an airtight container in the fridge for up to 5 days or frozen for up to a month.

NUTRITIONAL INFO (per serving)

| calories | fat | protein | carbs | fiber |
|----------|-----|---------|-------|-------|
| 303 | 22g | 26g | 2g | 0.3g |
| | 64% | 33% | 3% | |

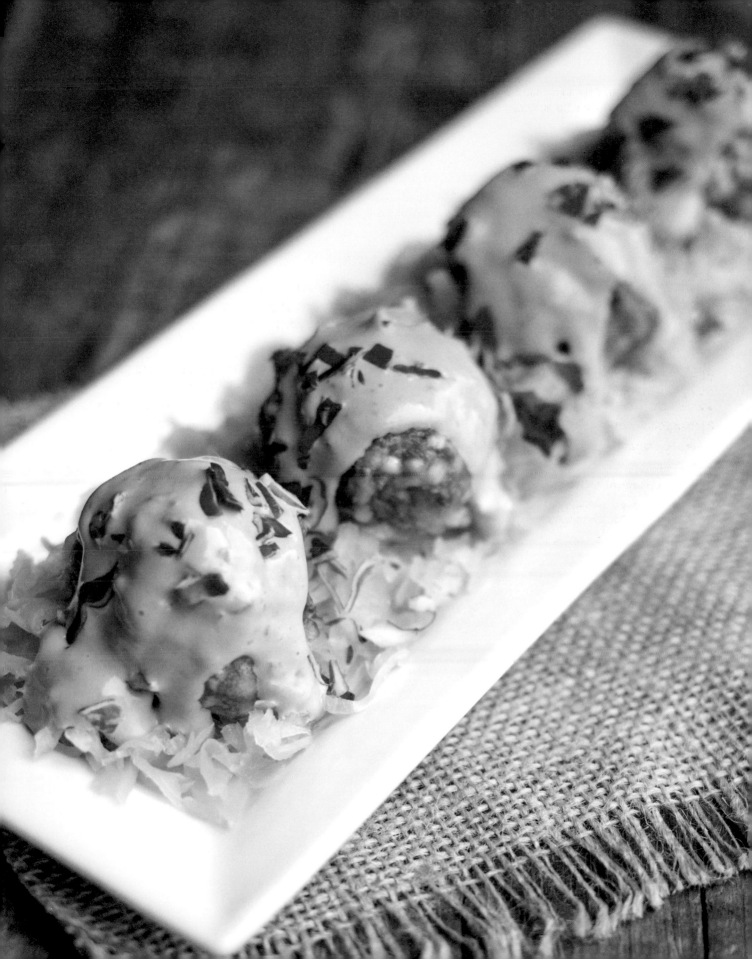

# spicy mexican meatballs

prep time: 10 minutes (not including time to make the dressing)
cook time: 35 minutes • yield: 8 servings

1 tablespoon coconut oil

¼ cup chopped onions

2 cloves garlic, minced

1 jalapeño pepper, seeded and finely chopped

1 teaspoon fine sea salt

2 pounds 80% lean ground beef or 1 pound each ground beef and ground pork (see note)

1 cup finely chopped mushrooms

½ teaspoon ground cumin

1 large egg

Lettuce leaves, for serving

Creamy Mexican Dressing (page 116), for serving

Lime wedges, for serving

1. Preheat the oven to 350°F.

2. Heat the oil in a skillet over medium heat. Add the onions, garlic, and jalapeño and season them with the salt; cook until the onions are translucent, about 5 minutes. Transfer the onion mixture to a small bowl and set aside to cool.

3. Put the ground beef, chopped mushrooms, cumin, and egg in a mixing bowl. When the onion mixture is no longer hot to the touch, add it to the bowl with the meat and work everything together with your hands.

4. Shape the meat mixture into 2-inch balls and place them on a rimmed baking sheet. Bake for 30 minutes, or until cooked through.

5. Place the meatballs on lettuce leaves and drizzle with the dressing. Serve with lime wedges.

6. The meatballs are best served fresh, but extras can be stored in an airtight container in the fridge for up to 5 days or frozen for up to a month.

note: *Because ground pork contains more fat than ground beef, using a 50/50 combination of ground pork and ground beef results in a more keto recipe than using all ground beef.*

NUTRITIONAL INFO (per serving)

| calories | fat | protein | carbs | fiber |
|----------|-----|---------|-------|-------|
| 318 | 25g | 21g | 2g | 1g |
| | 71% | 26% | 3% | |

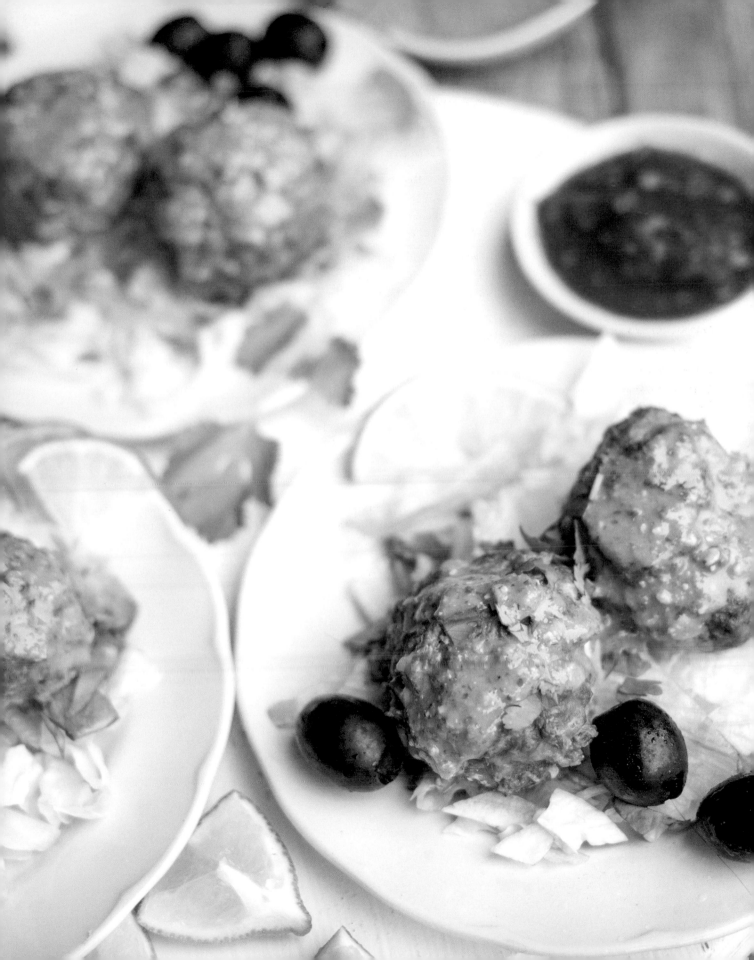

# herbes de florence meatballs

L M H KETO / prep time: 10 minutes (not including time to make the sauce)
cook time: 30 minutes • yield: 8 servings

The trick to getting moist meatballs is to either add a little liquid to the meatball mixture or include an ingredient that releases water, like mushrooms. In this recipe, the mushrooms not only help keep the meatballs moist but also add umami flavor, which makes for very tasty meatballs. The trick to getting meatballs with a crispy exterior and a tender, moist interior is to use a high-heat oven, as here. I like to serve these meatballs over Zoodles (page 262) or with a side salad.

1 tablespoon coconut oil or avocado oil

¼ cup chopped onions

1 teaspoon fine sea salt

2 pounds 80% lean ground beef or 1 pound each ground beef and ground pork (see note)

1 cup finely chopped mushrooms

1 large egg

2 teaspoons Herbes de Florence (page 113) or Italian seasoning

Herbes de Florence Red Sauce (page 130), for serving

Fresh basil leaves, for garnish

1. Preheat the oven to 425°F.

2. Heat the oil in a skillet over medium heat. Add the onions and season them with the salt; cook until the onions are translucent, about 5 minutes. Transfer the onions to a small bowl and set aside to cool.

3. Put the ground beef, mushrooms, egg, and Herbes de Florence in a mixing bowl. When the onions are no longer hot to the touch, add them to the bowl with the meat and work everything together with your hands.

4. Shape the meat mixture into 2-inch balls and place them on a rimmed baking sheet. Bake for 22 to 25 minutes, until cooked through.

5. Meanwhile, gently warm the red sauce in a saucepan over medium-low heat.

6. When the meatballs are ready to come out of the oven, pour the red sauce into a serving bowl. Remove the meatballs from the oven and place them in the bowl with the sauce. Garnish with fresh basil leaves. These meatballs are best served fresh, but extras can be stored in an airtight container in the fridge for up to 5 days or frozen for up to a month.

note: *Because ground pork contains more fat than ground beef, using a 50/50 combination of ground pork and ground beef results in a more keto recipe than using all ground beef.*

NUTRITIONAL INFO (per serving)

| calories | fat | protein | carbs | fiber |
|----------|-----|---------|-------|-------|
| 355 | 28g | 22g | 4g | 1g |
|  | 71% | 25% | 4% |  |

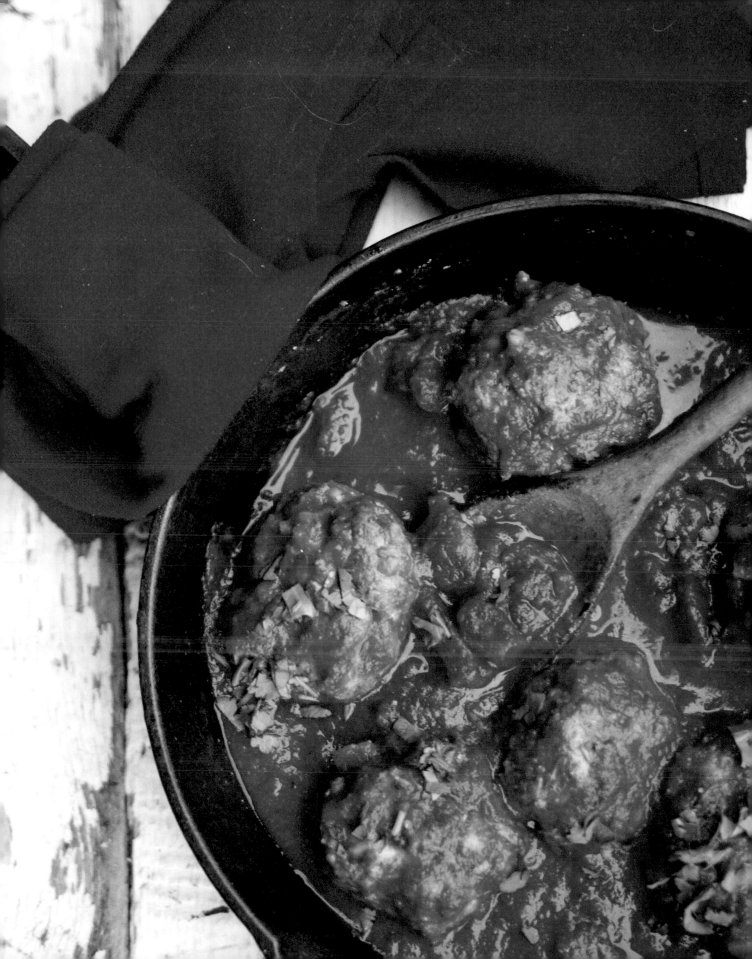

# slow cooker short rib and chorizo stew

L M H
KETO prep time: 10 minutes • cook time: 4½ hours • yield: 12 servings

1 pound bone-in short ribs

1 (20-ounce) box diced tomatoes with juices, or 3 tomatoes, chopped, with juices

1 cup tomato sauce

¼ cup chopped onions

1 red bell pepper, chopped

2 green chiles, chopped

½ cup beef bone broth, homemade (page 108) or store-bought

2 teaspoons minced garlic

2 tablespoons chili powder

2 teaspoons dried oregano leaves

1 teaspoon ground cumin

½ teaspoon cayenne pepper

½ teaspoon paprika

½ teaspoon fine sea salt

½ teaspoon fresh ground black pepper

4 slices bacon, diced

1 pound 80% lean ground beef

1 pound Mexican-style fresh (raw) chorizo, removed from casings

**for garnish:**

Sliced green onions

Chopped fresh cilantro

Lime wedges

1. Place the short ribs in a 4-quart (or larger) slow cooker. Pour in the diced tomatoes and tomato sauce. Add the onions, red bell pepper, chiles, and beef broth. Season with the garlic, chili powder, oregano, cumin, cayenne pepper, paprika, salt, and black pepper. Stir to combine, then cover. Cook on low until the meat is falling off the bone, about 4 hours.

2. When the ribs are nearly done, cook the rest of the meat on the stovetop: Heat a large sauté pan over medium-high heat. Fry the diced bacon in the pan until crispy, then remove the bacon from the pan and set aside, leaving the fat in the pan. Crumble the ground beef and chorizo into the hot pan and cook until evenly browned. Remove the pan from the heat.

3. When the ribs are done, remove them from the slow cooker and place them in a large bowl or casserole dish (to catch the juices as you work). Remove the meat from the bones, discard the bones, then shred the meat using two forks. Return the shredded meat and any juices to the slow cooker. Add the ground beef, chorizo, and bacon. Cover and cook on low for at least 20 minutes, then taste and add more salt, pepper, or chili powder, if desired. The longer the stew simmers, the better it will taste.

4. Serve garnished with sliced green onions and chopped cilantro, with lime wedges on the side. Store extras in an airtight container in the fridge for up to 4 days.

tip: *When using a slow cooker, do not be tempted to stir! Every time you remove the lid, you add about 20 minutes to the cooking time because you are releasing a lot of heat and moisture.*

NUTRITIONAL INFO (per serving)

| calories | fat | protein | carbs | fiber |
|---|---|---|---|---|
| 411 | 31g | 25g | 7g | 2g |
| | 68% | 25% | 7% | |

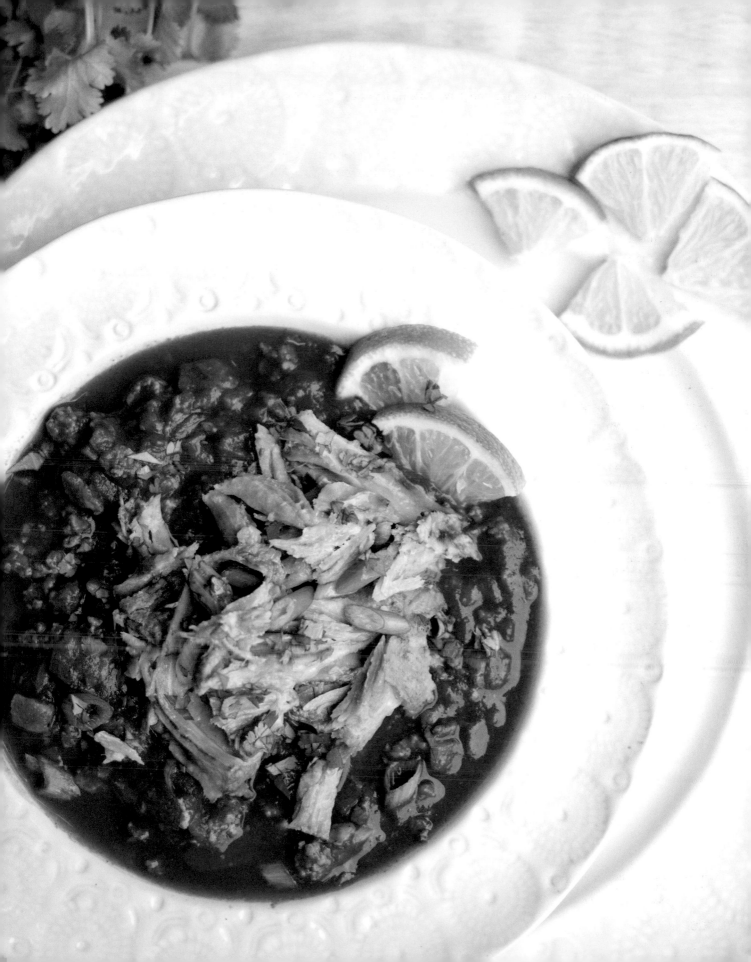

# slow cooker ropa vieja

L M H KETO · prep time: 15 minutes · cook time: 6 hours · yield: 6 servings

This is also known as Cuban shredded beef. I find that using brisket instead of the traditional flank steak works better—it has more collagen to keep it moist and is less chewy. I add anchovies to give it extra umami flavor. Don't worry, you won't even know they're in there!

1 red bell pepper, sliced ½ inch thick

1 green bell pepper, sliced ½ inch thick

½ cup thinly sliced onions

1 jalapeño pepper, thinly sliced (with seeds)

1 (2-ounce) can anchovies, chopped

1 large tomato, diced

½ cup beef bone broth, home-made (page 108) or store-bought

¼ cup tomato sauce

1 tablespoon coconut or apple cider vinegar

2 teaspoons minced garlic

2 teaspoons dried oregano leaves

2 teaspoons ground cumin

2 pounds beef brisket, cut across the grain into 2-inch-long strips

1 teaspoon fine sea salt

3 tablespoons chopped green olives

## for garnish:

Chopped fresh cilantro

Pitted whole green olives

Lime wedges or slices

Salsa

1. Place the bell peppers, onions, and jalapeño pepper on the bottom of a 6-quart slow cooker. Top with the anchovies, diced tomato, broth, tomato sauce, vinegar, garlic, oregano, and cumin. Add the brisket slices and sprinkle them with the salt.

2. Cover and cook on low for 6 hours, or until the brisket is falling apart and shreds easily. Shred the brisket with two forks, then stir in the olives.

3. Transfer the meat to a serving platter and garnish with cilantro, green olives, lime wedges, and a large spoonful of salsa.

| NUTRITIONAL INFO (per serving) | | | | |
|---|---|---|---|---|
| calories | fat | protein | carbs | fiber |
| 397 | 29g | 29g | 5g | 1g |
| | 66% | 29% | 5% | |

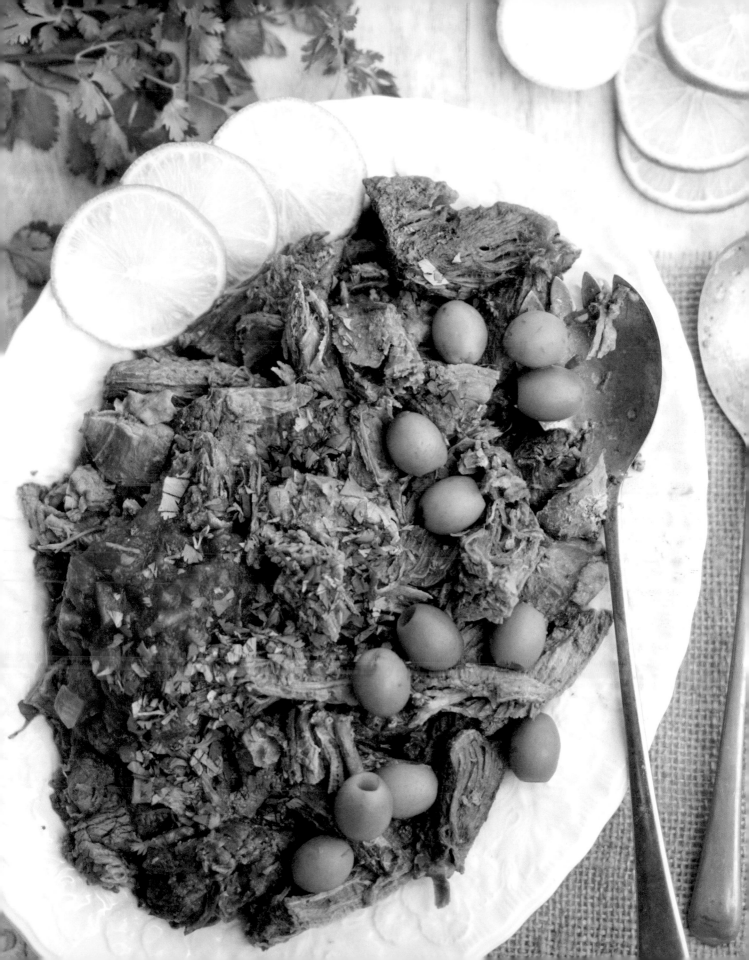

# chili-stuffed peppers

L M H T KETO

prep time: 10 minutes (not including time to cook the bacon) • cook time: 2 hours 10 minutes
yield: 12 servings (½ stuffed pepper per serving)

2 pounds 80% lean ground beef

1 pound Italian sausage, hot or sweet, removed from casings

2 (26-ounce) boxes diced tomatoes with juices

1 (6-ounce) jar tomato paste

1 large yellow onion, chopped

3 stalks celery, chopped

1 red bell pepper, chopped

1 green bell pepper, chopped

2 green chiles, chopped

4 slices bacon, fried until crispy and crumbled

1 cup beef bone broth, homemade (page 108) or store-bought

¼ cup chili powder

1 tablespoon minced garlic

1 tablespoon dried oregano leaves

2 teaspoons ground cumin

2 teaspoons hot sauce, homemade (page 134) or store-bought

1 teaspoon dried basil

1 teaspoon cayenne pepper

1 teaspoon paprika

1 teaspoon fine sea salt

1 teaspoon ground fresh black pepper

3 tablespoons Swerve confectioners'-style sweetener or equivalent amount of liquid or powdered sweetener (see page 81) (optional)

6 bell peppers, any color

1. Preheat a stockpot over medium-high heat. Crumble the ground beef and sausage into the hot pot and cook until evenly browned, about 8 minutes, stirring frequently to break up the meat.

2. Pour in the diced tomatoes and tomato paste. Add the onion, celery, chopped bell peppers, chiles, crumbled bacon, and beef broth. Season with the chili powder, garlic, oregano, cumin, hot sauce, basil, cayenne pepper, paprika, salt, black pepper, and sweetener, if using. Stir to blend, then cover and simmer over low heat for at least 2 hours, stirring occasionally. After 2 hours, taste and add more salt, pepper, or chili powder, if desired. The longer the chili simmers, the better it will taste.

3. When you're ready to serve the chili, slice the 6 bell peppers in half lengthwise and remove the cores and seeds. You can serve the peppers raw, blanch them, or bake them.

   *To blanch:* Bring a large pot of water to a boil. Blanch the peppers in the boiling water for 3 minutes. Drain the peppers in a colander and rinse with ice-cold water (this will preserve the bright color).

   *To bake:* If you'd like to soften the peppers, bake in a 350°F oven until tender, about 20 minutes.

4. Serve the chili in the peppers, or cover and refrigerate for up to 4 days or freeze for up to a month.

note: *Since we also eat with our eyes, I love to make food fun for my family. Here's how to make your peppers into jack-o'-lanterns, as shown: After Step 2, when the chili is ready to serve, carve the top off each pepper, as you would a pumpkin. Scrape out the seeds and ribs. Using a small sharp knife, carve eyes, a nose, and a mouth in the pepper. Blanch the peppers or bake to soften as in Step 3, or leave raw. Fill each pepper with chili and serve, or refrigerate or freeze as in Step 4.*

NUTRITIONAL INFO (per serving)

| calories | fat | protein | carbs | fiber |
|----------|-----|---------|-------|-------|
| 385 | 27g | 23g | 10g | 4g |
|  | 63% | 24% | 13% |  |

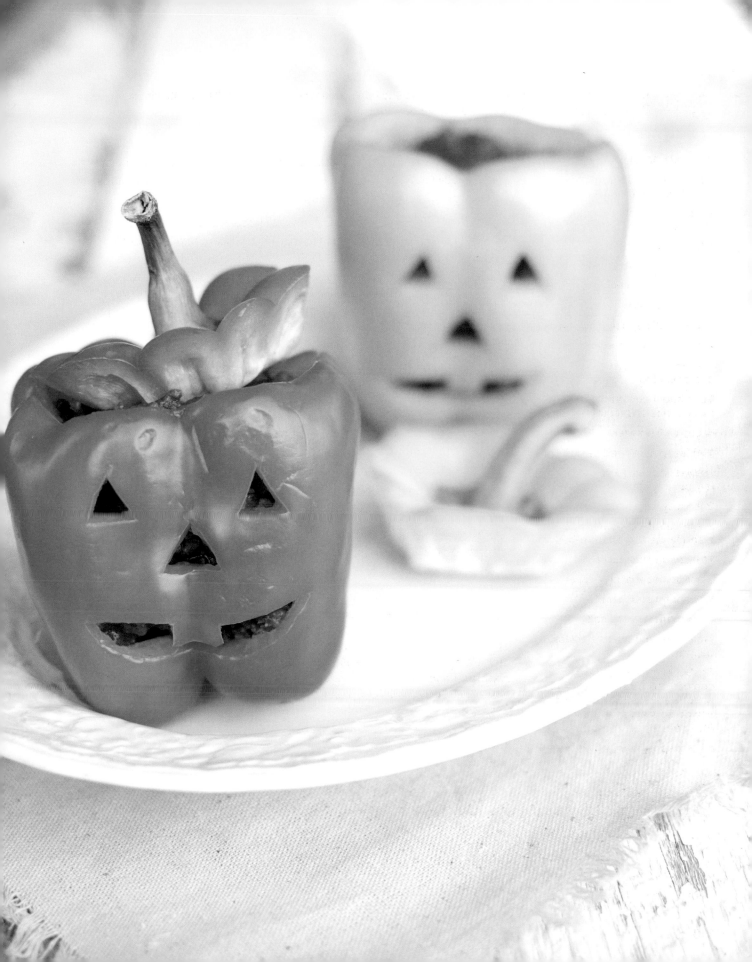

# slow cooker mole short ribs

LÂH KETO  prep time: 5 minutes • cook time: 6 to 8 hours • yield: 8 servings

This recipe uses the same mole sauce that's included in the sauces chapter. The difference is that the sauce in the sauces chapter is made on the stovetop, while this recipe has the slow cooker do the work for you—so you can make the entire meal in one step and in one pot. If you already have a batch of mole sauce made, you can use it here. Simply pour the prepared sauce into the slow cooker, add the ribs, and start cooking.

**mole sauce:**

2 tablespoons MCT oil

¼ cup finely chopped onions

1 clove garlic, minced

1 tablespoon chopped fresh cilantro

1 tablespoon unsweetened cocoa powder

1 teaspoon ground cumin

1 cup tomato sauce

1 (4-ounce) can diced green chiles

8 bone-in beef short ribs (4 pounds)

1. Place the ingredients for the sauce in a 4-quart (or larger) slow cooker. Stir to combine.

2. Place the short ribs in the slow cooker, arranging them in a single layer. Cover and cook on low for 6 to 8 hours, until the meat is tender and easily pulls away from the bone.

3. Transfer the short ribs to serving plates. Serve with the sauce. Store extras in an airtight container in the fridge for up to 4 days.

NUTRITIONAL INFO (per serving)

| calories | fat | protein | carbs | fiber |
|---|---|---|---|---|
| 612 | 54g | 27g | 4g | 1g |
| | 80% | 17% | 3% | |

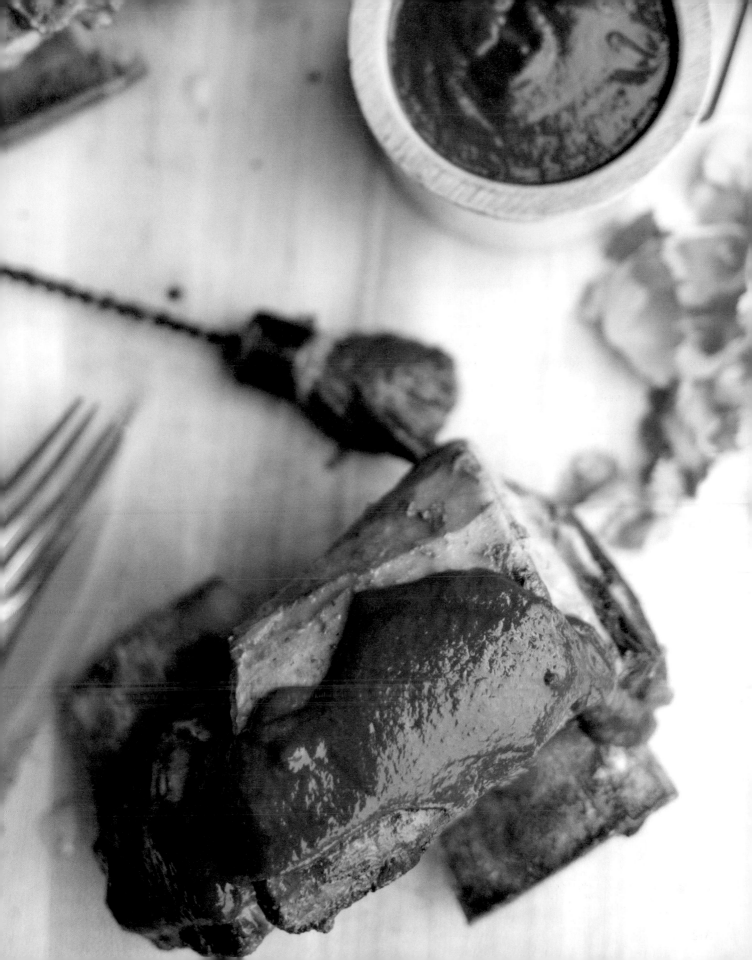

# texts beef sausage

KETO
prep time: 20 minutes, plus 3 to 4 hours to chill the meat, soak the casings, and rest the sausage • cook time: 10 minutes • yield: 12 sausages (1 per serving)

½ pound pork fatback

½ cup coconut vinegar

6 feet medium hog casings

2½ pounds 80% lean ground beef

⅓ cup ice-cold beef bone broth, homemade (page 108) or store-bought

3 cloves garlic, crushed to a paste

2 tablespoons smoked paprika

1 tablespoon whole mustard seeds

1 tablespoon fine ground sea salt

1 tablespoon fresh ground black pepper

1½ teaspoons cayenne pepper

1½ teaspoons red pepper flakes

½ teaspoon ground bay leaves

¼ teaspoon whole anise seeds

¼ teaspoon ground coriander

¼ teaspoon ground dried thyme

Lard or coconut oil, for cooking

Keto dipping sauce(s) of choice, such as Garlic and Herb Aioli (page 128) or Dairy-Free Ranch Dressing (page 115), for serving

## special equipment:

Meat grinder (or grinder attachment on stand mixer)

Sausage stuffer (optional)

1. Line a rimmed baking sheet with parchment paper. Cut the fatback into 1-inch cubes and spread out on the baking sheet. Freeze for 1 hour.

2. Fill a large bowl with the coconut vinegar and 2 quarts of water. Soak the casings in the liquid for 30 minutes.

3. Remove the fatback from the freezer and grind it using the coarse disk of a meat grinder (I use my KitchenAid food grinder attachment).

4. In a large bowl, place the ground pork fat, ground beef, broth, garlic, paprika, mustard seeds, salt, black pepper, cayenne pepper, red pepper flakes, ground bay leaves, anise seeds, coriander, and thyme; mix everything together until it's evenly combined. Cook up a small dab in a skillet over medium heat so that you can taste the sausage. Add more seasoning, if desired, before stuffing the casings.

5. Load a sausage stuffer (I used my KitchenAid sausage stuffer attachment) with the presoaked casings and stuff the sausages by pushing the meat mixture through the attachment. Twist the sausages into links about 5 inches in length. *Note:* If you do not have a sausage stuffer, you can form the meat into 12 large patties.

6. Refrigerate the sausages for a few hours to allow the flavors to meld. Cook within 3 days.

7. To cook the sausages, melt 1 tablespoon of lard or coconut oil in a large skillet over medium heat. Poke a few small holes into each sausage link. Cook the sausages for 10 minutes, until the internal temperature reaches 160°F. Serve with the keto dipping sauces of your choice. The cooked sausages will keep in an airtight container in the fridge for up to 5 days or in the freezer for up to a month.

## tips for making sausage:

Liquid is needed to bind protein to fat. The more liquid you add, the more fat you can add.

For great flavor and added nutrients, homemade bone broth is best for the liquid. But good-quality store-bought broth will work.

If the sausage pops out of the casing when you bite into it, you cooked it too fast and at too high a heat.

Use cold meat and fat when making sausage, so it won't turn mushy. (In fact, commercial sausage makers often add dry ice to the meat to keep it cold.) After cubing the meat, either place it in the freezer for 1 hour or refrigerate it for 4 hours or overnight before grinding. After grinding, place the bowl in the freezer for 30 minutes to keep meat cold while stuffing.

busy family tip: *Make a double batch and freeze for easy meals.*

NUTRITIONAL INFO
(per 4½-ounce sausage)

| calories | fat | protein | carbs | fiber |
|---|---|---|---|---|
| 377 | 32g | 18g | 4g | 1g |
|  | 77% | 19% | 4% |  |

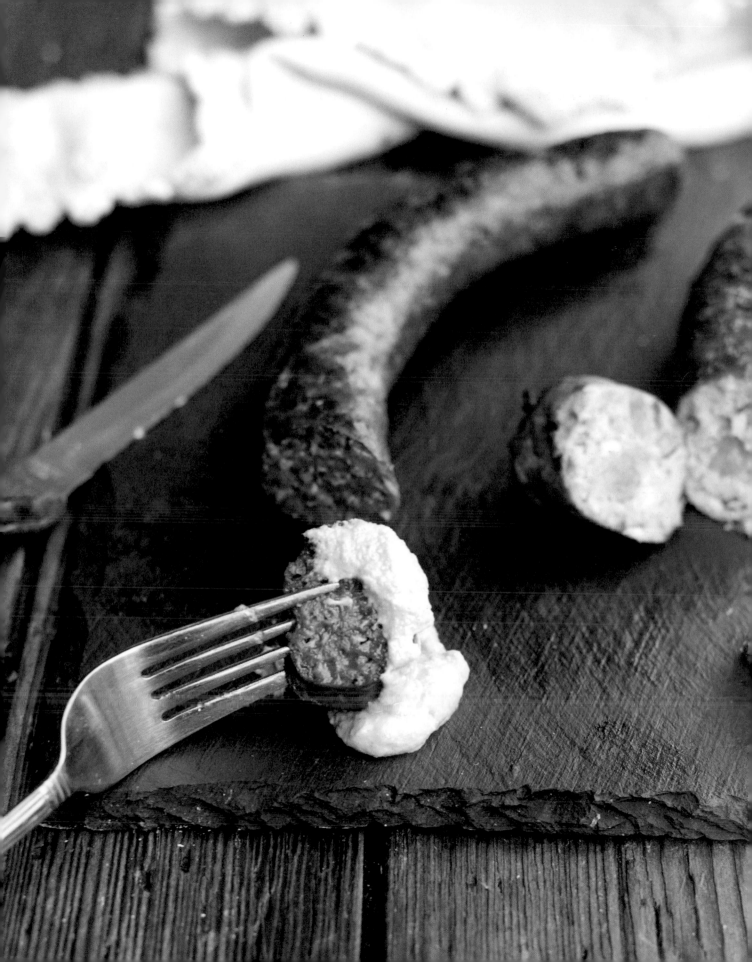

# deconstructed BLT filet mignons

prep time: 5 minutes (not including time to make the dressing)
cook time: 10 minutes • yield: 2 servings

1 tablespoon Paleo fat, such as lard, coconut oil, or avocado oil

2 (4-ounce) filet mignons

1½ teaspoons fine sea salt

½ teaspoon fresh ground black pepper

2 slices bacon

2 tablespoons minced shallots

¼ cup Bacon Marmalade (page 122), for serving

**salad:**

2 cups mixed greens

4 cherry tomatoes, cut in half

¼ cup Onion-Infused Dressing (page 120)

1. Heat a cast-iron skillet over medium-high heat; once hot, place the fat in the pan. While the pan is heating, prepare the filets: Pat the filets dry and season them well with the salt and pepper. Wrap a piece of bacon around the sides of each filet and secure with a toothpick.

2. When the fat is hot, place the bacon-wrapped filets and shallots in the pan and sear for 3 minutes, then flip them over and sear the other side for 3 minutes. Remove from the skillet for a rare filet, or continue to cook until done to your liking (see the chart below). Thicker filets will take longer. Using tongs, hold the filets on their sides to cook the bacon, rolling them to cook the bacon all the way around.

3. Remove the filets from the pan and set aside on a cutting board to rest while you prepare the salad.

4. Place the greens and tomatoes in a bowl and toss lightly with the dressing.

5. Place the filets on plates and top each with 2 tablespoons of Bacon Marmalade. Serve the salad on the side.

busy family tip: *For easy additions to meals, my fridge door is always filled with homemade dressings and sauces, two of which are Bacon Marmalade (page 122) and the Onion-Infused Dressing (page 120) used here.*

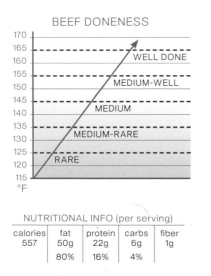

BEEF DONENESS

| °F | |
|---|---|
| 170 | |
| 165 | |
| 160 | WELL DONE |
| 155 | |
| 150 | MEDIUM-WELL |
| 145 | |
| 140 | MEDIUM |
| 135 | |
| 130 | MEDIUM-RARE |
| 125 | |
| 120 | RARE |
| 115 | |

NUTRITIONAL INFO (per serving)

| calories | fat | protein | carbs | fiber |
|---|---|---|---|---|
| 557 | 50g | 22g | 6g | 1g |
| | 80% | 16% | 4% | |

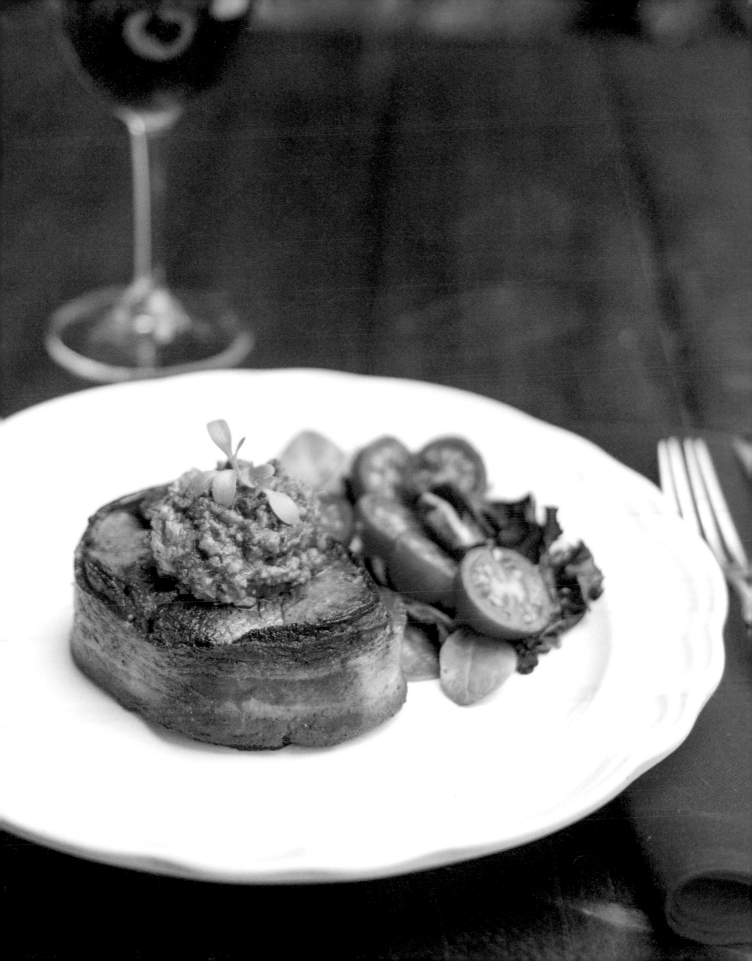

# steak au poivre for two

L ↻ H KETO · prep time: 5 minutes · cook time: 15 minutes · yield: 2 servings

¼ cup plus 1 tablespoon Paleo fat, such as lard, coconut oil, or avocado oil, divided

1 (8-ounce) rib-eye steak

1 tablespoon coarsely ground black peppercorns, plus more for garnish (optional)

1½ teaspoons fine sea salt

2 tablespoons chopped green onions or shallots

¼ cup beef bone broth, home-made (page 108) or store-bought

¼ cup full-fat coconut milk

1. Heat a cast-iron skillet over medium-high heat; once hot, place 1 tablespoon of the fat in the pan. While the pan is heating, prepare the steak: Pat the steak dry and season it well with the pepper and salt.

2. When the fat is hot, place the steak in the pan and sear for 3 minutes, then flip it over and sear the other side for 3 minutes. Remove from the skillet for a rare steak, or continue to cook until done to your liking (see the chart below). Thicker steaks will take longer.

3. When done to your liking, remove the steak from the pan and set on a cutting board to rest while you make the sauce. Leave the drippings in the pan.

4. Add the green onions to the pan and sauté over medium heat in the reserved drippings for 2 minutes. Add the remaining ¼ cup of fat and, using a whisk, scrape up the brown bits from the bottom of the pan. Add the broth and coconut milk and simmer for 5 minutes, whisking often. Once thickened a bit, remove from the heat.

5. Cut the steak into ½-inch slices. Place on a serving platter and pour the sauce over the steak. Garnish with coarsely ground peppercorns, if desired.

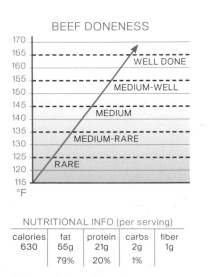

BEEF DONENESS

| °F | |
|---|---|
| 170 | |
| 165 | |
| 160 | WELL DONE |
| 155 | |
| 150 | MEDIUM-WELL |
| 145 | |
| 140 | MEDIUM |
| 135 | |
| 130 | MEDIUM-RARE |
| 125 | |
| 120 | RARE |
| 115 | |

NUTRITIONAL INFO (per serving)

| calories | fat | protein | carbs | fiber |
|---|---|---|---|---|
| 630 | 55g | 21g | 2g | 1g |
| | 79% | 20% | 1% | |

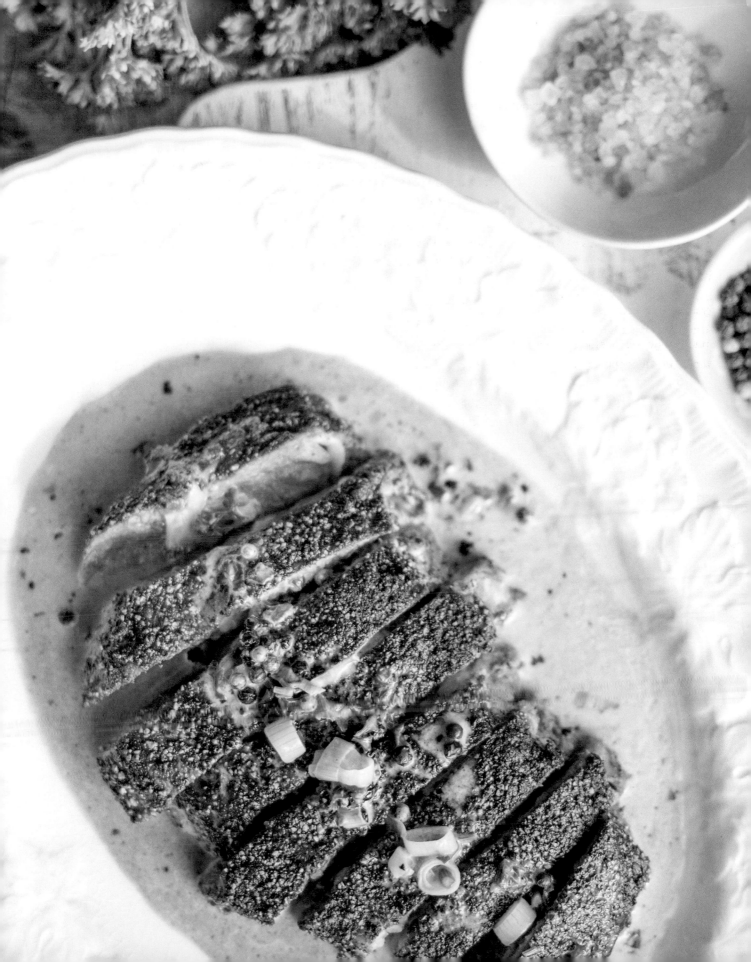

# steak diane

L M H KETO  prep time: 10 minutes • cook time: 15 minutes • yield: 4 servings

4 tablespoons Paleo fat, such as lard, coconut oil, or avocado oil, divided

4 (4-ounce) beef or venison tenderloins

1¼ teaspoons fine sea salt, plus more for the sauce

½ teaspoon fresh ground black pepper, plus more for the sauce

¼ cup minced shallots or onions

1 teaspoon minced garlic

½ pound button mushrooms, sliced ¼ inch thick (small mushrooms can be left whole)

¼ cup beef bone broth, home-made (page 108) or store-bought

¼ cup full-fat coconut milk

2 teaspoons Dijon mustard

1. Heat a cast-iron skillet over medium-high heat; once hot, place 1 tablespoon of the fat in the pan. While the pan is heating, prepare the tenderloins: Pat the tenderloins dry and season them well with the salt and pepper.

2. When the fat is hot, place the tenderloins in the skillet and sear for 3 minutes, then flip them over and sear for another 3 minutes. Remove from the skillet for rare meat, or continue to cook until done to your liking (see the chart below). Allow to rest for 10 minutes before slicing or serving.

3. While the meat is resting, make the pan sauce: Add the remaining 3 tablespoons of fat to the pan, then add the shallots, garlic, and mushrooms, season with a couple pinches each of salt and pepper, and sauté until the mushrooms are golden brown on both sides, about 6 minutes. (Add the mushrooms to the pan in batches if necessary to avoid overcrowding.) Pour in the broth and, using a whisk, scrape up the brown bits from the bottom of the pan to incorporate them into the sauce. Add the coconut milk and mustard, stir to combine, and heat until simmering. Simmer over low heat until thickened, about 3 minutes. Season to taste with salt and pepper.

4. Serve the steaks with the sauce.

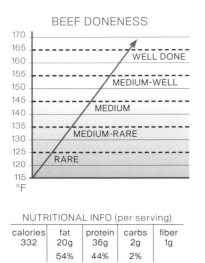

BEEF DONENESS

| °F | |
|---|---|
| 170 | |
| 165 | |
| 160 | WELL DONE |
| 155 | |
| 150 | MEDIUM-WELL |
| 145 | |
| 140 | MEDIUM |
| 135 | |
| 130 | MEDIUM-RARE |
| 125 | |
| 120 | RARE |
| 115 | |

NUTRITIONAL INFO (per serving)

| calories | fat | protein | carbs | fiber |
|---|---|---|---|---|
| 332 | 20g | 36g | 2g | 1g |
| | 54% | 44% | 2% | |

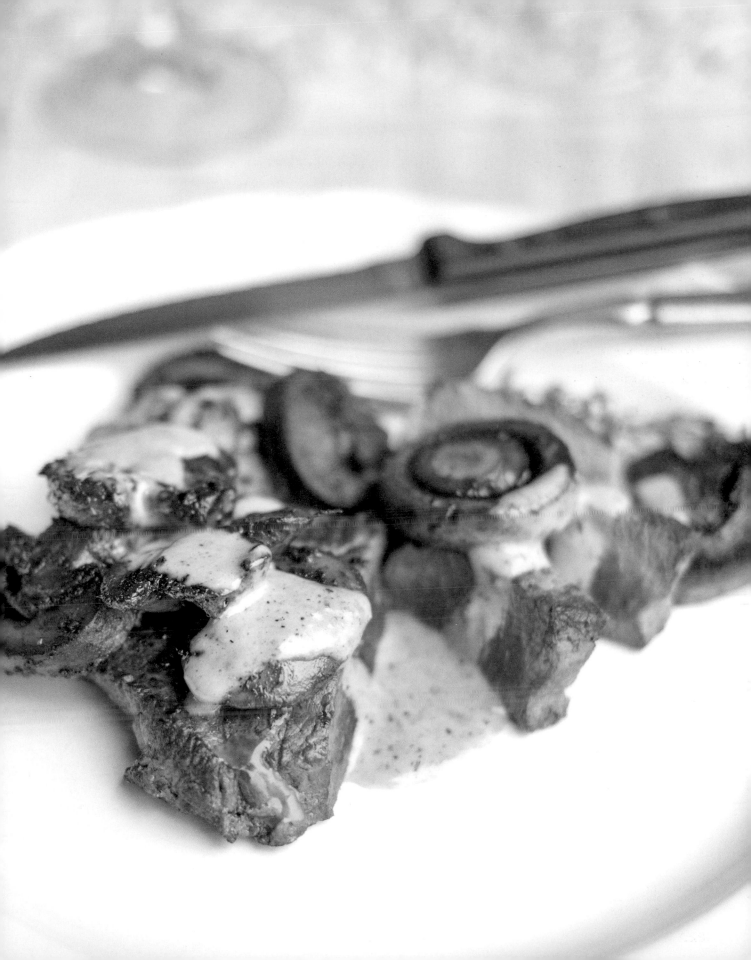

# hunan beef–stuffed peppers

L M H KETO ▢ ⊘ ⊘ prep time: 7 minutes, plus 2 hours to marinate the beef • cook time: 15 minutes • yield: 4 servings

## marinade:

½ cup beef bone broth, home-made (page 108) or store-bought (see notes)

¼ cup coconut aminos or wheat-free tamari

3 tablespoons MCT oil

1 tablespoon minced garlic

1 tablespoon grated fresh ginger

1 tablespoon fresh ground black pepper

1 teaspoon fish sauce (optional, for umami)

4 dried Thai chiles

¼ teaspoon guar gum (optional; see notes)

1 pound flank steak, sliced very thinly against the grain

2 bell peppers, any color, cored and cut in half lengthwise, for serving (see notes)

¼ cup coconut oil

½ cup thinly sliced onions

1 red bell pepper, cut into thin strips

1 green bell pepper, cut into thin strips

Fine sea salt, as needed

1. Place the ingredients for the marinade, except for the guar gum, in a shallow bowl. Give them a stir to combine, then add the steak to the marinade and toss to coat well. Cover and refrigerate for at least 2 hours and up to overnight.

2. Remove the beef and reserve the marinade. If you used store-bought beef broth in the marinade, sift the guar gum into the marinade. (It will help thicken the sauce as it cooks.)

3. To blanch the peppers, bring a large pot of water to a boil. Blanch the peppers in the boiling water for 3 minutes. Drain the peppers in a colander and rinse with ice-cold water (this will preserve their bright color).

4. Heat a wok or large skillet over high heat, then put the coconut oil in the wok. When the oil is hot, sear the slices of beef for 10 seconds, then remove from the pan and set aside.

5. Place the onions and bell peppers in the hot oil and stir-fry for 5 minutes. Add the beef and marinade, bring to a boil, and cook until the marinade has thickened, 5 to 7 minutes. Taste and add salt, if needed.

6. Serve the stir-fry in the blanched bell pepper halves. Store extras in an airtight container in the fridge for up to 5 days or in the freezer for up to a month.

notes: *Homemade beef bone broth is preferred for this recipe because it naturally creates a thick sauce. If you use store-bought broth, you will need to add a small amount of guar gum to thicken the sauce.*

*I cut the bell peppers into decorative designs for a cute holiday photo, but most days I keep it simple and serve the stir-fry in bell pepper "bowls," or halved peppers, as described above. To save a step, you can omit the blanched peppers and eat the stir-fry as is.*

NUTRITIONAL INFO (per serving)

| calories | fat | protein | carbs | fiber |
|----------|-----|---------|-------|-------|
| 480 | 34g | 27g | 17g | 7g |
| | 64% | 22% | 14% | |

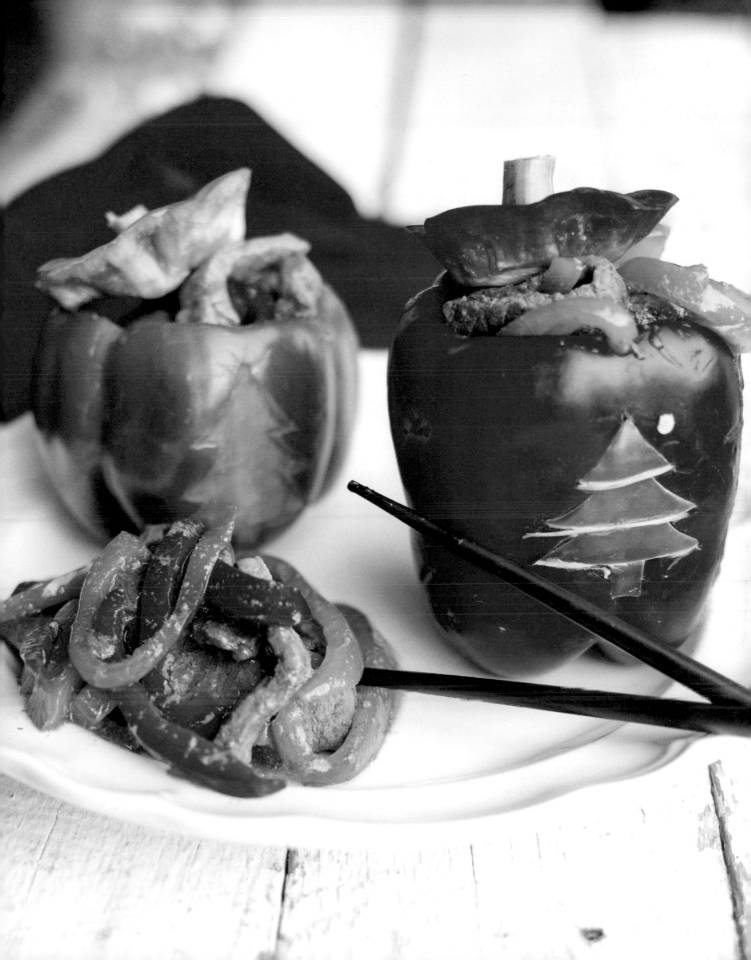

# slow cooker short rib tacos

L⟶M⟶H KETO ⊘ ⊘ ⊘   prep time: 5 minutes (not including time to make the guacamole)
cook time: 6 to 8 hours • yield: 12 servings

## ribs:

¼ cup diced onions

4 pounds boneless beef short ribs

1 cup green or red salsa

1 cup beef or chicken bone broth, homemade (page 108) or store-bought

2 cloves garlic, minced

2 teaspoons fine sea salt

1 teaspoon fresh ground black pepper

## for serving:

Purple cabbage, radicchio, or lettuce leaves, for "shells"

Guacamole (page 140)

Salsa verde

Lime wedges

Chopped fresh cilantro

1. Place the onions in a 6-quart (or larger) slow cooker. Set the ribs on top of the onions. Add the rest of the ingredients and stir to combine the seasonings. Cover and cook on low until the meat is fork-tender and falls apart easily, 6 to 8 hours.

2. Remove the ribs from the slow cooker. Pull the meat off the bones, discard the bones, and use two forks to shred the meat. Place the meat in a serving bowl.

3. Serve with purple cabbage, radicchio, or lettuce wraps for taco "shells," along with guacamole, salsa verde, lime wedges, and cilantro. Store extras in an airtight container in the fridge for up to 4 days.

NUTRITIONAL INFO (per serving)

| calories | fat | protein | carbs | fiber |
|----------|-----|---------|-------|-------|
| 296 | 16g | 32g | 6g | 2g |
| | 49% | 43% | 8% | |

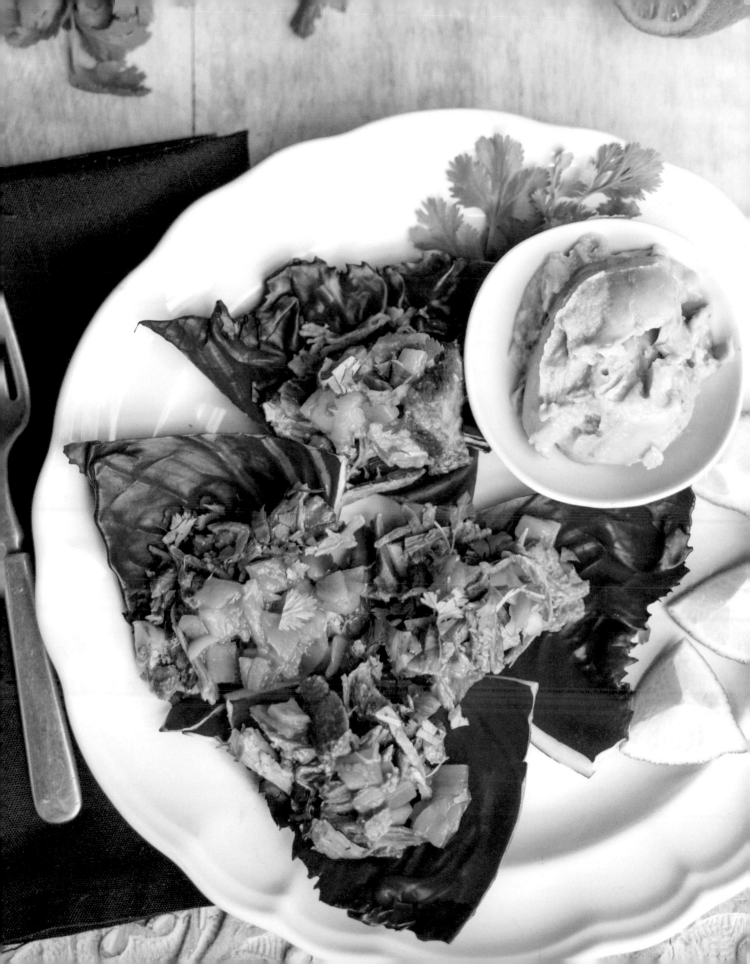

main dishes:
pork

# deconstructed egg rolls

1 pound ground pork

1 tablespoon untoasted, cold-pressed sesame oil

6 cups finely shredded cabbage

2 teaspoons minced garlic

1 tablespoon minced fresh ginger

1 tablespoon coconut aminos or wheat-free tamari

1 teaspoon fish sauce (optional)

¼ cup chopped green onions, for garnish

1. Place the pork and oil in a large cast-iron skillet over medium-high heat and cook, crumbling the meat with a wooden spoon, until cooked through, about 10 minutes. (Do not drain the drippings from the pan.)

2. Add the cabbage, garlic, ginger, coconut aminos, and fish sauce, if using, to the skillet. Sauté until the cabbage is soft, 3 to 5 minutes.

3. Divide among six plates or bowls and serve garnished with the green onions.

NUTRITIONAL INFO (per serving)

| calories | fat | protein | carbs | fiber |
|---|---|---|---|---|
| 250 | 19g | 14g | 6g | 3g |
| | 68% | 22% | 10% | |

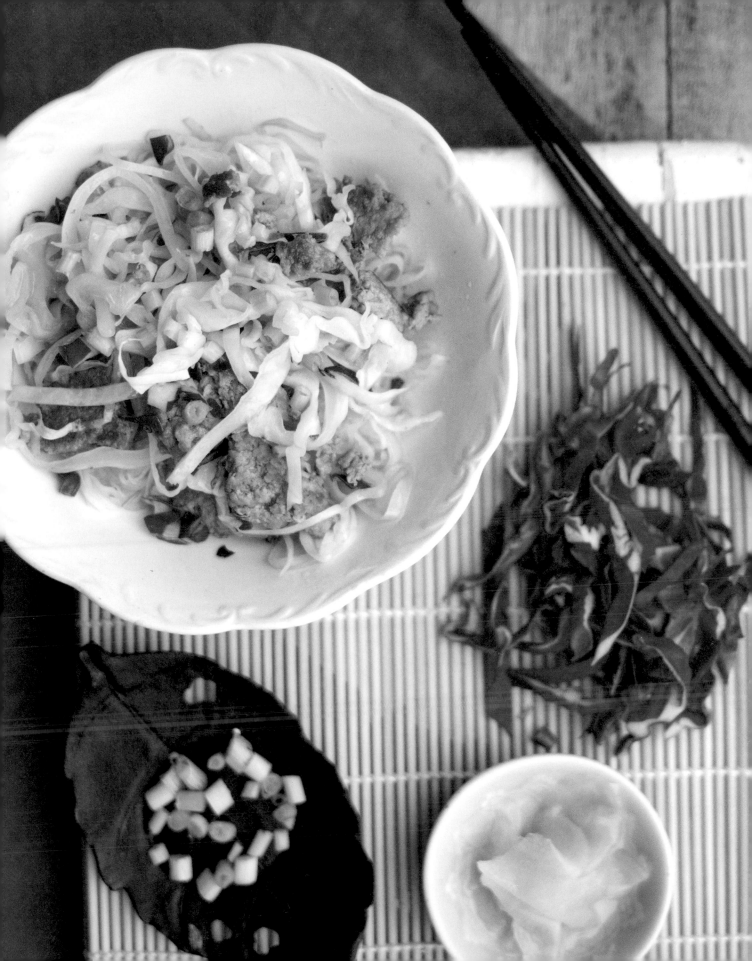

# pizza meatballs in red gravy

L M H KETO prep time: 10 minutes • cook time: 40 minutes • yield: 36 meatballs (4 per serving)

I love to watch cooking shows with my little boys on rainy days. On one of the shows they talked about "red gravy." What in the world is red gravy? Well, in Philly, that's what they call pizza sauce. My boys and I now call my Pizza Meatballs in Red Sauce, Pizza Meatballs in Red Gravy!

1 tablespoon coconut oil

¼ cup chopped onions

1 teaspoon fine sea salt

1 cup finely chopped mushrooms

¼ cup diced red bell peppers

2 pounds ground pork

1 cup finely chopped black olives (optional)

1 large egg

1 teaspoon dried basil

1 teaspoon dried oregano leaves

1 teaspoon garlic powder

1 teaspoon red pepper flakes

## for serving:

2 cups store-bought pizza sauce (aka "red gravy"), warmed (see note)

1 recipe Italian Marinated Mushrooms (page 208) (optional)

1. Preheat the oven to 350°F.

2. Heat the oil in a skillet over medium heat. Add the onions, season with the salt, and cook for 3 minutes. Add the mushrooms and bell peppers and cook for 5 more minutes, or until the onions are translucent. Remove to a bowl to cool.

3. Put the ground pork, olives (if using), egg, herbs, and spices in a mixing bowl. When the onion mixture is no longer hot to the touch, add it to the bowl with the meat and work everything together with your hands.

4. Shape the meat mixture into 1½-inch balls (about the size of golf balls) and place on a rimmed baking sheet. Bake for 30 minutes, or until cooked through.

5. Remove the meatballs from the oven and place on serving plates. Cover with warm red gravy and serve with marinated mushrooms, if desired.

6. Store extras in an airtight container in the fridge for up to 3 days. To reheat, place the meatballs and sauce in a skillet and warm over medium heat.

note: *When purchasing pizza sauce, check the ingredients list for added sugars and soybean or canola oil.*

NUTRITIONAL INFO (per serving)

| calories | fat | protein | carbs | fiber |
|---|---|---|---|---|
| 369 | 29g | 20g | 7g | 1g |
| | 71% | 22% | 7% | |

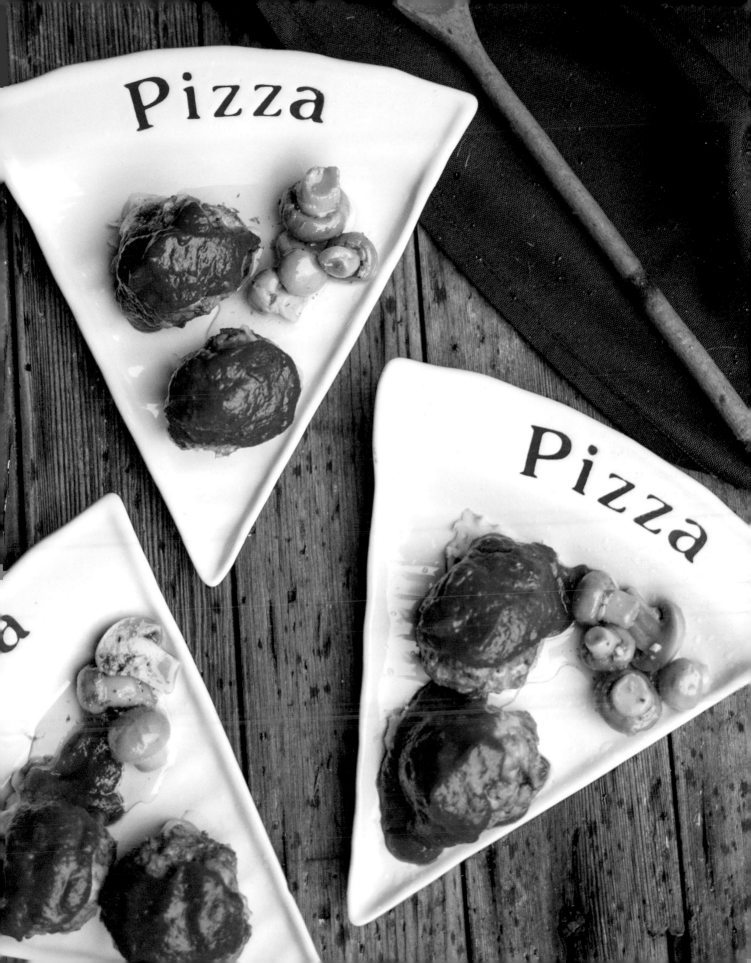

# sloppy ottos

L M H
KETO · ⊘ · ⊘ · ⊘ option

prep time: 8 minutes (not including time to make the buns or dressing)
cook time: 10 minutes • yield: 6 servings

A sloppy otto is a German take on a sloppy joe, which suits my German heritage just fine. This is my ketogenic spin on the sloppy joe's lesser-known cousin! Just make sure *not* to use Bavarian-style sauerkraut because it is typically sweetened.

1 pound ground pork

1 teaspoon fine sea salt

½ teaspoon fresh ground black pepper

¼ cup diced onions

6 Keto Buns (page 256) (or lettuce wraps for egg-free)

Paleo fat, such as bacon fat, for the buns

1 cup sauerkraut (not Bavarian-style), warmed

¾ cup Dairy-Free Thousand Island Dressing (page 118)

Pickles, for serving

1. Crumble the pork into a cast-iron skillet over medium heat. Season the meat with the salt and pepper and add the onions. Sauté until the pork is cooked through, about 6 minutes, stirring from time to time to break up the clumps of meat.

2. Meanwhile, slice the keto buns in half. In a large skillet, pan-fry them cut side down in Paleo fat until golden brown. (*Note*: Fry only the buns you plan to consume right away.)

3. To serve, place about one-sixth of the pork on a bun, then top with a large spoonful of sauerkraut and 2 tablespoons of the Thousand Island dressing. Repeat with the remaining ingredients. Serve with pickles.

4. Store extra buns and filling separately in airtight containers in the fridge for up to 3 days. To reheat, place the pork and sauerkraut in a skillet and warm over medium heat. Pan-fry the split keto buns to go with the meat and sauerkraut, following the instructions in Step 2.

NUTRITIONAL INFO (per serving)

| calories | fat | protein | carbs | fiber |
|---|---|---|---|---|
| 418 | 37g | 19g | 3g | 0.4g |
|  | 80% | 18% | 2% |  |

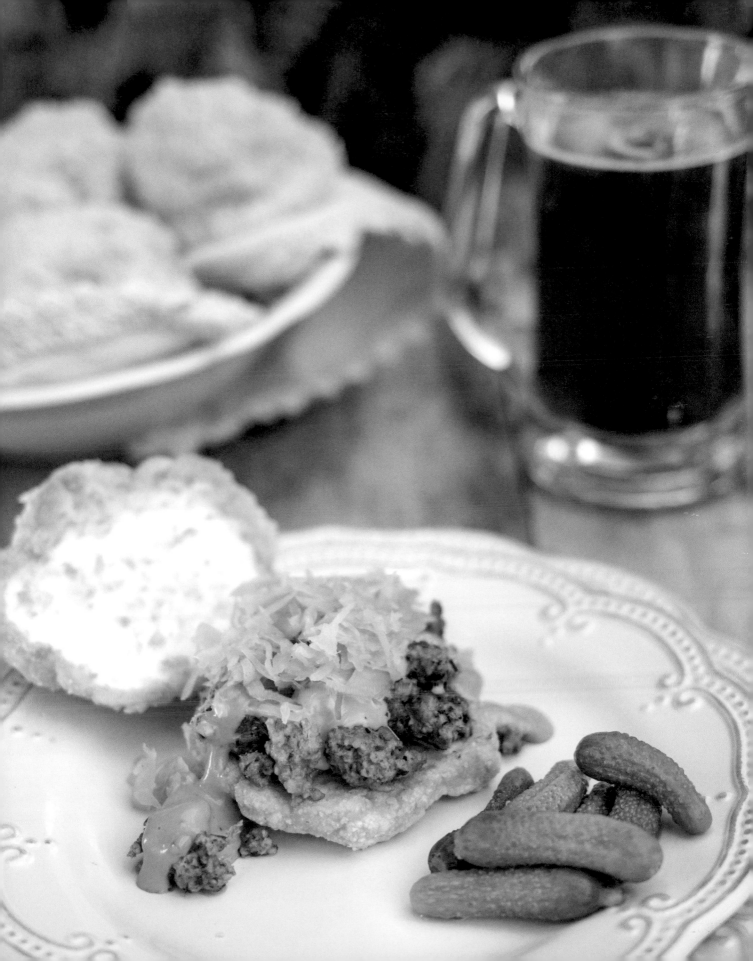

# reuben pork chops

L⌢M H KETO · option · prep time: 10 minutes (not including time to make the dressing)
cook time: 15 minutes • yield: 4 servings

2 tablespoons coconut oil or other Paleo fat

4 (5-ounce) bone-in pork chops, about ¾ inch thick

Fine sea salt and fresh ground black pepper

**for serving:**

1 cup sauerkraut, warmed

1 recipe Dairy-Free Thousand Island Dressing (page 118), preferably made with Copycat Baconnaise (page 124) (or Egg-Free Keto Mayo, page 125, for egg-free)

1 cup chopped red cabbage (optional)

1. Preheat a large cast-iron skillet over medium-high heat; once hot, place the oil in the pan. While the pan is heating, prepare the chops: pat the pork chops dry and season both sides liberally with salt and pepper.

2. When the oil is hot, place the chops in the skillet and sear for about 3½ minutes, then flip them over and sear the other side until the chops are cooked through, about 3½ more minutes (the cooking time will depend on the thickness of the chops). Do not overcrowd the pan; if necessary, cook the chops in batches.

3. Serve each chop with ¼ cup sauerkraut and 3 tablespoons of the dressing. Serve with chopped red cabbage, if desired.

4. Store extras in an airtight container in the fridge for up to 3 days. To reheat, place the chops and kraut in a skillet over medium heat and sauté for 3 minutes per side, or until warmed.

busy family tip: *The dressing can be made up to 1 week ahead and stored in an airtight container in the refrigerator. Shake well before using.*

| NUTRITIONAL INFO (per serving) | | | | |
|---|---|---|---|---|
| calories | fat | protein | carbs | fiber |
| 670 | 55g | 40g | 4g | 0.5g |
| | 74% | 24% | 2% | |

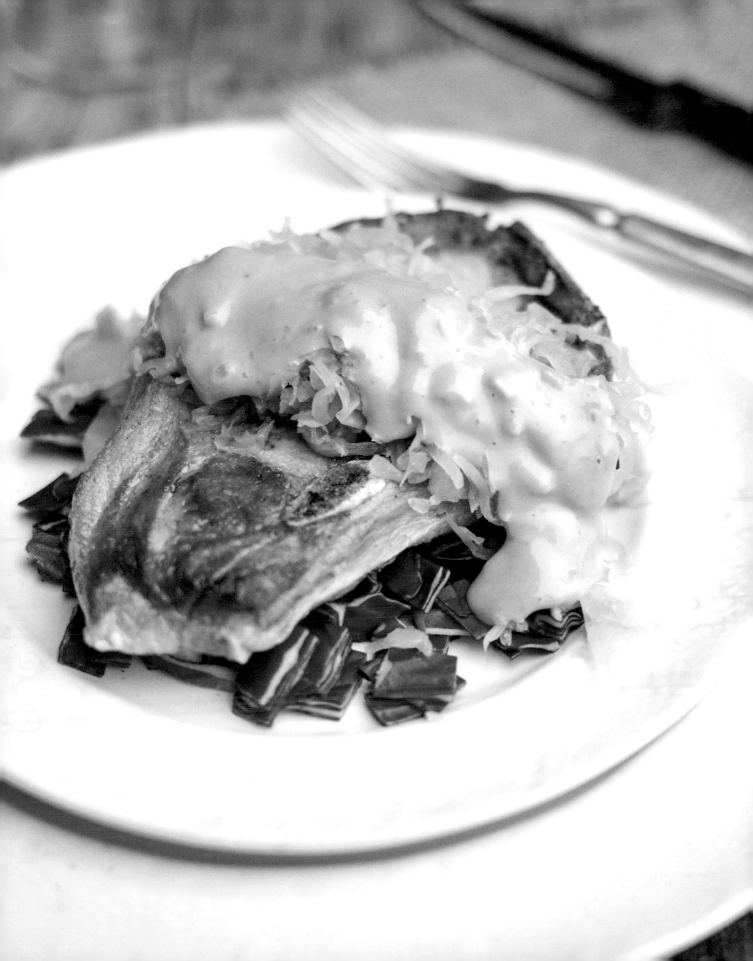

# slow cooker hot 'n' spicy country-style ribs

L ⌂ H M KETO 🗌 ⌀ ⌀   prep time: 10 minutes (not including time to make the hot sauce)
cook time: 6 to 8 hours • yield: 8 servings

¼ cup diced onions

4 pounds boneless country-style pork ribs

1 cup tomato sauce

1 cup beef or chicken bone broth, homemade (page 108) or store-bought

1 to 2 tablespoons hot sauce, homemade (page 134) or store-bought

2 cloves garlic, minced

2 teaspoons liquid smoke

2 teaspoons fine sea salt

1 teaspoon fresh ground black pepper

Red pepper flakes, for garnish

1. Place the onions in a 6-quart slow cooker. Place the ribs on top of the onions. Add the rest of the ingredients, except for the red pepper flakes, to the slow cooker and stir to combine. Place the lid on the slow cooker and cook on low until the meat is fork-tender and falls apart easily, 6 to 8 hours.

2. Serve topped with sauce from the slow cooker and garnished with red pepper flakes.

NUTRITIONAL INFO (per serving)

| calories | fat | protein | carbs | fiber |
|---|---|---|---|---|
| 370 | 19g | 47g | 3g | 1g |
| | 47% | 50% | 3% | |

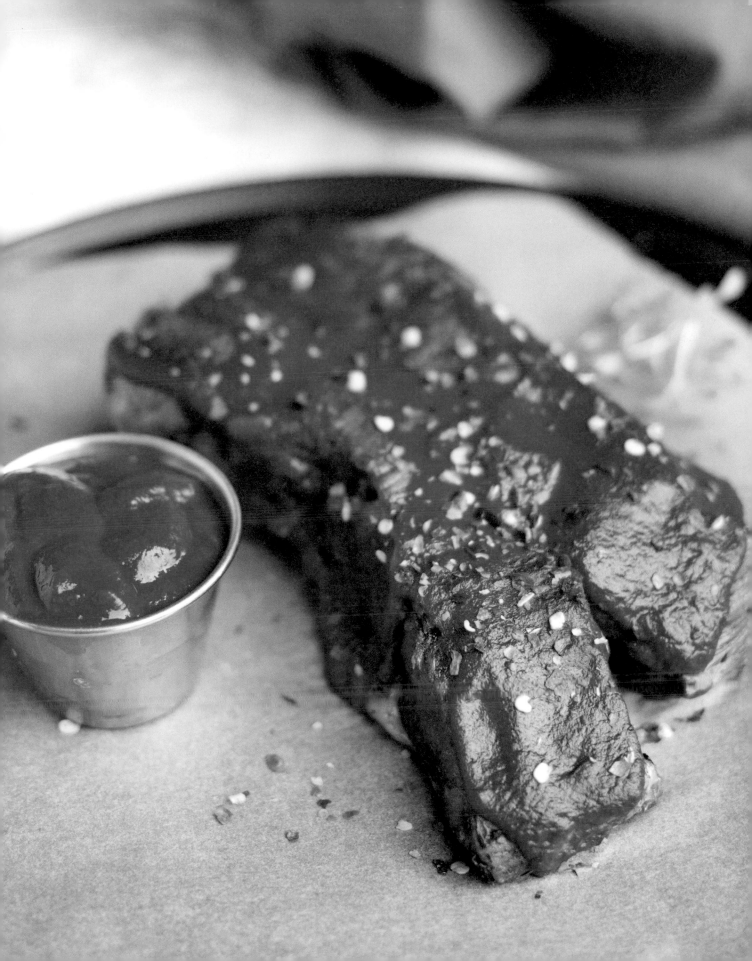

# chive panna cotta with bacon marmalade

prep time: 10 minutes, plus 2 hours to chill (not including time to make the marmalade)
cook time: 3 minutes • yield: 6 servings

2 teaspoons grass-fed powdered gelatin

1 cup unsweetened, unflavored cashew milk (homemade, page 106, or store-bought) or almond milk (or hemp milk for nut-free)

1 cup full-fat coconut milk

1 teaspoon minced garlic

1 tablespoon chopped fresh chives

½ teaspoon fine sea salt

1 cup Bacon Marmalade (page 122)

1. Pour ¼ cup of water into a small bowl. Sprinkle the gelatin over the water and allow to soften for 3 minutes.

2. Meanwhile, put the cashew milk, coconut milk, garlic, chives, and salt in a saucepan. Place the pan over medium heat and gently heat to a bare simmer.

3. Add the softened gelatin to the hot mixture in the saucepan and stir well to dissolve.

4. Pour the mixture into six 4-ounce ramekins and place them in the fridge for at least 2 hours or up to 4 hours to set.

5. Serve each panna cotta with about 2½ tablespoons Bacon Marmalade. Store extras in an airtight container in the fridge for up to 3 days.

gelatin tip: *Using gelatin is an easy way to make tasty treats, but foods made with gelatin can easily get too rubbery if they sit in the fridge overnight. If you plan on making this recipe ahead of time and not serving it the same day it is made, I suggest using ¼ teaspoon less gelatin than called for; this quantity will create a perfect creamy texture even after a day or two of resting in the fridge.*

busy family tip: *Can be made up to 3 days ahead (with caveat—see gelatin tip above).*

NUTRITIONAL INFO (per serving)

| calories | fat | protein | carbs | fiber |
|----------|-----|---------|-------|-------|
| 210 | 18g | 10g | 2g | 0.2g |
| | 77% | 19% | 4% | |

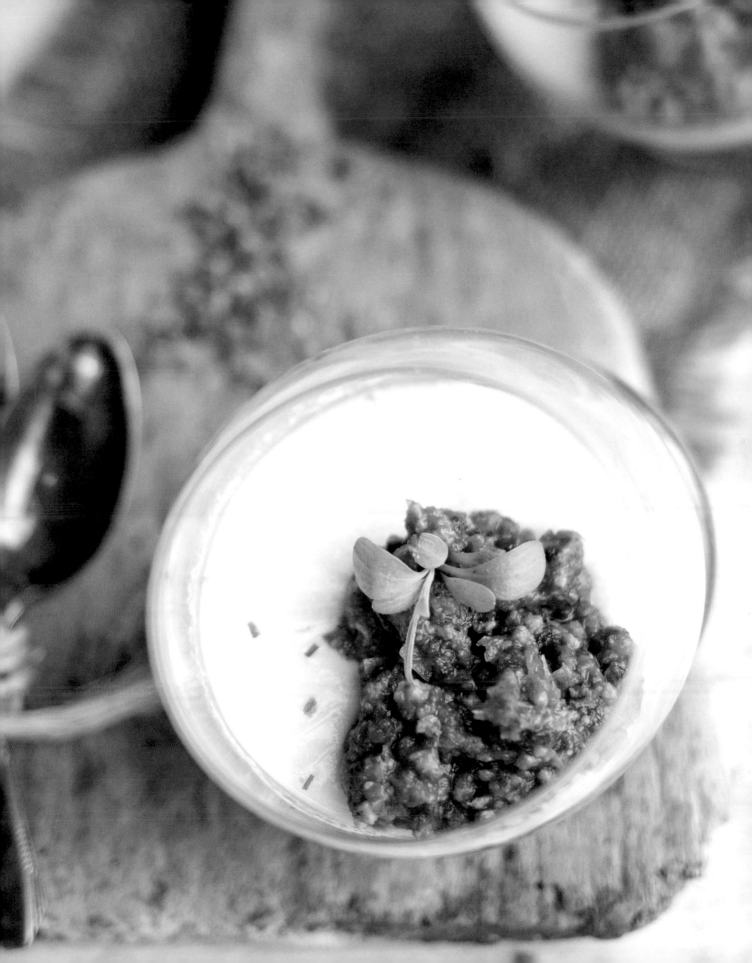

# slow cooker pastrami-style pork ribs

L⤳M⤳H KETO 🍶 🚫🥛 🚫🥚  prep time: 5 minutes • cook time: 7 to 8 hours • yield: 8 servings

When you think of pastrami, you probably think of beef. But I like to think outside the box. In this recipe, I use traditional pastrami seasonings to transform pork ribs into a tasty and easy dinner!

## pastrami seasoning:

½ cup fresh ground black pepper

1 tablespoon ground coriander

1 tablespoon dry mustard

1 tablespoon smoked paprika

2 teaspoons fine sea salt

½ teaspoon cayenne pepper

4 pounds boneless country-style pork ribs

½ cup water or beef bone broth, homemade (page 108) or store-bought

## sauce:

¾ cup Dijon mustard

¼ cup coconut vinegar or apple cider vinegar

¼ cup Swerve confectioners'-style sweetener or equivalent amount of liquid or powdered sweetener (see page 81)

2 tablespoons coconut aminos or wheat-free tamari

## for serving (optional):

Sauerkraut, warmed

Cornichons

1. Combine the pastrami seasoning ingredients and rub over the surface of the ribs.

2. Place the ribs in a 4-quart (or larger) slow cooker, standing them on their edge with the meaty side out.

3. Add the water or broth to the slow cooker. Cover and cook on low until the meat is falling apart and very tender, 7 to 8 hours.

4. Meanwhile, make the sauce: Place all the ingredients in a small bowl and stir to combine.

5. When the meat is done, preheat the oven to broil. Place the ribs on a rimmed baking sheet and spoon the sauce all over the top of the ribs. Broil for 3 to 5 minutes, until charred to your liking.

6. Serve with sauerkraut and cornichons, if desired. Store extras in an airtight container in the fridge for up to 4 days.

| NUTRITIONAL INFO (per serving) | | | | |
|---|---|---|---|---|
| calories | fat | protein | carbs | fiber |
| 353 | 18g | 47g | 1g | 1g |
| | 46% | 53% | 1% | |

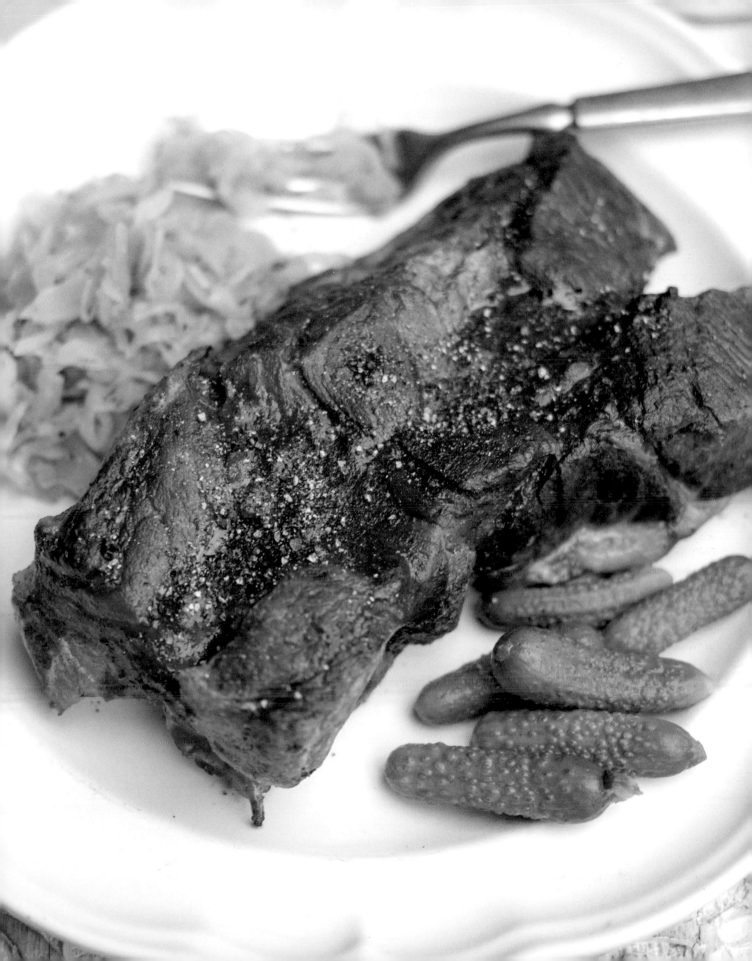

# mexican-style chorizo sausage

prep time: 20 minutes, plus 3 to 4 hours to chill the meat, soak the casings, and rest the sausage • cook time: 10 minutes • yield: 12 sausages (1 per serving)

When making sausage, homemade bone broth is much preferable to store-bought broth, but store-bought broth will work. Serve with the keto dipping sauces of your choice.

2½ pounds pork shoulder

½ pound pork fatback

½ cup coconut vinegar

6 feet medium hog casings

⅓ cup ice-cold pork, chicken, or beef bone broth, homemade (page 108) or store-bought

3 cloves raw garlic, smashed with the side of a knife, or 1 head Garlic Confit (page 142)

6 tablespoons ancho chili powder

1½ tablespoons fine sea salt

1 teaspoon dried Mexican oregano

½ teaspoon ground cinnamon

½ teaspoon ground cumin

½ teaspoon fresh ground black pepper

⅛ teaspoon ground cloves

Lard or coconut oil, for cooking

## special equipment:

Meat grinder (or grinder attachment on stand mixer)

Sausage stuffer (or sausage stuffer attachment on stand mixer) (optional)

busy family tip: *Make a double batch and freeze for easy meals.*

1. Cut the pork and pork fat into 1-inch cubes and spread out on a parchment-lined baking sheet. Freeze for 1 hour.

2. Fill a large bowl with the coconut vinegar and 2 quarts of water. Place the casings in the liquid to soak for 30 minutes.

3. Remove the pork and pork fat from the freezer and grind it using the coarse disk of a meat grinder (I use my KitchenAid food grinder attachment). In a large bowl, place the ground pork and fat, broth, garlic, ancho chili powder, salt, Mexican oregano, cinnamon, cumin, pepper, and cloves; combine well.

4. Fry up a small dab of the sausage mixture in a skillet over medium heat to taste it; add more seasoning if desired.

5. Load a sausage stuffer (I use my KitchenAid sausage stuffer attachment) with the presoaked casings and stuff the sausages by pushing the meat mixture through the attachment. Twist the sausages into links about 5 inches long.

6. Refrigerate the sausages in an airtight container for a few hours to allow the flavors to meld. Cook within 3 days, or freeze for up to 2 months. To cook: Place 1 tablespoon of lard or coconut oil in a large pan over medium heat. Sauté the sausages for 10 minutes, until the internal temperature reaches 160°F.

note: *If you do not have a sausage stuffer, you can form the sausage mixture into 12 large patties.*

tips for making the best sausage:
- *Liquid is needed to bind protein to fat; the more liquid you add, the more fat you can add (to a point).*
- *For great flavor and added nutrients, homemade bone broth is best for the liquid.*
- *If the sausage pops out of the casing when you bite into it, you cooked it too fast and at too high a heat.*
- *Use cold meat and fat so the sausage won't turn mushy. (In fact, commercial sausage makers often add dry ice to the meat to keep it cold.) After cubing the meat, place it in the freezer for 1 hour or in the fridge for 4+ hours before grinding. After grinding, place the bowl in the freezer for 30 minutes to keep the meat cold while stuffing.*

NUTRITIONAL INFO (per serving)

| calories | fat | protein | carbs | fiber |
|---|---|---|---|---|
| 345 | 30g | 18g | 1g | 0.2g |
| | 78% | 21% | 1% | |

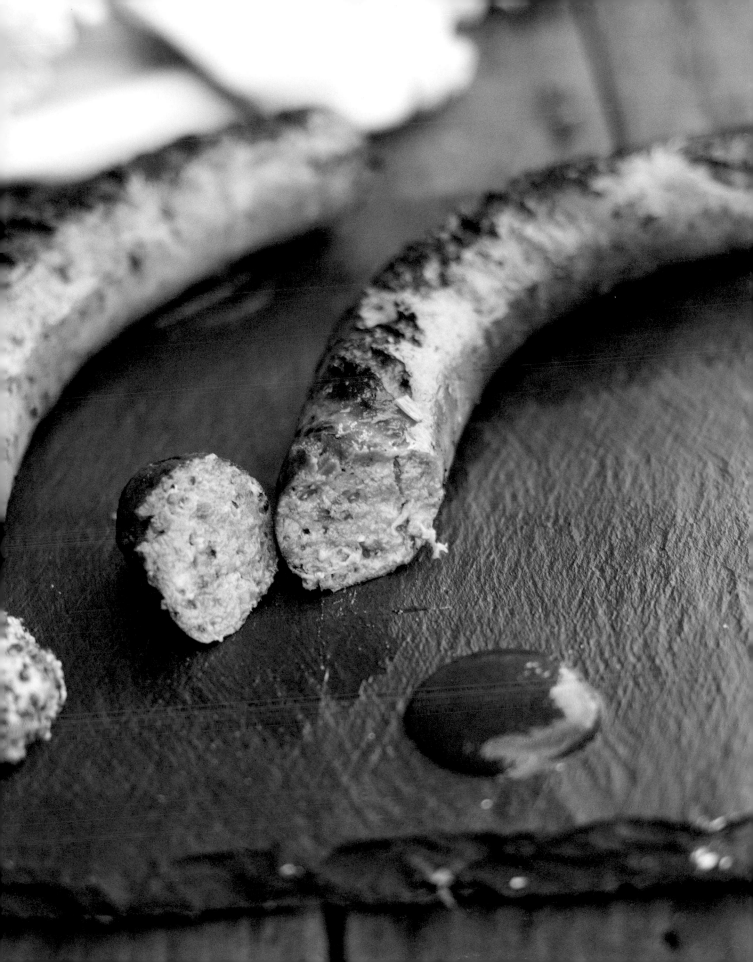

# easy smoked ham hocks
# with smoky whole-grain mustard

L—M—H KETO

prep time: 5 minutes, plus time to rest the mustard
cook time: 10 minutes • yield: 4 servings

This recipe is extremely easy to make. It uses smoked ham hock steaks. Because they're already cooked, all you need to do is heat them up until their skin gets crispy (though they taste great cold, too). Just remember to make the mustard the day before you plan to eat the hocks. It needs time in the fridge to allow the flavors to develop.

**smoky whole-grain mustard:**

¼ cup prepared yellow mustard

¼ cup brown mustard seeds

2 tablespoons Swerve confectioners'-style sweetener or equivalent amount of liquid or powdered sweetener (page 81)

¼ cup coconut vinegar or apple cider vinegar

2 teaspoons chili powder

½ teaspoon fresh ground black pepper

2 tablespoons coconut oil, melted

½ teaspoon liquid smoke


4 (3-ounce) smoked ham hock steaks

2 cups sauerkraut, warmed, for serving

Cornichons or other pickles of choice, for serving

1. To make the mustard: In a small bowl, stir together the prepared mustard, mustard seeds, sweetener, vinegar, chili powder, and pepper. Stir in the melted coconut oil and liquid smoke; mix well to combine. Refrigerate overnight to allow the flavors to blend before using.

2. Preheat the oven to 425°F. Place the smoked ham hocks on a rimmed baking sheet and bake for 10 minutes, or until the skin gets crispy.

3. Place each ham hock on a plate with ½ cup sauerkraut and 2 to 4 tablespoons of the smoky mustard.

4. Store extras in an airtight container in the fridge for up to 3 days. To reheat, place in a skillet over medium heat and sauté for 3 minutes per side, or until warmed to your liking.

tip: *To save money and time spent running to the market, I get a whole pasture-raised pig from a local farmer to keep in our chest freezer. One of the best parts is that I get to choose the cuts of meat my family likes best and have them readily available in my freezer whenever I need them! Of course, you don't need to purchase a pig to make this dish—just stop by your local butcher to purchase smoked ham hock steaks to store in your freezer for easy breakfasts or dinners.*

NUTRITIONAL INFO (per serving)

| calories | fat | protein | carbs | fiber |
|---|---|---|---|---|
| 228 | 17g | 10g | 9g | 3g |
| | 67% | 18% | 15% | |

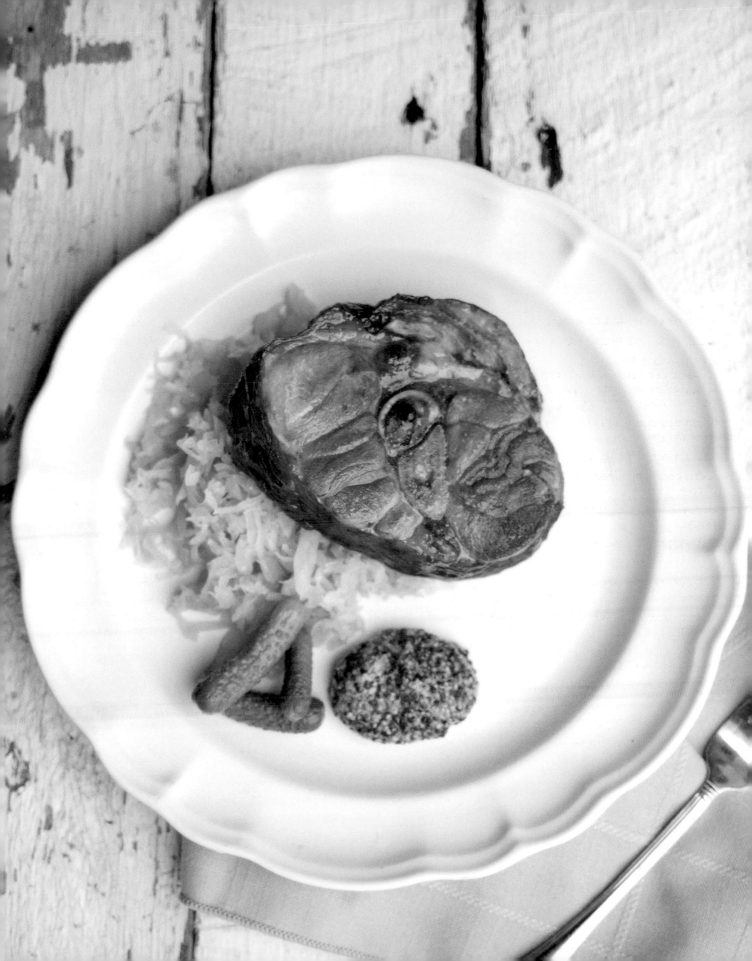

# porchetta

L M H KETO   prep time: 10 minutes, plus overnight to chill the pork belly and 10 minutes to rest
cook time: 4 hours • yield: 40 servings

It was a little difficult to get my butcher to understand what I was looking for when I called to request a ten-pound pork belly for making porchetta. He said, "You don't want that. It's too fatty. We will roll you up a nice pork loin with a little skin on the side." I just smiled and replied, "No thank you. A European cut of pork belly is what I'm looking for—a large slab of pork from the belly with the skin and fat still on the cut." Serve with a salad of mixed greens or on a Keto Bun (page 256) for a tasty sandwich.

1 (10-pound) fresh pork belly, skin on

½ cup fine sea salt, divided

3½ tablespoons baking soda, divided

4 cloves garlic, minced, divided

2 sprigs fresh rosemary, leaves removed and finely chopped, divided

busy family tip: *This recipe makes a lot of food. I suggest that you divvy it up into dinner-sized portions and freeze them. All you have to do is take one container out at a time for easy dinners for you and your family.*

1. Place a wire rack in a large rimmed baking sheet.

2. Cut the pork belly in half, slicing lengthwise down the middle so that you have 2 large slabs. Liberally season the meat side of one of the belly pieces with half of the salt. Flip the belly over and rub half of the baking soda evenly into the skin. Repeat with other half of the pork belly and the remaining salt and baking soda.

3. Place both pork belly halves on the wire rack in the baking sheet and place in the fridge, uncovered, overnight.

4. Preheat the oven to 400°F.

5. Remove the belly from the fridge and, with a very sharp knife, make diagonal cuts across the skin side, about 2 inches apart, to score the skin and expose the fat, but without piercing the fat. Repeat in the opposite direction to create a crisscross pattern.

6. Flip the pieces over so that the skin side is down, then evenly spread the garlic and chopped rosemary over the meat of both pieces.

7. Take one of the pieces and, starting with the long end, tightly roll up the belly and tie it closed with butcher's twine at 2-inch intervals. Repeat with the other piece so you have two roasts. Place the roasts on the wire rack set inside the baking sheet.

8. Place the roasts in the oven for 40 minutes. After 40 minutes, lower the oven temperature to 325°F. Continue to cook for 3 hours, or until the interior is tender and starting to fall apart just a touch.

9. At that point, increase the oven temperature to 500°F to crisp the skin. Broil the roasts for 20 minutes, or until the skin is crispy.

10. Remove from the oven and allow to rest for 10 minutes. To serve, slice into 1½-inch-thick pieces.

11. Store extras in an airtight container in the fridge for up to 3 days or in the freezer for up to 1 month. To reheat, place in a lightly greased skillet over medium heat until warmed.

## NUTRITIONAL INFO (per serving)

| calories | fat | protein | carbs | fiber |
|---|---|---|---|---|
| 321 | 28g | 17g | 0.1g | 0g |
| | 79% | 21% | 0% | |

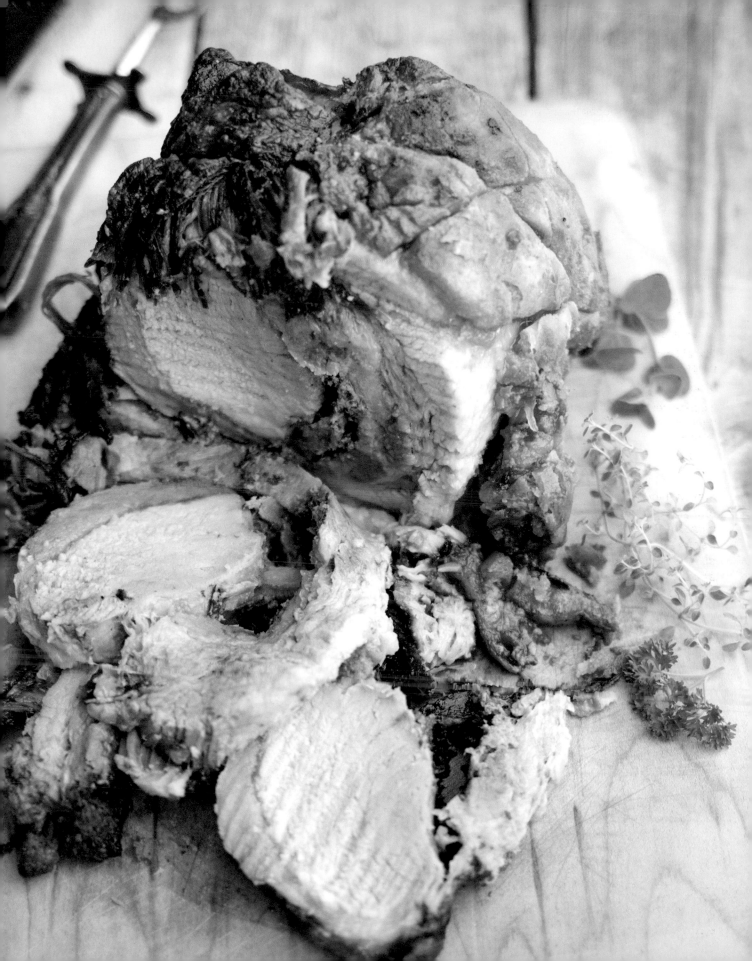

# chorizo sausage and mushroom casserole

LMH KETO · prep time: 10 minutes • cook time: 10 minutes • yield: 4 servings

¼ cup Paleo fat, such as coconut oil or lard

1 pound Mexican-style fresh (raw) chorizo, removed from casings

1 pound baby portobello or button mushrooms, quartered

¼ cup diced onions

1½ teaspoons fine sea salt

½ teaspoon fresh ground black pepper

**sausage vinaigrette:**

1 clove garlic

2 ounces dry-cured Spanish-style chorizo, casing removed, chopped

½ cup coconut vinegar

2 teaspoons smoked paprika

1 teaspoon lemon juice

¼ teaspoon ground coriander

¼ cup MCT oil or extra-virgin olive oil

2 tablespoons beef bone broth, homemade (page 108) or store-bought

1 teaspoon fine sea salt

Chopped fresh flat-leaf parsley or cilantro, for garnish (optional)

1. Heat the Paleo fat in a large skillet over medium heat. Add the fresh chorizo, mushrooms, and onions and sauté, breaking up the chorizo with a spoon as it cooks, until the sausage is cooked through and the mushrooms are tender and browned, about 10 minutes. Season with the salt and pepper.

2. Meanwhile, make the vinaigrette: In a blender, puree the garlic, cured chorizo, coconut vinegar, paprika, lemon juice, and coriander until smooth. With the blender running, drizzle in the oil and broth until well combined. Season the vinaigrette with the salt.

3. Pour the vinaigrette into the skillet with the chorizo mixture and toss to coat. Divide among four plates and garnish with parsley, if desired.

4. Store extras in an airtight container in the fridge for up to 4 days. To reheat, place in a skillet over medium heat until warmed.

NUTRITIONAL INFO (per serving)

| calories | fat | protein | carbs | fiber |
|----------|-----|---------|-------|-------|
| 596 | 56g | 17g | 7g | 1g |
| | 85% | 11% | 4% | |

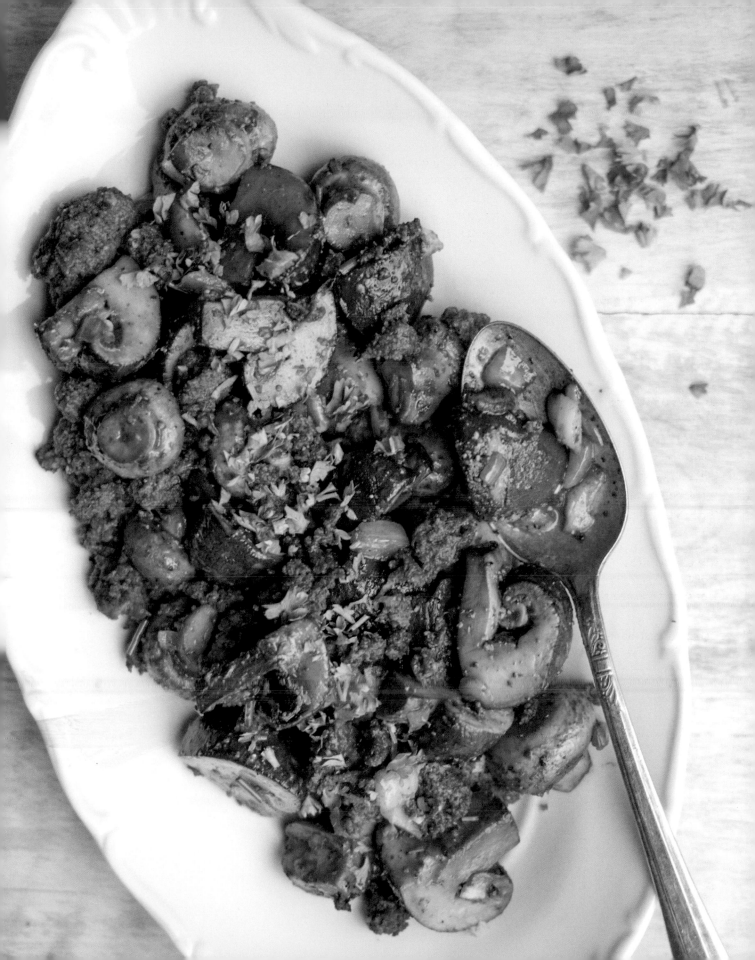

# slow cooker asian pulled pork lettuce cups

L M H KETO · prep time: 10 minutes · cook time: 7 to 8 hours · yield: 8 servings

**asian pulled pork:**

1 (4-pound) boneless pork shoulder

¾ cup coconut aminos or wheat-free tamari

½ cup beef bone broth, homemade (page 108) or store-bought

⅓ cup Swerve confectioners'-style sweetener or equivalent amount of liquid or powdered sweetener (see page 81)

2 tablespoons unseasoned rice vinegar

6 cloves garlic, minced

2 teaspoons grated fresh ginger

3 teaspoons fish sauce (optional)

3 to 5 drops orange oil or orange extract

Bibb lettuce cups, for serving

Sliced green onions, for garnish

Finely chopped red cabbage, for garnish

1. Place the pork shoulder in a 4-quart (or larger) slow cooker. Add the rest of the ingredients for the pulled pork. Cover and cook on low until the meat is fork-tender and falls apart easily, 7 to 8 hours. When ready to serve, use two forks to shred the meat in the slow cooker and stir well to incorporate the flavorful sauce.

2. Serve in lettuce cups garnished with green onions and red cabbage.

3. Store extras in an airtight container in the fridge for up to 4 days.

NUTRITIONAL INFO (per serving)

| calories | fat | protein | carbs | fiber |
|----------|-----|---------|-------|-------|
| 548 | 41g | 40g | 5g | 5g |
| | 67% | 29% | 4% | |

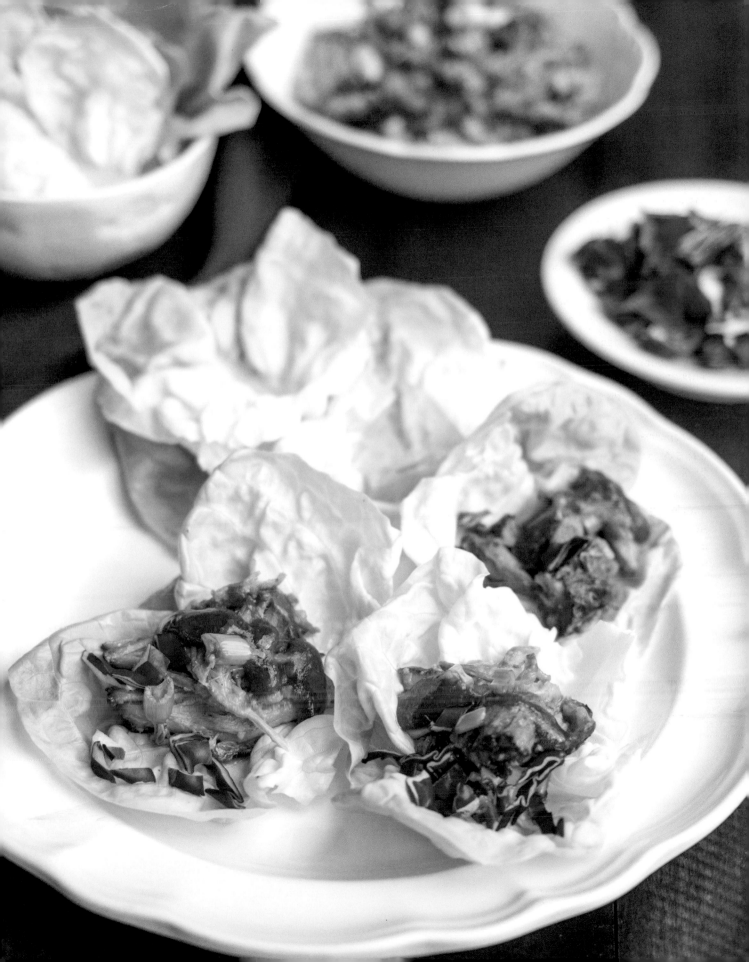

# greek meatballs

L M H KETO  prep time: 10 minutes • cook time: 30 minutes • yield: 8 servings

These meatballs are made with a blend of ground pork and ground lamb: the pork makes them more keto, and the lamb gives them a signature Greek flavor. I use a high-heat oven for meatballs with a crispy exterior and a tender, moist interior. Adding a little water or an ingredient that releases moisture helps the fat bind into the meatballs, which also keeps them moist. Mushrooms are a great choice: not only do they release water, but they also have a special umami flavor that creates very tasty meatballs.

1 tablespoon coconut oil

¼ cup chopped onions

2 cloves garlic, minced

1¼ teaspoons fine sea salt

1 pound ground lamb

1 pound ground pork

1 cup finely chopped mushrooms

1 large egg

1 tablespoon grated lemon zest

1 tablespoon chopped fresh oregano leaves

## for serving (optional):

Dairy-Free Yogurt (page 178), unsweetened

Sliced cucumbers

Greek olives

Extra-virgin olive oil, for drizzling

1. Preheat the oven to 425°F.

2. Heat the coconut oil in a skillet over medium heat. Add the onions and garlic and season them with the salt; cook until the onions are translucent, about 5 minutes. Transfer the onion mixture to a small bowl and set aside to cool.

3. Put the lamb, pork, mushrooms, egg, lemon zest, and oregano in a mixing bowl. When the onion mixture is no longer hot to the touch, add it to the bowl with the meat and work everything together with your hands.

4. Shape the meat mixture into 2-inch balls and place on a rimmed baking sheet. Bake for 20 to 25 minutes, until cooked through.

5. Serve the meatballs with yogurt, sliced cucumbers, Greek olives, and a drizzle of olive oil, if desired. They are best served fresh, but extras can be stored in an airtight container in the fridge for up to 5 days or frozen for up to a month.

NUTRITIONAL INFO (per serving)

| calories | fat | protein | carbs | fiber |
|----------|-----|---------|-------|-------|
| 320 | 26g | 20g | 2g | 0.2g |
|  | 73% | 25% | 2% |  |

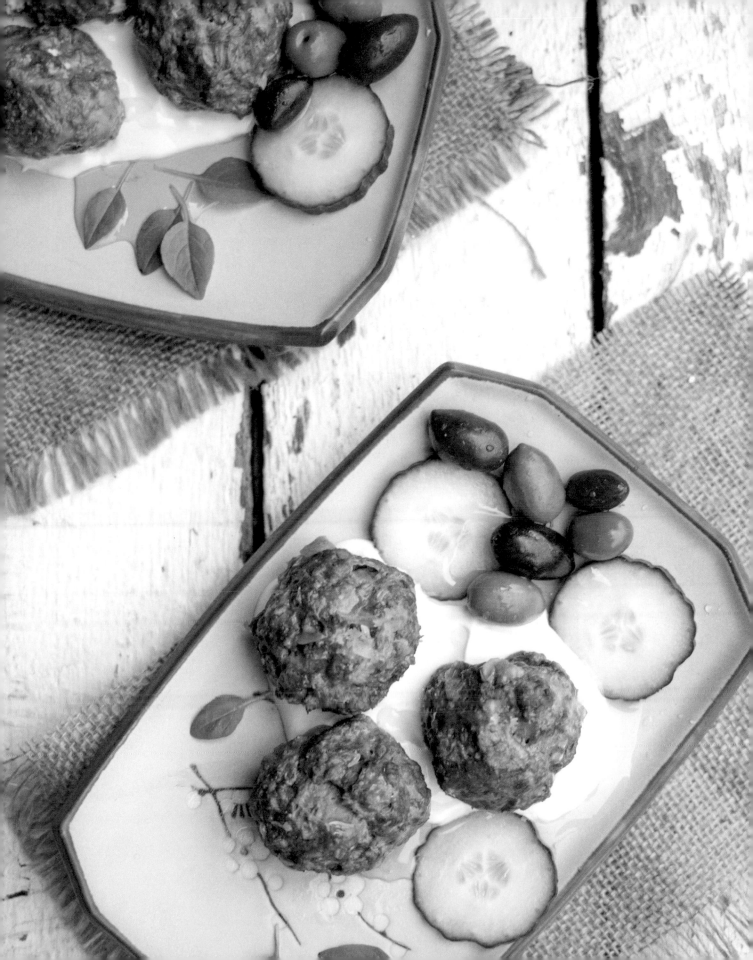

# keto BLTs with soft-boiled eggs

L M H KETO · option · prep time: 7 minutes · cook time: 15 minutes · yield: 12 wraps (2 per serving)

My son insists on soft-boiled eggs with his Keto BLTs. A boy after my own heart! For the tastiest BLT, salt the tomatoes with a flaky sea salt.

12 slices bacon

6 large eggs (omit for egg-free)

Coarse sea salt and fresh ground black pepper

12 thick slices tomato (about 3 tomatoes)

12 large lettuce leaves, such as romaine, green leaf, or Boston

¾ cup mayonnaise and/or baconnaise, homemade (page 124) or store-bought (or Egg-Free Keto Mayo, page 125, for egg-free)

1. If using standard-sliced bacon, preheat the oven to 400°F; if using thick-cut bacon, preheat the oven to 375°F. Place the bacon on a wire rack set inside a rimmed baking sheet. Bake until crispy, 10 to 15 minutes, depending on how thick the bacon is.

2. Meanwhile, make the soft-boiled eggs: Place the eggs in a pot of simmering (not boiling) water, cover, and simmer for 6 minutes. Immediately rinse the eggs under cold water. Peel the eggs, then cut them in half and place on a large serving platter. Sprinkle the eggs with flaky sea salt and pepper.

3. Place the tomato slices on the serving platter with the eggs and sprinkle them with flaky sea salt. Then add the cooked bacon to the platter.

4. Place the lettuce leaves in a bowl and have mayo out for serving.

5. Let everyone assemble their wraps!

NUTRITIONAL INFO (per serving)

| calories | fat | protein | carbs | fiber |
|---|---|---|---|---|
| 461 | 42g | 16g | 5g | 1g |
| | 82% | 14% | 4% | |

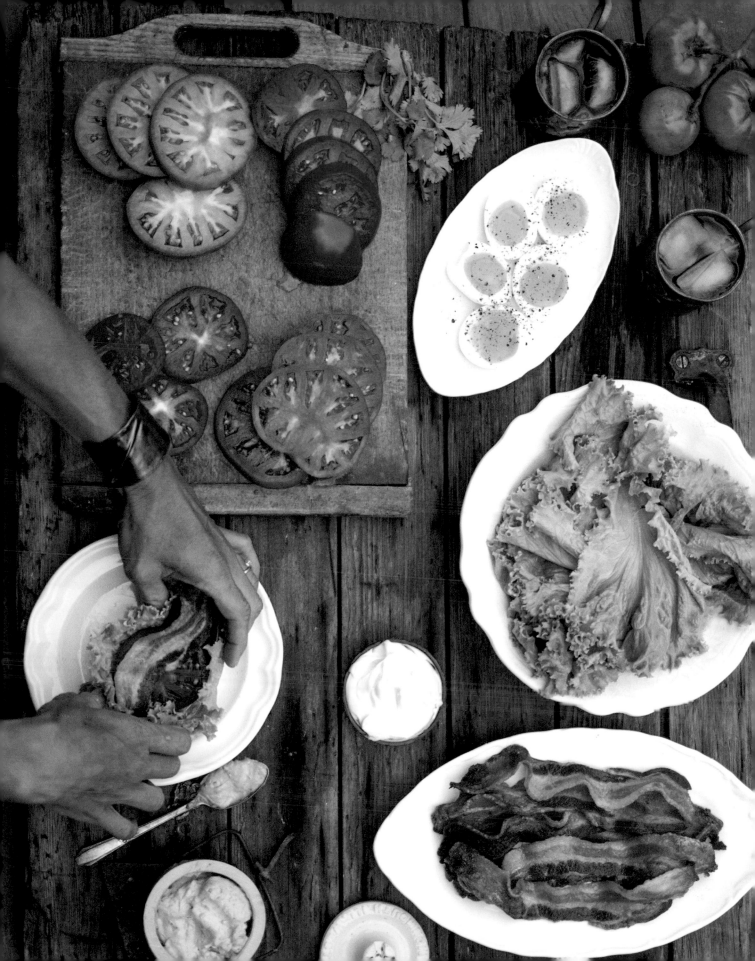

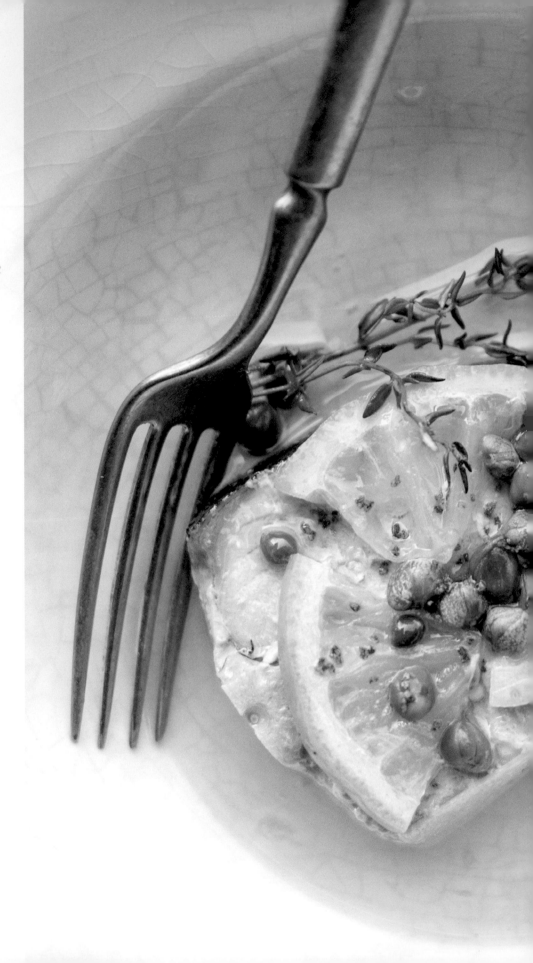

main dishes:
fish and
seafood

# spicy tuna stacks

KETO · option · prep time: 10 minutes · yield: 2 servings

¼ cup mayonnaise, homemade (page 124) or store-bought (or Egg-Free Keto Mayo, page 125, for egg-free

1 teaspoon medium-hot hot sauce, homemade (page 134) or store-bought

1 (6-ounce) can tuna

¼ teaspoon fine sea salt

Pinch of fresh ground black pepper

1 avocado

1 teaspoon lime or lemon juice

¼ cup chopped purple cabbage

¼ cup diced cucumbers

Black sesame seeds, for garnish (optional)

## variation:
**Spicy Salmon Stacks.**

*Out of tuna? You can make this dish with salmon. Simply swap the canned tuna for an equivalent amount of canned salmon.*

1. In a medium bowl, combine the mayonnaise and hot sauce. Place 2 tablespoons of the mixture in a small resealable plastic bag (for drizzling at the end).

2. Gently fold the tuna, salt, and pepper into the rest of the spicy mayo. Taste for seasoning and add more salt and pepper, if desired.

3. Cut the avocado into ½-inch dice and drizzle with the lime juice to keep it from discoloring.

4. Divide the diced avocado between two serving plates. Use your hands to cup the avocado pieces together to form a 3- or 4-inch-wide circle. Mound each avocado circle with half of the cabbage, followed by half of the spicy tuna salad. Top the stacks with the diced cucumbers, dividing them equally between the stacks.

5. Cut a tiny hole in the corner of the plastic bag containing the reserved spicy mayo and squirt some of the mayo over each stack. Garnish with black sesame seeds, if desired.

6. Store extras in an airtight container in the refrigerator for up to 3 days.

NUTRITIONAL INFO (per serving)

| calories | fat | protein | carbs | fiber |
|----------|-----|---------|-------|-------|
| 466 | 37g | 27g | 7g | 4g |
| | 71% | 23% | 6% | |

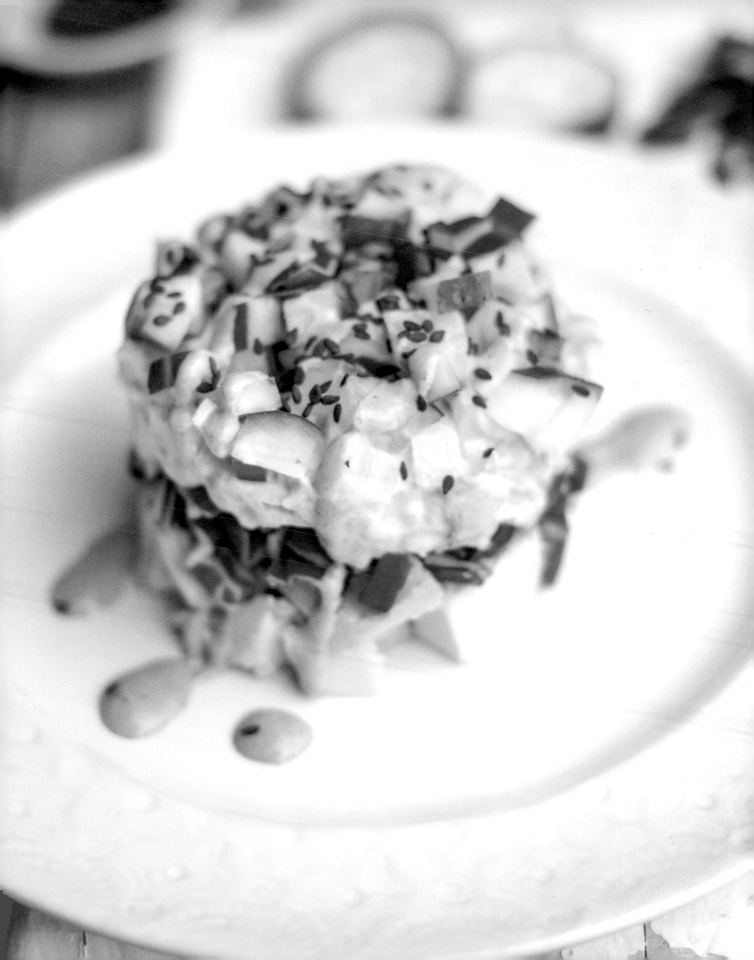

# peel-and-eat garlic shrimp

L M H KETO

prep time: 20 minutes (not including time to make the bread and garlic confit)
cook time: 5 minutes • yield: 8 servings

I grew up in the middle of Wisconsin. Not the best place for seafood, as you can imagine! So I thought I didn't like shrimp, crab, or lobster. But then I had the opportunity to visit Monterey, California, with Craig on one of his work trips. He encouraged me to try "good shrimp." I don't know if it was the beautiful view, the ambiance, or his company, but it was the best-tasting dish I ever had. I will never forget my first tasty bite of garlicky shrimp on the coast of California!

Leaving the shells on protects the shrimp from drying out. To make this dish even easier to prepare, you can purchase extra jumbo shrimp already butterflied and deveined at your local seafood market.

2 pounds extra jumbo shrimp (with shells on), deveined and butterflied (see note)

1 cup chilled lard

4 cloves Garlic Confit (page 142) or raw garlic, peeled

Juice of 1 lemon

1 teaspoon fine sea salt

1 teaspoon fresh thyme leaves or other herb of choice

8 slices Keto Bread (page 256), toasted in Paleo fat in a skillet, for serving

1. Place an oven rack in the top position and preheat the broiler to high.

2. Arrange the shrimp in a single layer on a rimmed baking sheet.

3. Place the cold lard, garlic, lemon juice, salt, and thyme in the bowl of a food processor; pulse until very smooth. Crumble the cold fat over the shrimp.

4. Bake the shrimp for 5 minutes, or until opaque.

5. Place the pan with the shrimp in the middle of the table. Peel and eat the shrimp, then dip the bread into the sauce in the bottom of the pan.

6. Store extras in an airtight container in the fridge for up to 3 days. To reheat, place in a lightly greased skillet over medium heat and sauté until warmed.

note: *To butterfly shrimp, hold a shrimp with the back side exposed and slice gently from the head to the tail. If a black vein appears, remove that.*

NUTRITIONAL INFO
(per serving, with bread)

| calories | fat | protein | carbs | fiber |
|----------|-----|---------|-------|-------|
| 369 | 28g | 28g | 1g | 0.3g |
| | 69% | 30% | 1% | |

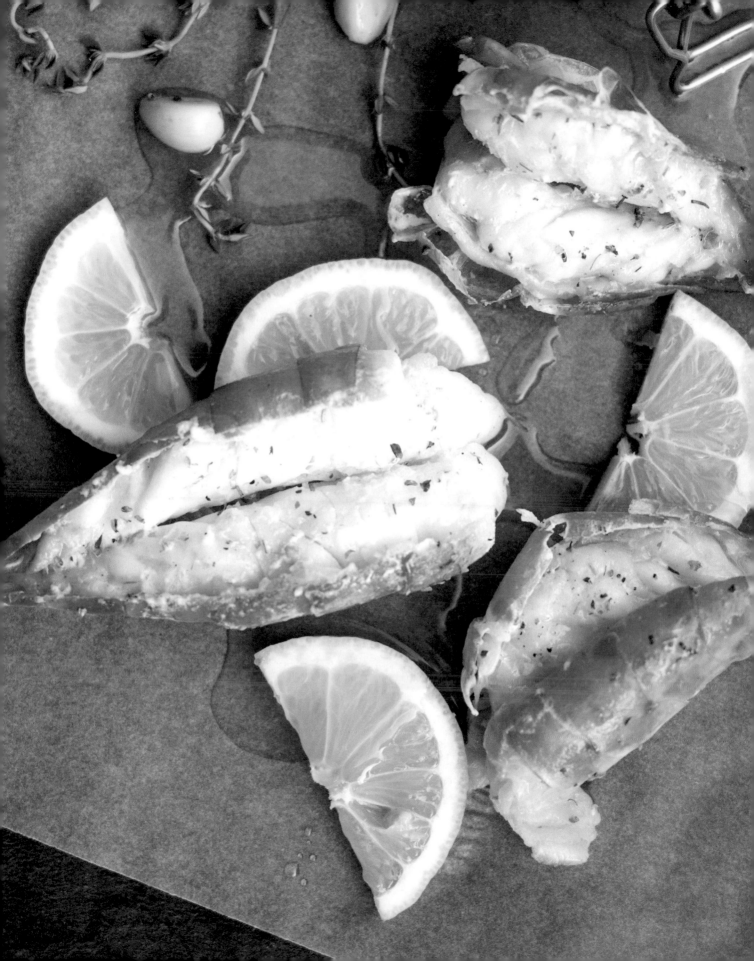

# hawaiian delight

L ⟩ H M KETO  prep time: 15 minutes (not including time to make the aioli) • yield: 4 servings

I call this crab dish Hawaiian Delight because I enjoyed one like it in Maui. If you really want to impress your guests, serve them this dish. They will assume that you slaved away in the kitchen, but in reality you don't even have to turn on the stove!

**sauce:**

¼ cup coconut aminos or wheat-free tamari

2 teaspoons unseasoned rice vinegar

2 teaspoons toasted sesame oil

1 tablespoon Swerve confectioners'-style sweetener or equivalent amount of liquid or powdered sweetener (see page 81)

¼ teaspoon grated fresh ginger

¼ teaspoon garlic paste

⅛ teaspoon guar gum

**crab:**

8 ounces canned lump crabmeat

1 tablespoon lime juice

4 ounces gravlax

1 avocado, halved, peeled, and pitted

½ cup Garlic and Herb Aioli (page 128), made with chopped chives instead of thyme leaves, for garnish

1. To make the sauce: Combine the coconut aminos, vinegar, oil, sweetener, ginger, and garlic paste in a small bowl. Whisk in the guar gum and set aside to thicken, about 5 minutes. Place the sauce in a squeeze bottle (or use a spoon) and drizzle in a zigzag pattern over four plates.

2. To make the crab: Place the crabmeat and lime juice in a small bowl and gently stir to coat the crab in the juice. Form the mixture into 4 balls. Wrap the gravlax around each ball, overlapping the ends of the gravlax at the bottom of the ball. Place the balls on top of the drizzled sauce in the center of each plate.

3. Place the aioli in a resealable plastic bag with a tiny corner cut off. Gently squeeze the bag to squirt dots of aioli around the perimeter of each plate.

4. Slice the avocado lengthwise into 4 pieces. Thinly slice each fourth, but leave the top 1 inch or so intact so you can fan it. Place a sliced avocado quarter on top of each ball, fanning them out for a pretty appearance. (*Easy option:* Slice the whole avocado and place 4 thin slices over each ball.)

5. This dish is best served fresh, but extras can be stored in an airtight container in the fridge for up to 3 days (the avocado will brown).

notes: *To make this dish egg-free, use my Egg-Free Keto Mayo (page 125) to make the aioli.*

*Because this dish is slightly sweetened, it's best not to make it while you're becoming keto-adapted and learning to curb your sweet tooth.*

busy family tip: *The sauce and aioli can be made up to 1 week ahead of time and stored in the fridge.*

NUTRITIONAL INFO (per serving)

| calories | fat | protein | carbs | fiber |
|----------|-----|---------|-------|-------|
| 398 | 33g | 17g | 9g | 6g |
| | 75% | 17% | 9% | |

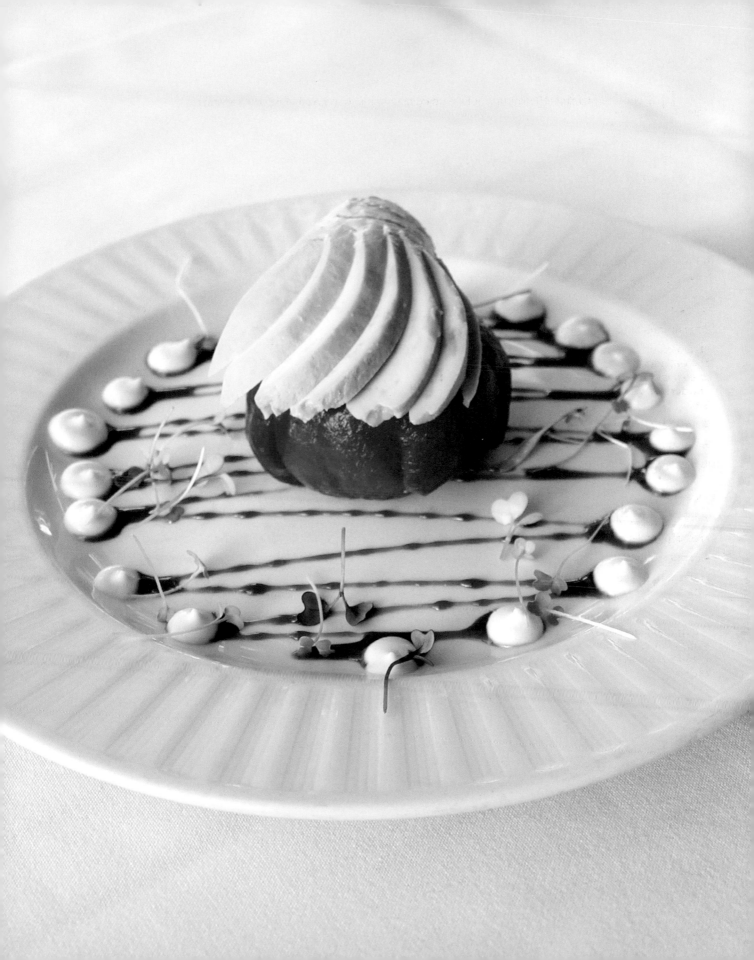

# spicy grilled shrimp with mojo verde

L M H KETO  prep time: 20 minutes • cook time: 8 minutes • yield: 4 servings

Leaving the shells on protects the shrimp from drying out. To make this dish even easier to prepare, you can purchase extra jumbo shrimp already butterflied and deveined at your local seafood market.

½ cup lime or lemon juice

3 teaspoons minced garlic

¼ red onion, thinly sliced

12 jumbo shrimp (peels on), deveined and butterflied (see note, page 360)

2 teaspoons cayenne pepper

1 teaspoon ground cumin

1 teaspoon fine sea salt

## dipping sauce:

3 loosely packed cups fresh cilantro leaves

½ cup MCT oil or extra-virgin olive oil

2 tablespoons minced garlic

2 teaspoons coconut vinegar

1 teaspoon fine sea salt

½ teaspoon ground cumin

1. Preheat a grill to medium-high heat. Place 4 wooden skewers in water to soak while you prepare the ingredients.

2. Place the lime juice in a shallow baking dish. Add the garlic, onion, and shrimp and let marinate for 15 minutes while you prepare the spices and dipping sauce.

3. Place the cayenne pepper, cumin, and salt in a small dish and stir well to combine. Set aside.

4. Make the dipping sauce: Place all the sauce ingredients in a food processor or blender and pulse until smooth. Add more salt to taste, if needed.

5. Remove the shrimp from the marinade and liberally sprinkle them with the spice mixture. Thread 3 shrimp onto each skewer. Grill for 3 to 4 minutes per side, or until the shrimp are pink and cooked through. Remove from the grill and serve each skewer with ¼ cup of the sauce.

6. This dish is best served fresh, but extras can be stored in an airtight container in the fridge for up to 3 days. It can be served cold. To reheat, place the shrimp in a skillet over medium heat and sauté until warmed.

| NUTRITIONAL INFO (per serving) | | | | |
|---|---|---|---|---|
| calories | fat | protein | carbs | fiber |
| 365 | 29g | 21g | 5g | 1g |
| | 72% | 23% | 5% | |

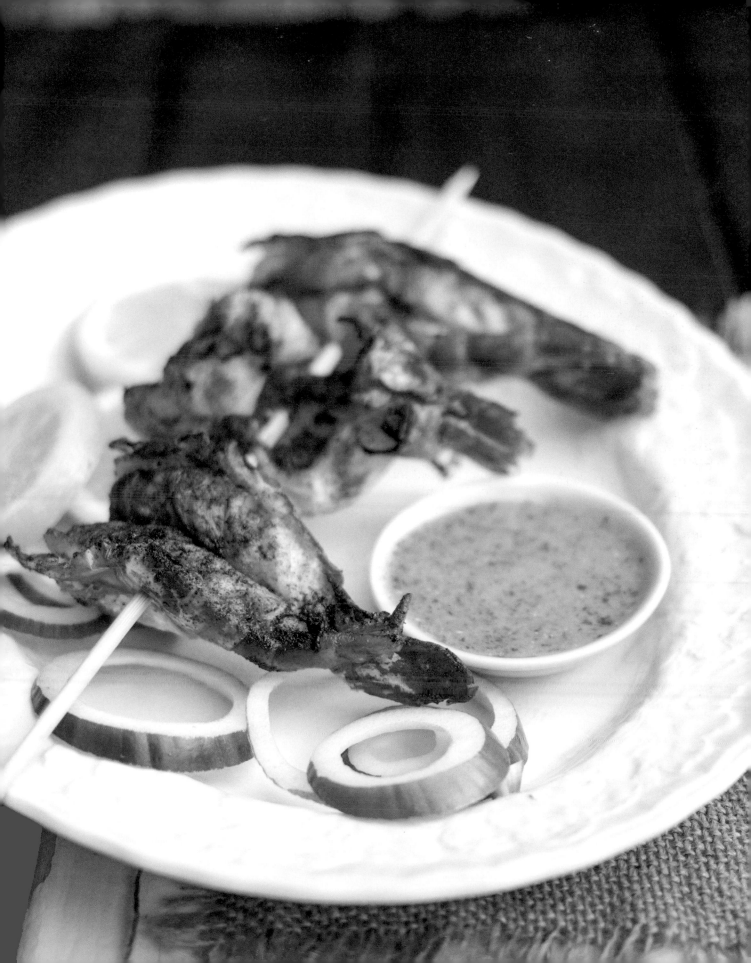

# seafood sausage with leek confit

L M H KETO (icons) prep time: 30 minutes (not including time to make the mostarda)
cook time: 45 minutes • yield: 6 sausages (1 per serving)

¼ cup coconut vinegar

3 feet medium hog casings

## leek confit:

¼ cup Paleo fat, such as lard

2 large leeks (white and pale green parts only), halved lengthwise and rinsed well, then cut crosswise into ¼-inch-thick slices (about 2 cups)

2 tablespoons fish or chicken bone broth, homemade (page 108) or store-bought, or water

½ teaspoon fine sea salt

12 ounces medium shrimp (about 14 shrimp), peeled and deveined

4 ounces fresh scallops

4 ounces smoked salmon

1 cup peeled, seeded, and diced Roma tomatoes (about 4 ounces), divided

1 ounce fresh basil leaves (about ¾ cup), cut into ribbons, divided

2 teaspoons lemon juice

1 teaspoon fine sea salt

½ teaspoon fresh ground white pepper

2 tablespoons MCT oil

1 recipe Keto Lemon Mostarda (page 138), for serving

## special equipment:

Sausage stuffer (or sausage stuffer attachment on stand mixer)

1. Fill a large bowl with the coconut vinegar and 1 quart of water. Place the casings in the liquid to soak for 30 minutes.

2. To make the confit: Melt the ¼ cup of fat in a large pot over medium-low heat. Add the leeks and stir to coat in the fat. Stir in the broth and ½ teaspoon of salt. Cover the pot and reduce the heat to low. Cook until the leeks are tender, stirring often, about 25 minutes. Uncover and cook to evaporate the excess water, 2 to 3 minutes.

3. Dice the shrimp, scallops, and salmon into ¼-inch pieces. Place the seafood in a mixing bowl along with the tomatoes, basil, lemon juice, salt, and pepper and mix well.

4. Load a sausage stuffer (I used my KitchenAid sausage stuffer attachment) with the presoaked casings and stuff the sausages by pushing the seafood mixture through the attachment. Twist the sausages into links about 6 inches long.

5. Poach the sausages in a large pot of simmering water for 10 minutes, or until firm; do not overcook.

6. To brown the sausages, heat the MCT oil in a skillet over medium heat. Brown the sausages on all sides, about 3 minutes. Place the sausages on serving plates (1 sausage per person) and serve with the leek confit and Keto Lemon Mostarda.

7. Store extras in an airtight container for up to 3 days. To reheat, place in a skillet over medium heat until warmed.

busy family tip: *The leek confit can be made up to 1 week ahead. Rewarm before using. The Keto Lemon Mostarda can be made up to 5 days ahead.*

| NUTRITIONAL INFO (per serving) | | | | |
|---|---|---|---|---|
| calories | fat | protein | carbs | fiber |
| 469 | 36g | 30g | 6g | 1g |
| | 69% | 26% | 5% | |

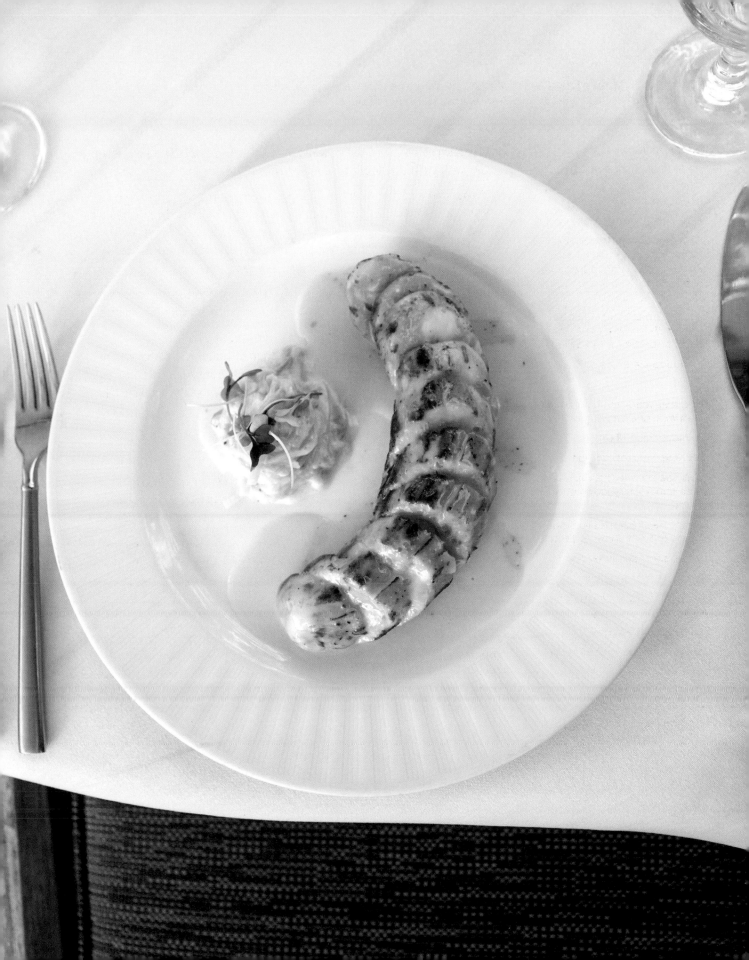

# lemon-thyme poached halibut

L M H KETO · prep time: 5 minutes · cook time: 15 minutes · yield: 4 servings

1 lemon, thinly sliced

½ cup extra-virgin olive oil or MCT oil, plus more for drizzling

4 (6-ounce) halibut steaks

1 teaspoon fine sea salt

½ teaspoon fresh ground black pepper

1 sprig fresh thyme or other herb of choice

Coarse sea salt, for garnish (preferably Hawaiian alaea sea salt for color)

1 tablespoon capers, for garnish (optional)

1. Line the bottom of a large enameled cast-iron skillet with the lemon slices. Pour the oil over the top of the lemon slices. Place the halibut steaks in the skillet and add enough water to cover the fish. Season the poaching liquid with the salt and pepper, then add the sprig of thyme.

2. Heat on medium-low until the poaching liquid is steaming but not boiling (about 165°F). Once the liquid is steaming, poach the halibut steaks until they are cooked through and opaque, 10 to 12 minutes (depending on thickness). Remove the steaks from the poaching liquid.

3. Serve with a drizzle of olive oil and garnished with coarse sea salt and capers, if desired.

4. Store extras in an airtight container in the fridge for up to 3 days. To reheat, place the halibut in a heat-safe dish with a few tablespoons of water, cover, and place in a preheated 350°F oven until warmed.

NUTRITIONAL INFO (per serving)

| calories | fat | protein | carbs | fiber |
|----------|-----|---------|-------|-------|
| 305 | 29g | 9g | 2g | 1g |
| | 86% | 12% | 2% | |

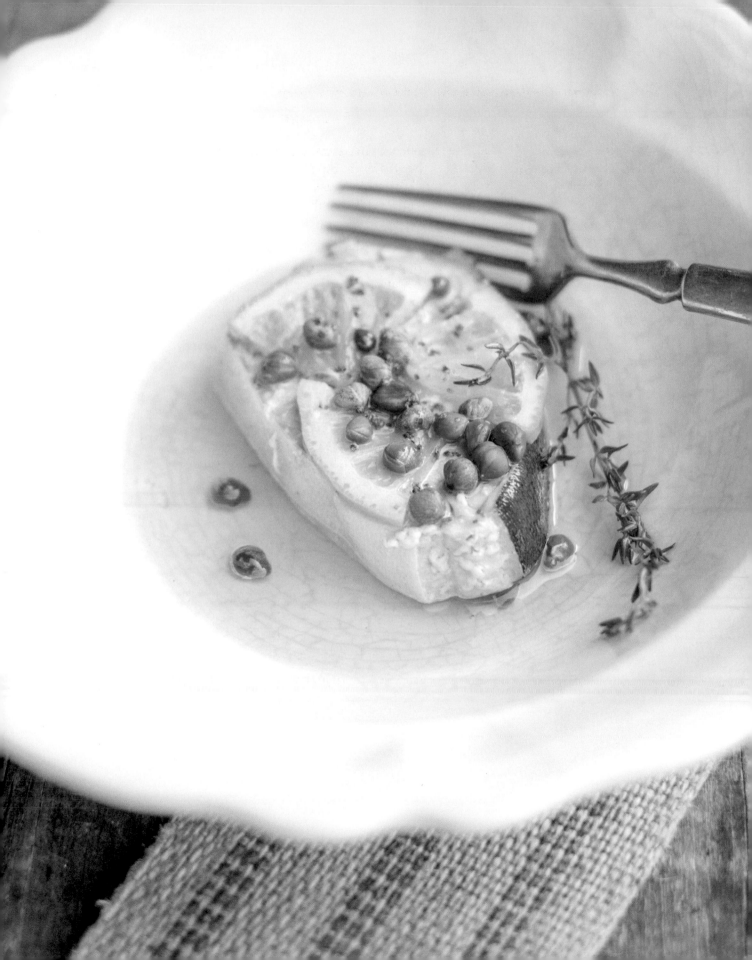

# fried catfish with cajun keto mustard

L⤳H / KETO M · 🗋 ⊘ ⊘   prep time: 7 minutes • cook time: 6 minutes • yield: 4 servings

I wasn't sure if my kids were going to like this meal since I wasn't a fan of fish when I was a child, but after I made this the first night, they asked for it again the next three nights in a row!

**cajun keto mustard:**

¼ cup plus 2 tablespoons bacon fat or duck fat, at room temperature

¼ cup prepared yellow mustard

2 tablespoons Cajun Seasoning (page 112)

4 (4-ounce) catfish fillets

3 tablespoons Paleo fat, such as coconut oil, divided

¼ cup Cajun Seasoning (page 112)

1. To make the mustard: Place the softened bacon fat in a small bowl. Add the mustard and Cajun seasoning and stir well to combine; set aside.

2. Place the catfish fillets on a clean surface and pat dry. Melt 1 tablespoon of the Paleo fat and brush it over each side of the fish. Cover each fillet evenly with about 1 tablespoon of Cajun seasoning. Use your hands to rub the spice mix into the fillets.

3. Heat the remaining 2 tablespoons of Paleo fat in a large cast-iron skillet over medium-high heat. Fry the fish in the hot oil. Place another heavy cast-iron skillet on top of the fillets and press down to create a very crispy exterior (or press down with a spatula). Fry for 3 minutes per side, or until the fish is cooked through (the cooking time will depend on how thick your fillets are).

4. Place each fillet on a serving plate with 2 tablespoons of the Cajun Keto Mustard.

5. Store extras in an airtight container in the fridge for up to 3 days. To reheat, place the fillets in a lightly greased skillet over medium heat until warmed.

NUTRITIONAL INFO (per serving)

| calories | fat | protein | carbs | fiber |
|----------|-----|---------|-------|-------|
| 361 | 33g | 16g | 0g | 0g |
| | 82% | 18% | 0% | |

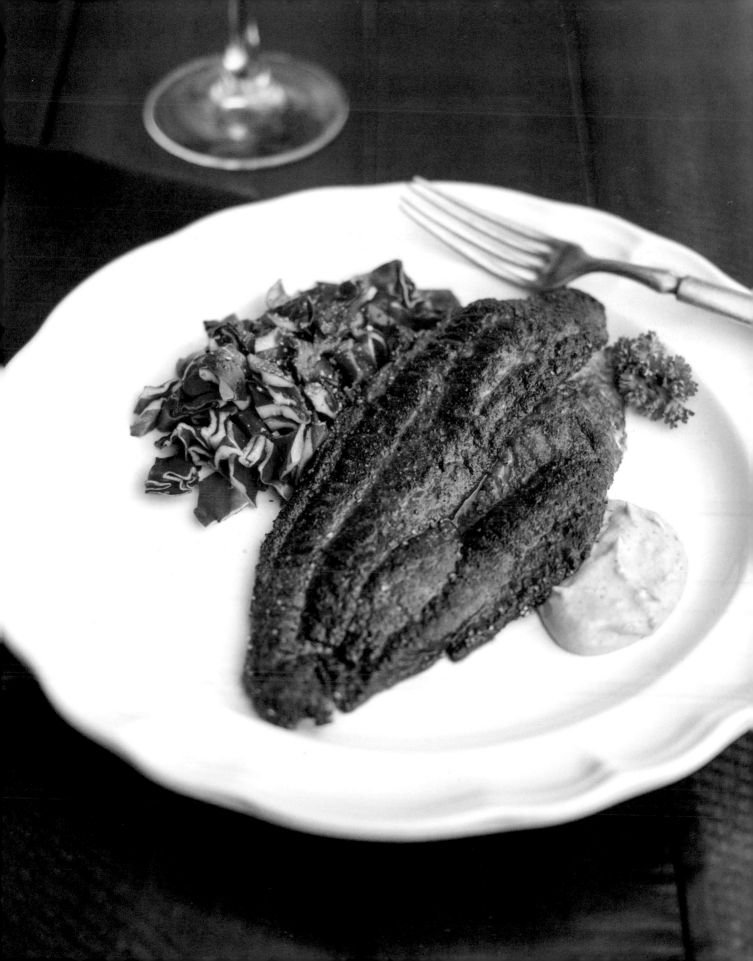

# grilled trout with hollandaise

 prep time: 8 minutes (not including time to make the hollandaise)
cook time: 15 minutes • yield: 4 servings

2 whole trout with skin, scaled, gutted, and butterflied (see note)

1 tablespoon avocado oil or MCT oil

1 teaspoon fine sea salt, divided

½ teaspoon fresh ground black pepper, divided

4 sprigs fresh thyme

4 sprigs fresh rosemary

2 slices lemon

2 teaspoons capers

2 teaspoons lard, coconut oil, or duck fat

1 cup Easy Dairy-Free Hollandaise (page 136), for serving

Olives, for garnish

Capers, for garnish

1. Preheat a grill to medium heat.

2. Drizzle the outside of the fish generously with the oil and season with half of the salt and pepper.

3. Open the trout up. Season the insides with the remaining salt and pepper. Place half of the herbs, lemon slices, capers, and lard in the center of each trout.

4. Close the trout and place them on the grill. Cook until the fish is flaky, 13 to 15 minutes (depending on how thick your fish are), flipping them over halfway through cooking.

5. Remove the fish from the grill and serve with the hollandaise. Garnish with olives and capers.

6. Store extras, without the hollandaise, in an airtight container in the fridge for up to 3 days. Reheat in a skillet over medium heat until warmed.

note: *Whole trout often comes butterflied, ready for stuffing. If you're not sure if the trout you are buying has already been butterflied, ask your fishmonger to do it for you.*

NUTRITIONAL INFO (per serving)

| calories | fat | protein | carbs | fiber |
|----------|-----|---------|-------|-------|
| 515 | 48g | 19g | 2g | 1g |
| | 84% | 15% | 1% | |

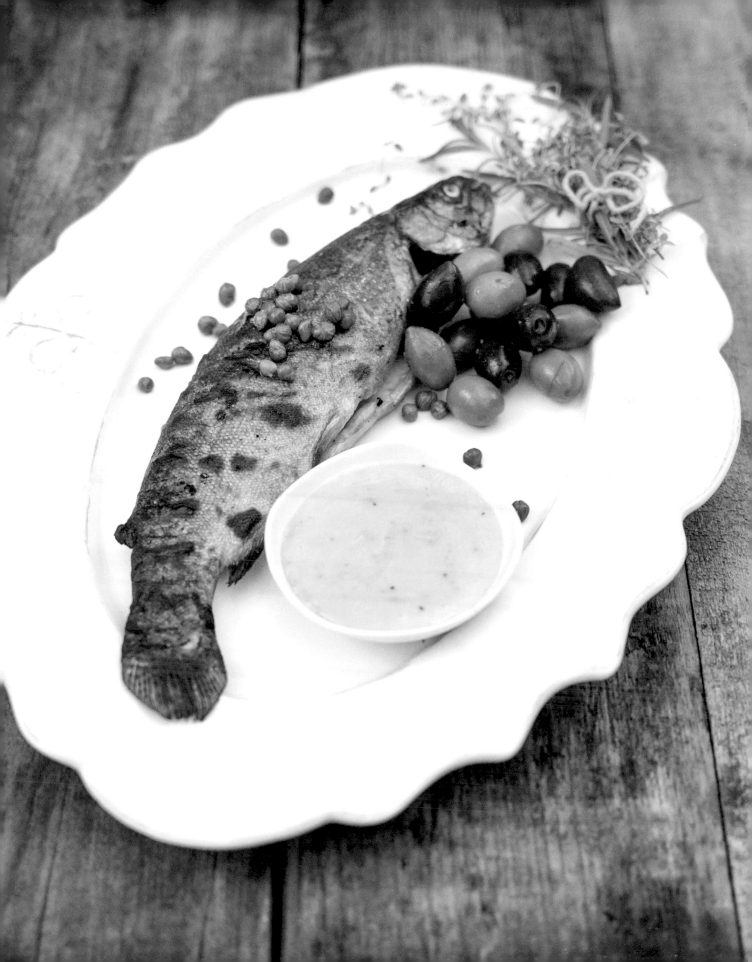

# tom ka plaa (thai coconut fish)

prep time: 10 minutes (not including time to make the zoodles)
cook time: 25 to 45 minutes • yield: 4 servings

I grew up in a small town in north-central Wisconsin, which is lovely but doesn't exactly have exotic Thai cuisine. My first taste of tom ka plaa was in Hawaii, and I have been in love with this dish and Thai cuisine ever since! Traditionally, tom ka plaa is eaten as a soup, but here, I've made my keto version of it a bit more substantial—think of it as a meal with copious amounts of a wonderful sauce.

1 tablespoon avocado oil, MCT oil, or extra-virgin olive oil

3 shallots, chopped

1½ tablespoons red curry paste

1½ cups chicken bone broth, homemade (page 108) or store-bought

1 (13½-ounce) can full-fat coconut milk

¼ teaspoon fine sea salt, plus more for the fish

1 pound halibut fillets, cut into 2-inch pieces

¼ cup fresh cilantro leaves, chopped, plus more for garnish

2 green onions, cut into ½-inch pieces, plus more for garnish

Juice of 1 lime

2 cups Zoodles (page 262), for serving (optional)

1. Heat the oil in a cast-iron skillet over medium heat. Add the shallots and sauté until tender, about 2 minutes. Reduce the heat to low. Whisk in the curry paste, broth, coconut milk, and salt. Simmer, uncovered, until thickened a bit, 20 to 40 minutes, depending on exactly how thick you would like the soup to be.

2. Sprinkle salt all over the fish pieces and add to the soup. Cover the skillet and poach the fish until it is cooked through and opaque and flakes easily, 4 to 5 minutes, depending on how thick your pieces are.

3. Once the fish is cooked through, stir in the cilantro, green onions, and lime juice. Immediately remove from the heat and place in serving bowls over zoodles, if desired. Garnish with additional sliced green onions and cilantro leaves.

4. Store extras in an airtight container in the fridge for up to 3 days. Store any leftover zoodles separately to keep them from getting soggy. Reheat in a saucepan over medium heat for a few minutes or until warmed to your liking, then spoon over warmed zoodles.

NUTRITIONAL INFO (per serving)

| calories | fat | protein | carbs | fiber |
|---|---|---|---|---|
| 360 | 22.4g | 32g | 7g | 1g |
| | 56% | 37% | 7% | |

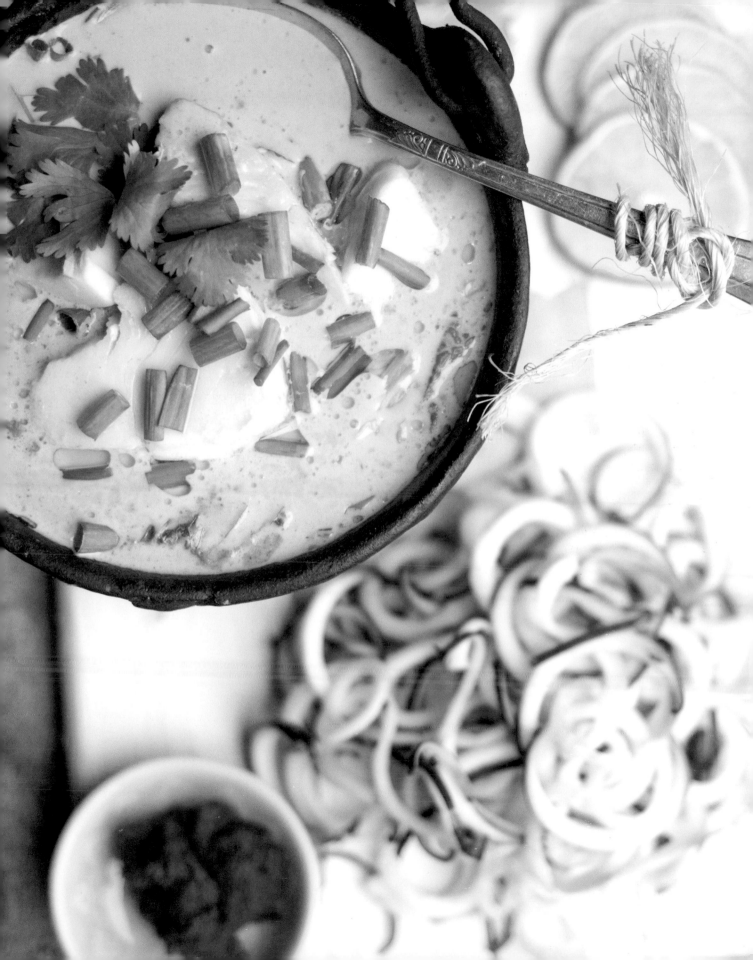

# spaghetti al tonno

prep time: 10 minutes (not including time to make the zoodles)
cook time: 17 minutes • yield: 4 servings

2 tablespoons MCT oil or coconut oil

1 anchovy fillet

2 tablespoons capers

4 cloves garlic, minced

½ cup chicken or fish bone broth, homemade (page 108) or store-bought

1½ cups chopped fresh tomatoes (about 2 medium)

1 tablespoon fresh oregano leaves, chopped, or ¼ teaspoon dried oregano leaves

⅛ teaspoon cayenne pepper

½ teaspoon fine sea salt

½ teaspoon fresh ground black pepper

1 tablespoon extra-virgin olive oil (optional)

½ teaspoon red pepper flakes (optional)

1 recipe Zoodles (page 262)

1 (7-ounce) can oil-packed tuna, drained

2 tablespoons chopped fresh flat-leaf parsley

Mixed olives, for garnish

1. Heat the MCT oil in a large skillet over medium heat. Add the anchovy, capers, and garlic and cook for 2 minutes, stirring often with a wooden spoon to break down the anchovy and work it into the oil.

2. Add the broth, tomatoes, oregano, cayenne pepper, salt, and black pepper to the skillet and cook until reduced by half, about 15 minutes.

3. If you desire a very spicy sauce, combine the olive oil and red pepper flakes in a small bowl; set aside.

4. Divide the zoodles among four serving bowls and top each bowl with an equal amount of the tuna, sauce, and parsley. Drizzle each bowl with red pepper oil, if using. Garnish with olives.

5. Store extra sauce and zucchini noodles separately in airtight containers in the refrigerator for up to 3 days. Reheat in a skillet over medium heat until warmed.

NUTRITIONAL INFO (per serving)

| calories | fat | protein | carbs | fiber |
|---|---|---|---|---|
| 275 | 17g | 20g | 11g | 3g |
| | 56% | 29% | 16% | |

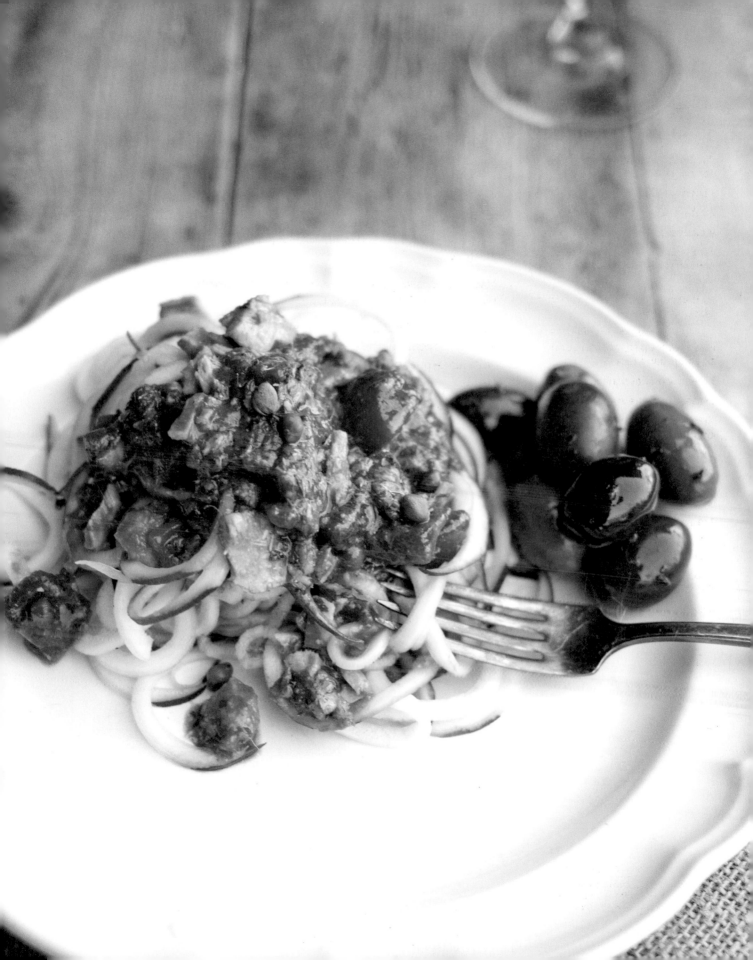

# zoodles in clam sauce

L→M→H KETO

prep time: 5 minutes (not including time to make the zoodles)
cook time: 7 minutes • yield: 2 servings

¼ cup MCT oil, duck fat, or bacon fat

2 tablespoons minced onions

2 cloves garlic, minced

1 (6½-ounce) can whole clams, drained and chopped

¼ teaspoon fine sea salt

⅛ teaspoon fresh ground black pepper

2 cups Zoodles (page 262)

Fresh basil leaves, for garnish (optional)

1. Heat the oil in a cast-iron skillet over medium heat. Add the onions and garlic and cook until the onions are translucent, about 4 minutes. Add the chopped clams and heat for 3 minutes. Season with the salt and pepper.

2. Serve over zoodles, garnished with basil, if desired.

3. Store extra sauce and zoodles separately in airtight containers in the fridge for up to 3 days. Reheat in a skillet over medium heat until warmed.

NUTRITIONAL INFO (per serving)

| calories | fat | protein | carbs | fiber |
|----------|-----|---------|-------|-------|
| 355 | 29g | 16g | 8g | 1g |
| | 73% | 18% | 9% | |

# pasta puttanesca

prep time: 10 minutes (not including time to make the zoodles)
cook time: 25 minutes · yield: 4 servings

¼ cup MCT oil

1 cup finely chopped onions

6 cloves garlic, minced

4 medium plum tomatoes, chopped, with juices

1 tightly packed cup pitted and halved Kalamata olives

2 tablespoons tomato paste

2 tablespoons capers

2 tablespoons minced anchovy fillets (about 8 fillets)

½ teaspoon dried crushed basil

½ teaspoon red pepper flakes

½ teaspoon fine sea salt

4 cups Zoodles (page 262)

Fresh basil leaves, for garnish (optional)

1. Heat the oil in a large pot over medium heat. Add the onions and sauté until soft and lightly caramelized, about 6 minutes. Add the garlic and cook for an additional 2 minutes. Add the remaining ingredients, except the zoodles, and simmer until the sauce has thickened and slightly reduced, about 15 minutes.

2. Adjust the seasoning to taste, then add the prepared zoodles to the pan and toss for 1 minute. Divide among four serving bowls and garnish with fresh basil leaves, if desired.

3. Store extra zucchini noodles and sauce separately in airtight containers in the fridge for up to 3 days. Reheat in a skillet over medium heat until warmed.

| NUTRITIONAL INFO (per serving) | | | | |
|---|---|---|---|---|
| calories | fat | protein | carbs | fiber |
| 275 | 20g | 5g | 19g | 5g |
| | 66% | 7% | 27% | |

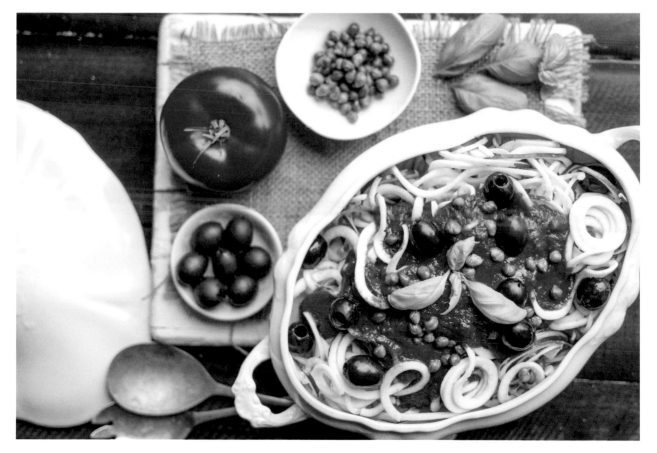

# poached salmon with creamy dill sauce

L—H M KETO · option

prep time: 15 minutes (not including time to make the mayo)
cook time: 12 minutes · yield: 4 servings

**creamy dill sauce:**

¼ cup mayonnaise, homemade (page 124) or store-bought (or Egg-Free Keto Mayo, page 125, for egg-free)

Grated zest of ½ lime

Juice of ½ lime

3 tablespoons diced cucumber

1 tablespoon chopped fresh chives

1 tablespoon chopped fresh dill

1 clove garlic, minced

¼ teaspoon fine sea salt

Pinch of fresh ground black pepper

1 lime, sliced thin

½ cup extra-virgin olive oil or MCT oil

4 (6-ounce) salmon fillets

1 teaspoon fine sea salt

½ teaspoon fresh ground black pepper

1 sprig fresh dill

Thinly sliced radish, for garnish

Thinly sliced cucumber, for garnish

1. To make the sauce: Place all the sauce ingredients in a small bowl and stir well to combine. Store in an airtight container in the fridge until ready to use.

2. To prepare the salmon: Line the bottom of an enameled cast-iron skillet with the lime slices. Pour the oil over the top of the lime. Place the salmon fillets in the skillet and add enough water to cover the fillets. Season the poaching liquid with the salt and pepper and add the sprig of dill.

3. Heat on medium-low until the poaching liquid is steaming but not boiling (about 165°F). Poach the fillets until the fish is cooked through and opaque, 10 to 12 minutes (depending on how thick your fillets are). Remove the salmon from the poaching liquid.

4. Serve each piece of fish with 2 tablespoons of the dill sauce. Garnish the plates with radish and cucumber slices.

5. Store leftover salmon and dill sauce separately in airtight containers in the fridge for up to 3 days. To reheat, place the salmon in a heat-safe dish with a few tablespoons of water, cover, and place in a preheated 350°F oven until warmed. Serve with the dill sauce.

busy family tip: *The dill sauce can be made up to 3 days ahead.*

NUTRITIONAL INFO (per serving)

| calories | fat | protein | carbs | fiber |
|----------|-----|---------|-------|-------|
| 439 | 32g | 34g | 4g | 1g |
| | 66% | 31% | 3% | |

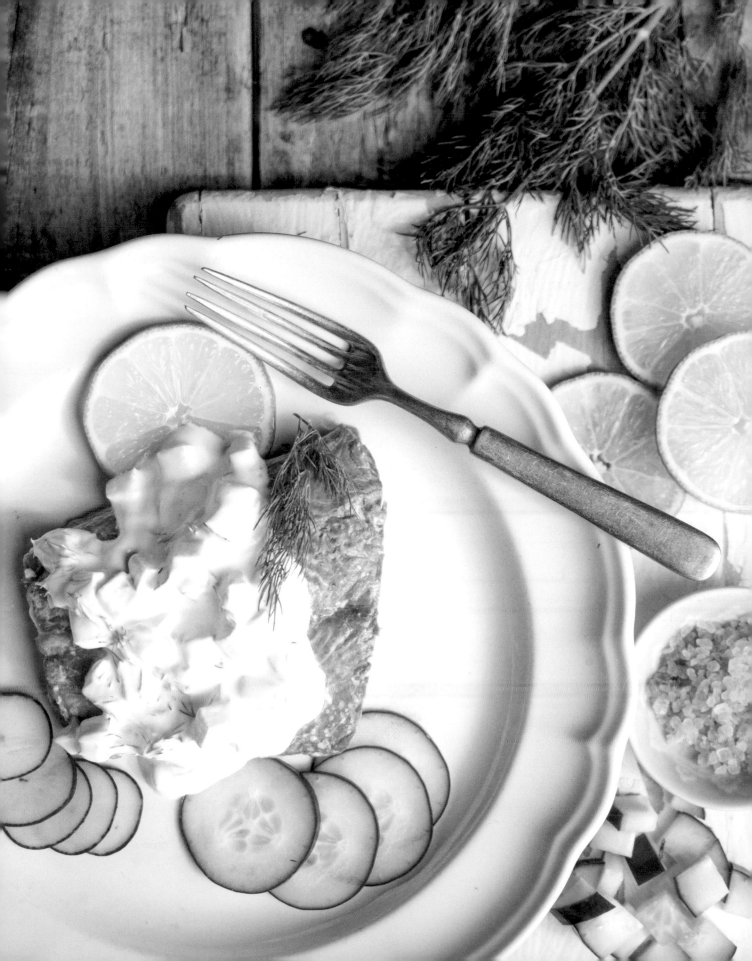

*I love food of all types—savory and sweet. And having keto treats available, like the ones in this chapter, keeps me from cheating. If you use a keto-friendly natural sweetener, such as stevia without additives such as maltodextrin, desserts will not take you out of ketosis. But for maximum results during the 30-Day Keto Cleanse, it's best to curb your sweet tooth and omit desserts, even keto sweets, altogether if you can.*

*If your cravings for sweets get too strong, I encourage you to use one of the recipes in this chapter rather than grabbing something that contains sugar or other nonketo sweeteners, which will take you out of ketosis. The treats in this chapter are absolutely keto and besides fixing a sweet tooth can also satisfy hunger. Of course, overeating can cause weight gain, so if you find these treats so tasty that you can't stop eating them, you may want to reserve them for special occasions. And remember that if you are following the Whole30 eating plan, no sugars of any type, even keto-friendly sweeteners, are allowed.*

A note on nuts and nut flours: *Many ketogenic dessert recipes use nuts and nut flours, especially blanched almond flour. However, not only is nut flour expensive, but nuts are hard on the gut as well as quite high in carbohydrates. After years of working with metabolically damaged clients as well as many type 1 diabetics, I'm convinced that eliminating nuts helps my clients heal faster. On rare occasions I do use coconut flour in this cookbook. The reason I prefer coconut flour over almond flour is that it's very absorptive; as a result, you need only a few tablespoons versus a few cups of almond flour for a recipe, which helps keep the carbohydrates down.*

keto treats

# keto mocha latte panna cotta

L M→H KETO | option | prep time: 10 minutes, plus 2 hours to chill • cook time: 5 minutes • yield: 4 servings

There is a popular drink called bulletproof coffee that many people consume when they adopt the ketogenic lifestyle. It might shock you to find out that I am not a fan of bulletproof coffee for those who are trying to lose weight. I often write about liquid calories and how they don't trigger the proper hormones that signal satiation and fullness. Chewing our calories helps signal to the brain that we have eaten, so satiety kicks in. In addition, drinking bulletproof coffee takes you out of fasting, and fasting is what helps accelerate weight loss. This is my "chewable" version of bulletproof coffee, designed for those of you who are trying to lose weight. But I don't mind bulletproof coffee for those who are *not* trying to lose weight.

## layer 1:

2 cups full-fat coconut milk, divided

1 tablespoon grass-fed powdered gelatin

¼ cup Swerve confectioners'-style sweetener or equivalent amount of liquid or powdered sweetener (see page 81)

Seeds scraped from 1 vanilla bean (about 6 inches long), split lengthwise, or 1 teaspoon vanilla extract

## layer 2:

1½ teaspoons grass-fed powdered gelatin

½ cup unsweetened, unflavored cashew milk, homemade (page 106) or store-bought, or water

1 cup decaf espresso (or strong-brewed coffee if not caffeine-sensitive)

¼ cup Swerve confectioners'-style sweetener or equivalent amount of liquid or powdered sweetener (see page 81)

2 teaspoons unsweetened cocoa powder

⅛ teaspoon fine sea salt

1. To make the first layer: Pour ½ cup of the coconut milk into a medium bowl. Sprinkle the 1 tablespoon of gelatin over the milk and let it soften while you prepare the rest of the ingredients.

2. Heat the remaining 1½ cups of coconut milk in a saucepan over medium heat for a few minutes, until hot. Alternatively, heat the milk in a microwave-safe container in the microwave for a minute.

3. Whisk the sweetener into the cool coconut milk–gelatin mixture until well combined. Pour the hot coconut milk into the gelatin mixture while stirring constantly. Add the vanilla and stir to blend.

4. Pour the custard into four 4-ounce serving cups. Place in the refrigerator to chill for 1 hour, or until the custard is set and is no longer jiggly. (*Note*: To make the panna cotta layers angled, as shown in the photo, prop up the cups at an angle with a dishtowel.)

5. To make the second layer: After the first layer has set, sprinkle the 1½ teaspoons of gelatin over the cashew milk.

6. Heat the espresso in a saucepan over medium heat. Whisk in the cashew milk mixture. Add the ¼ cup sweetener, cocoa powder, and salt and stir until well combined.

7. Pour the mocha mixture evenly over the vanilla layer in the four cups (making sure that the bottom layer has set up enough first). Place in the refrigerator for 1 hour, or until the custard is set. This is best served at room temperature but can be served cold. Store extras in the refrigerator, covered tightly, for up to 4 days.

tip: *Using gelatin is an easy way to make tasty treats, but foods made with gelatin can easily get too rubbery if they sit in the fridge overnight. If you plan on making this recipe in advance, I suggest using ¼ teaspoon less gelatin than called for in each layer; this quantity will create the perfect creamy texture even after a day or two of resting in the fridge.*

NUTRITIONAL INFO (per serving)

| calories | fat | protein | carbs | fiber |
|----------|-----|---------|-------|-------|
| 210 | 19g | 7g | 3g | 0.5g |
| | 81% | 13% | 6% | |

note: *I once made the mistake of preparing the mocha layer before the bottom vanilla layer had fully set. If you make this mistake, set the mocha layer aside and, once the vanilla layer is completely set, gently reheat the mocha mixture until it's hot and the gelatin melts.*

# chai ice lollies

KETO · option · prep time: 5 minutes, plus 3 hours to freeze • yield: 4 lollies (1 per serving)

If you don't normally sweeten your tea, this recipe is perfect for you without sweetener. But if you need a little sweetness, feel free to add 2 to 4 tablespoons of Swerve confectioners'-style sweetener or a few drops of stevia. Adjust the sweetness to your liking before freezing. During freezing, the tea and spices may separate, giving you a punch of concentrated flavor (that I love!) at the tops of your pops.

Vanilla beans are a great way to load up on phytonutrients on a ketogenic diet. The seeds also provide an amazing flavor! I always keep a large, tightly sealed pack in my fridge for additions to desserts.

You could also use my homemade Keto Chai (page 146) to make these pops.

2 to 3 chai tea bags

2 cups boiling water

½ cup unsweetened, unflavored cashew milk, homemade (page 106) or store-bought (or full-fat coconut milk for nut-free)

2 to 4 tablespoons Swerve confectioners'-style sweetener or equivalent amount of liquid or powdered sweetener (see page 81) (optional)

¼ teaspoon ground cinnamon

Seeds scraped from 1 vanilla bean, split lengthwise (optional)

### special equipment:

4 ice pop molds

1. Place the teabags in the boiling water and allow to steep for 3 minutes. Remove the teabags. Stir in the cashew milk, sweetener (if using), cinnamon, and vanilla seeds (if using). Allow to cool to room temperature.

2. Pour into ice pop molds and freeze until set, about 3 hours. Store in the freezer for up to 1 month.

NUTRITIONAL INFO (per serving)

| calories | fat | protein | carbs | fiber |
|---|---|---|---|---|
| 42 | 4g | 0.4g | 1g | 0.2g |
| | 86% | 4% | 10% | |

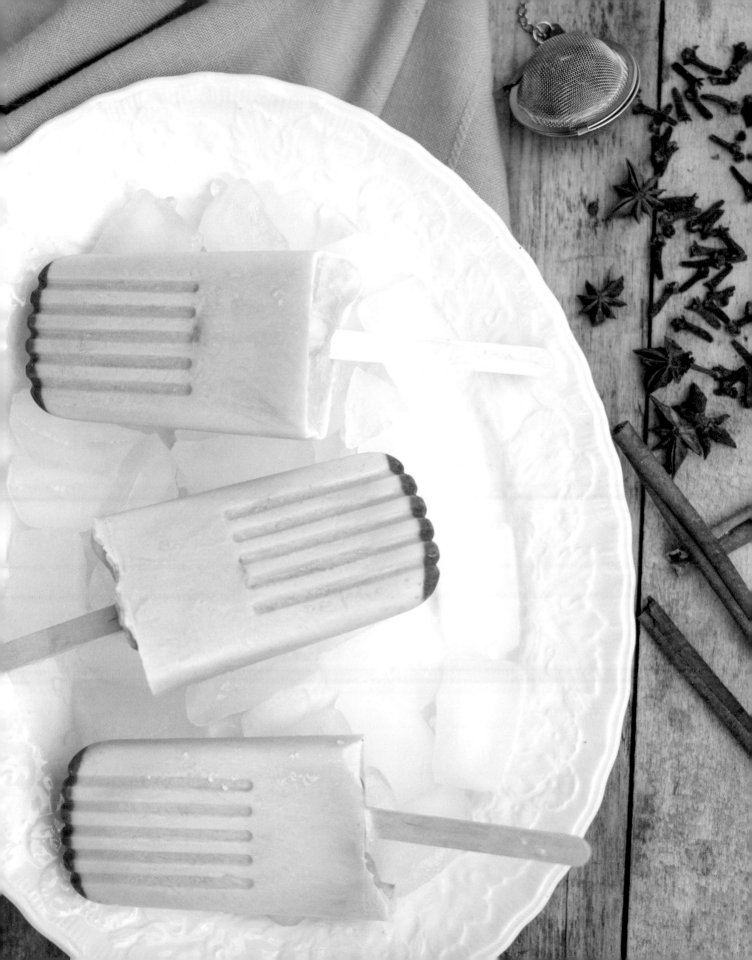

# bone broth ice pops

L M H KETO · prep time: 6 minutes, plus 4 hours to freeze • yield: 16 pops (1 per serving)

If you're trying to get rid of your sweet tooth but want a fun treat while eating keto, try these bone broth ice pops. You can experiment with different herbs and spices to your desired taste!

1 tablespoon grass-fed powdered gelatin

2 cups homemade bone broth, any type (page 108), warmed

**special equipment:**

2 (8-cavity) ice pop molds

1. Sprinkle the gelatin over the broth and whisk to combine.

2. Let cool to room temperature, then pour the liquid into the ice pop molds and freeze until set, at least 4 hours. Store in the freezer for up to 1 month.

NUTRITIONAL INFO (per serving)

| calories | fat | protein | carbs | fiber |
|---|---|---|---|---|
| 20 | 4g | 1.5g | 1.7g | 0g |
| | 60% | 19% | 21% | |

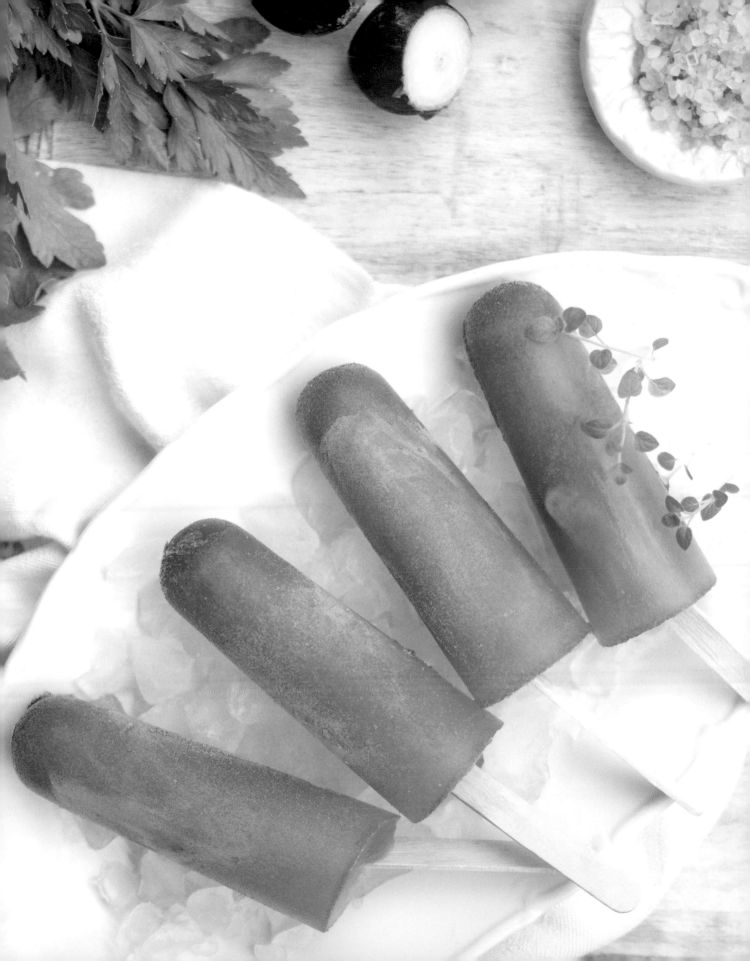

# no-bake grasshoppers in jars

L M H KETO · prep time: 8 minutes, plus 1 hour to chill · cook time: 7 minutes · yield: 8 servings

When I was a little girl, my parents often took me to High View, a restaurant in the small town of Medford, Wisconsin, that has Friday night fish fries. There is a cute little lake out in front where my brother and I would fish until our meal came to the table. After dinner, my parents often let us have nonalcoholic grasshopper drinks. The first taste of this creamy dessert took me back to fishing with my little brother at those Friday night fish fries.

In most mint-flavored recipes, the mint is used to infuse flavor, but to get the most benefit from the healing properties of mint, I puree it into this dessert. This also gives the dessert a lovely green color without the need for artificial dyes, such as those used to make crème de menthe so very green.

### chocolate bottom:

1 cup full-fat coconut milk

⅓ cup Swerve confectioners'-style sweetener or equivalent amount of liquid or powdered sweetener (see page 81)

Seeds scraped from 1 vanilla bean, split lengthwise, or 1 teaspoon vanilla extract

2 ounces unsweetened chocolate, finely chopped

### creamy mint filling:

2½ cups full-fat coconut milk, divided

2 teaspoons grass-fed powdered gelatin

½ cup chopped fresh mint

½ cup Swerve confectioners'-style sweetener or equivalent amount of liquid or powdered sweetener (see page 81)

½ teaspoon mint-flavored stevia (optional)

Pinch of fine sea salt

Fresh mint leaves, for garnish

1. Make the chocolate bottom: Place the coconut milk, sweetener, and vanilla bean seeds in a saucepan over medium heat. Once the mixture is simmering, remove from the heat and stir in the chopped chocolate until the chocolate is totally melted. Pour 2 tablespoons into each of eight 2-ounce jars or small glasses. Place in the fridge to harden a bit, about 30 minutes.

2. Meanwhile, make the filling: Place 1 cup of the coconut milk in a small saucepan. Sprinkle the gelatin over the milk and stir until dissolved. Add the mint and sweetener(s) and heat the mixture to a bare simmer. Remove from the heat and add the remaining 1½ cups of coconut milk and the salt.

3. Transfer the mixture to a blender and process until it is extremely smooth and the mint leaves are completely pureed.

4. Pour the mint filling over the chocolate bottom in the jars. Garnish with mint leaves and place in the fridge for 1 hour or until set. Store in an airtight container in the fridge for up to 3 days, until ready to serve.

gelatin tip: *Using gelatin is an easy way to make tasty treats, but foods made with gelatin can easily get too rubbery if they sit in the fridge overnight. If you plan on making this recipe ahead of time and not serving it the same day it is made, I suggest using ¼ teaspoon less gelatin than called for; this quantity will create a perfect creamy texture even after a day or two of resting in the fridge.*

busy family tip: *Can be made up to 3 days ahead (with caveat—see gelatin tip).*

| NUTRITIONAL INFO (per serving) | | | | |
|---|---|---|---|---|
| calories | fat | protein | carbs | fiber |
| 195 | 19g | 3g | 3g | 2g |
| | 88% | 6% | 6% | |

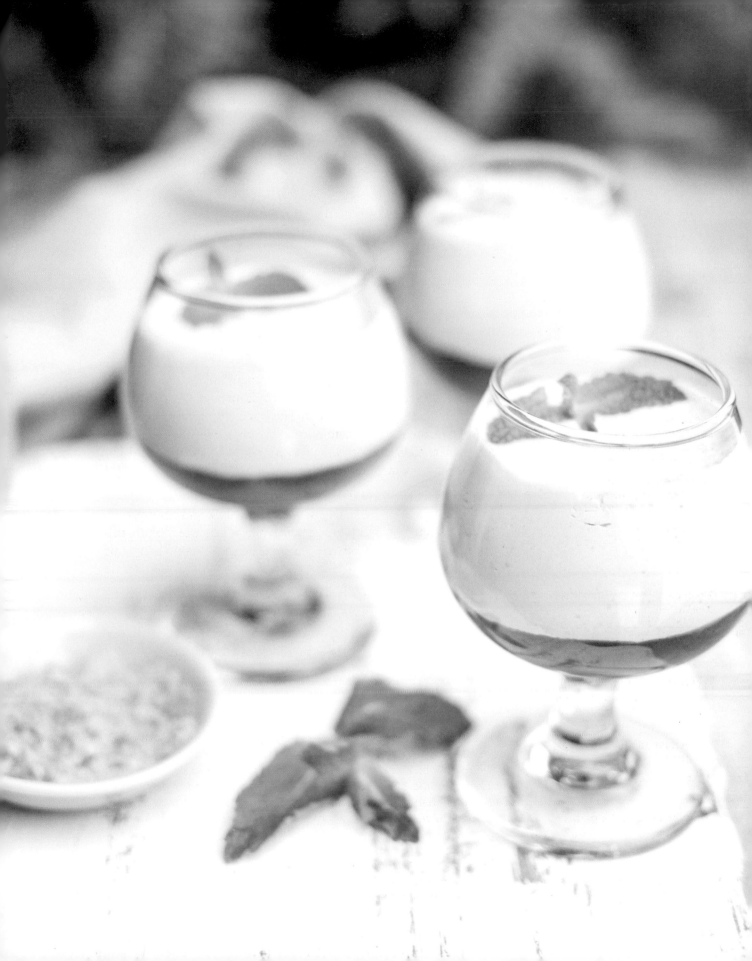

# no-bake vanilla bean petits fours

prep time: 5 minutes, plus 4 hours to chill • cook time: 5 minutes
yield: 12 petits fours (1 per serving)

I love an adorable French coffee shop in Minneapolis called Patisserie 46. You can often find my family riding bikes around the lakes of Minneapolis, then up the hill to this cute shop for decaf Americanos. They have the most amazing dessert case that is filled with works of art. I never thought I could create such beautiful desserts, but it really doesn't have to be hard! I've learned that all you need is the right mold.

2 tablespoons cold water

1 tablespoon grass-fed powdered gelatin (see note)

2 cups full-fat coconut milk

1 cup unsweetened almond milk (or hemp milk for nut-free)

⅓ cup Swerve confectioners'-style sweetener or equivalent amount of liquid or powdered sweetener (see page 81)

Seeds scraped from 1 vanilla bean, split lengthwise, or 1 teaspoon vanilla extract

⅛ teaspoon fine sea salt

Hot Fudge Sauce (page 403), thinned and warmed (optional)

## special equipment:

Silicone mold with 12 (1⅞-ounce) rectangular cavities (see page 85)

1. Place the cold water in a saucepan, then sprinkle the gelatin over the water and let sit for 1 minute to soften. Whisk in the coconut milk, almond milk, sweetener, vanilla bean seeds, and salt. Stir well to combine with the gelatin. Bring the mixture to a boil, then remove from the heat and let cool to room temperature.

2. Place a 12-cavity silicone mold on a baking sheet or other large flat surface for transporting to the fridge. Fill each mold just shy of the top with the mixture. Place in the fridge until set, about 2 hours, then transfer to the freezer for 2 hours for easy removal from the mold.

3. Remove the petits fours from the mold by pushing the bottom of the mold with your hands. Place on a serving platter, allow to thaw, and serve chilled, not frozen. Just before serving, drizzle with thinned, warm hot fudge sauce, if desired.

4. Store covered in the fridge for up to 5 days or in the freezer for up to 1 month.

note: *Gelatin gets gummier as time goes by. If you're not serving the petits fours the same day you make them, decrease the amount of gelatin to 2¼ teaspoons.*

variation: No-Bake Strawberry Petits Fours.

*Add 2 teaspoons of strawberry extract or a few drops of strawberry oil in Step 1 with the milks, sweetener, and salt. For additional depth of flavor and a pretty presentation, add the seeds scraped from 1 vanilla bean along with the strawberry extract or oil.*

NUTRITIONAL INFO (per serving, without hot fudge sauce)

| calories | fat | protein | carbs | fiber |
|---|---|---|---|---|
| 62 | 6g | 1g | 1g | 0.1g |
| | 86% | 7% | 7% | |

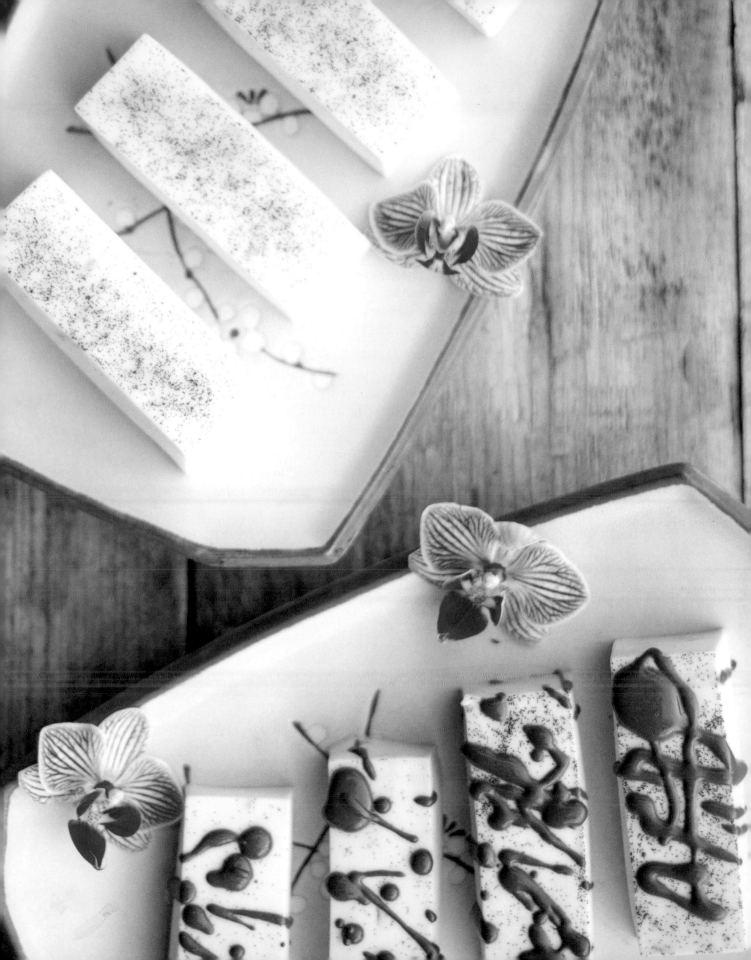

# tom ka gai savory ice cream

L M H KETO · prep time: 6 minutes, plus 2 hours to chill · yield: 8 servings

If a savory dessert sounds crazy to you, think about the tradition in some cultures to finish a meal with a salad or cheese course. I just morphed the salad/cheese course into a dessert that really and truly tastes like bowl of frozen tom ka gai soup! Also, many of my clients want to lose their sweet tooth yet still crave dessert, so I wanted to include a dessert for them.

1 stalk lemongrass, trimmed, tough outer leaves removed

¾ cup plus 2 tablespoons coconut oil, softened

¼ cup MCT oil

¼ cup chicken bone broth, homemade (page 108) or store-bought

¼ cup full-fat coconut milk

4 large whole eggs

4 large egg yolks

½ teaspoon fish sauce

1 teaspoon grated fresh ginger

1 teaspoon chopped fresh cilantro

Grated zest of 1 lime

Juice of 1 lime

½ teaspoon salt

2 tablespoons Swerve confectioners'-style sweetener or equivalent amount of liquid or powdered sweetener (see page 81) (optional)

## special equipment:

Ice cream maker

1. If you have a high-speed blender, cut the bottom half of the lemongrass stalk into two or three pieces and drop them into the blender jar; if you have a regular blender, grate the bottom third or so of the lemongrass stalk into the blender jar.

2. Add the coconut oil, MCT oil, broth, coconut milk, eggs, egg yolks, fish sauce, ginger, cilantro, lime zest and juice, salt, and sweetener to the blender and puree until very smooth.

3. Pour into an ice cream maker and churn, following the manufacturer's instructions, until set. Store in an airtight container in the freezer for up to 1 month.

note: *Making ice cream with oil and salt may seem unusual, but they play important roles: the oil gives the ice cream a smooth texture and the salt helps keep it soft.*

| NUTRITIONAL INFO (per serving) | | | | |
|---|---|---|---|---|
| calories | fat | protein | carbs | fiber |
| 350 | 36g | 5g | 2g | 0.3g |
| | 92% | 6% | 2% | |

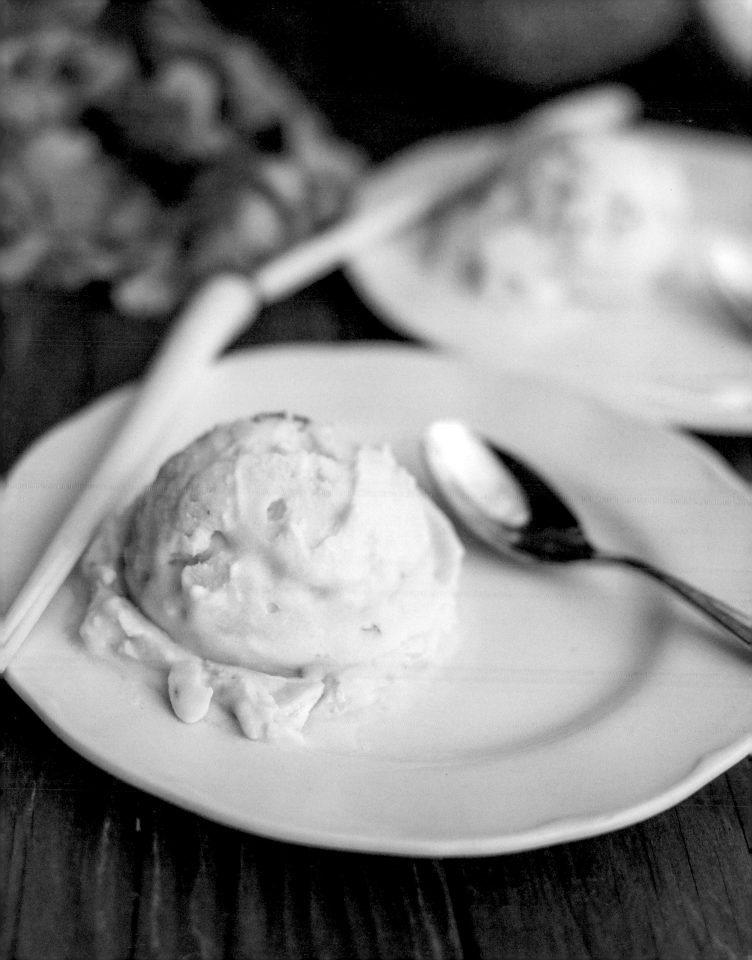

# vanilla bean bread pudding
# with vanilla bean crème anglaise

prep time: 12 minutes, plus time to cool the bread (not including time to make the crème anglaise) • cook time: 1 hour 45 minutes • yield: 12 servings

If you try making the bread for this dessert with a carton of egg whites, you will not end up with an airy bread. It is best to use real eggs and separate the whites from the yolks yourself. Egg whites from a carton do not whip as well, and you will end up with a soufflé-like bread instead of a fluffy and airy bread.

## bread:

½ cup unflavored egg white protein powder

½ cup Swerve confectioners'-style sweetener or equivalent amount of liquid or powdered sweetener (see page 81) (optional)

12 large egg whites

2 teaspoons cream of tartar

1 teaspoon vanilla extract

## pudding:

1 cup unsweetened, unflavored almond milk (or full-fat coconut milk for nut-free)

½ cup full-fat coconut milk

3 large eggs

⅔ cup Swerve confectioners'-style sweetener or equivalent amount of liquid or powdered sweetener (see page 81) (optional)

1 teaspoon ground cinnamon

½ teaspoon fine sea salt

Seeds scraped from 1 vanilla bean, split lengthwise, or 1 teaspoon vanilla extract

1½ recipes Vanilla Bean Crème Anglaise (page 404), warm or chilled

1. To make the bread: Preheat the oven to 350°F. Grease a 13 by 9-inch casserole dish. Sift the protein powder and sweetener together and set aside. In a large, scrupulously clean metal bowl, whip the egg whites until foamy (save the yolks for the crème anglaise). Add the cream of tartar and continue to beat until very stiff (when the whites are sufficiently whipped, you should be able to turn the bowl upside down and the whites won't fall out). Add the vanilla extract and whisk to combine. Quickly fold in the protein powder mixture. Pour into the prepared pan. Bake for 45 minutes, until light golden brown. Remove from the oven and let cool completely in the pan. Once completely cool, cut into 1-inch cubes and place in a mixing bowl (see tip).

2. To make the pudding: Preheat the oven to 350°F. Grease an 11 by 7-inch baking dish. Cover the cubed bread with the almond milk and coconut milk; set aside. In another bowl, combine the eggs, sweetener, cinnamon, salt, and vanilla; blend well. Pour the egg mixture over the soaked bread and stir to blend. Pour the bread cube mixture into the prepared baking dish.

3. Bake for 45 to 60 minutes, until set. Remove from the oven, allow to cool to room temperature, then cut into 12 pieces.

4. To serve, pour about 2 tablespoons of crème anglaise over each piece of bread pudding (only sauce pieces of pudding that you plan to serve right away). Store leftover bread pudding and crème anglaise separately in airtight containers in the fridge for up to 3 days.

busy family tip: *The bread can be made a day ahead, cooled to room temperature, and then placed in the fridge overnight. The next day, cube it and continue with the recipe. The crème anglaise can be made ahead of time as well.*

NUTRITIONAL INFO (per serving)

| calories | fat | protein | carbs | fiber |
|----------|-----|---------|-------|-------|
| 340 | 25g | 26g | 3g | 1g |
| | 66% | 31% | 3% | |

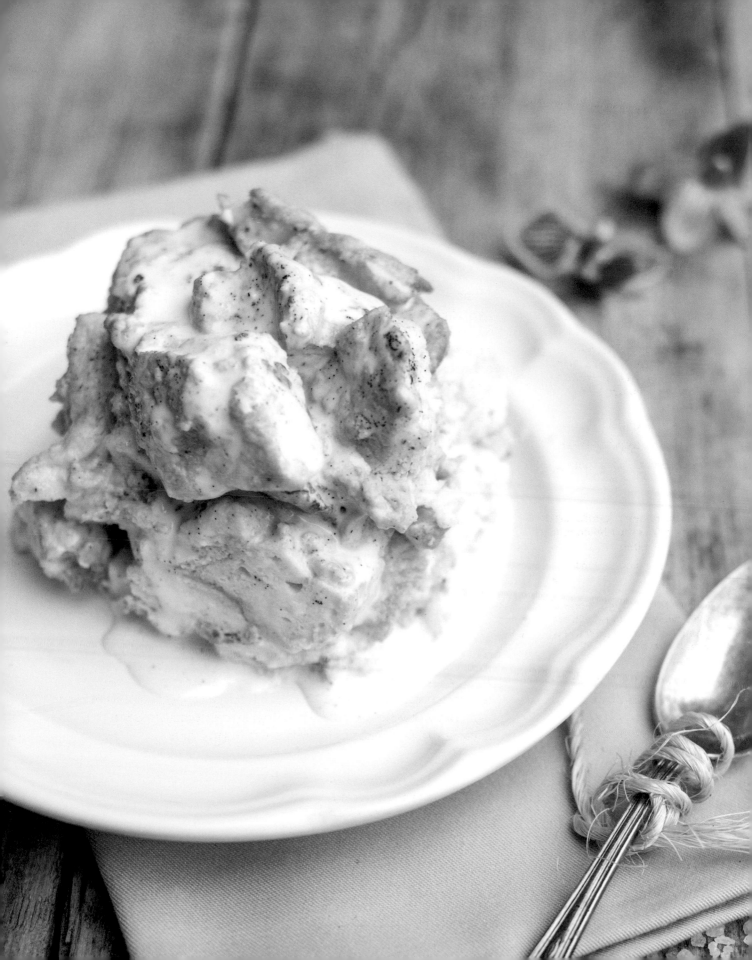

# chai fat bombs

prep time: 3 minutes, plus 20 minutes or 1 hour to chill (not including time to brew the tea)
yield: 6 fat bombs (1 per serving)

1 cup coconut oil, softened but not liquid

¾ cup strong-brewed chai tea, at room temperature

¾ cup Swerve confectioners'-style sweetener or equivalent amount of liquid or powdered sweetener (see page 81) (optional)

1 teaspoon ground cinnamon

**special equipment:**

Silicone mold with 12 (1⅞-ounce) rectangular cavities (see page 85)

1. Place the silicone mold on a rimmed baking sheet (to avoid spilling while transporting).

2. Place all the ingredients in a blender or food processor and puree until smooth.

3. Pour the pureed tea mixture into six of the cavities in the mold. (The pureed mixture will separate if it sits out and gets too hot; if that happens, puree it again before you pour the mixture into the mold.) Place the mold in the fridge or freezer to set, about 1 hour in the fridge or 20 minutes in the freezer.

4. Use your hands to push the hardened fat bombs from the mold. Store in an airtight container in the fridge for up to 6 days, or freeze for up to 1 month.

NUTRITIONAL INFO (per serving)

| calories | fat | protein | carbs | fiber |
|---|---|---|---|---|
| 335 | 37g | 0g | 1g | 0.4g |
| | 99% | 0% | 1% | |

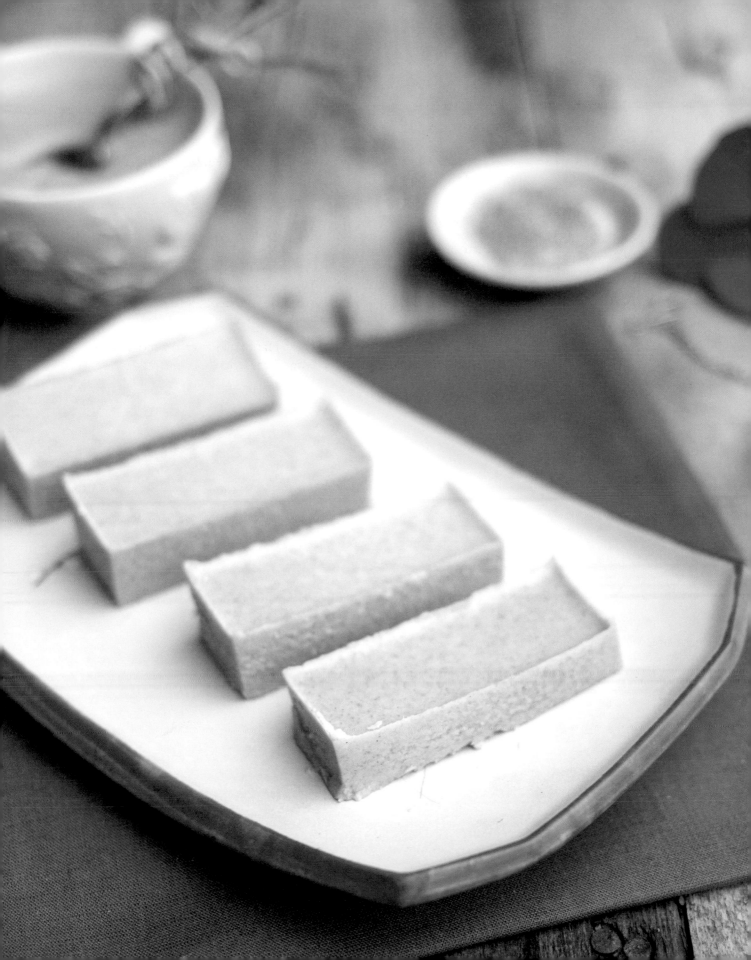

# lava cakes with mocha ice cream

prep time: 20 minutes, plus time to chill the ice cream • cook time: 15 minutes
yield: 8 cakes (1 per serving)

This is a fabulous dessert for a special occasion. It takes a little bit of time to pull together because there are two components—cake and ice cream—but since both components can be made ahead, it's really quite easy. The ice cream can be made up to a month in advance, and the batter for the cakes can be made a few days before a dinner party. You can pop the batter in the oven when needed to have perfect lava cakes, warm with gooey centers.

## mocha ice cream:

¾ cup plus 2 tablespoons coconut oil

½ cup strong-brewed decaf espresso, chilled

¼ cup MCT oil

4 large eggs

4 large egg yolks

Seeds scraped from 1 vanilla bean, split lengthwise, or 1 teaspoon vanilla extract

¼ cup Swerve confectioners'-style sweetener or equivalent amount of liquid or powdered sweetener (see page 81) (optional)

2 tablespoons unsweetened cocoa powder

½ teaspoon fine sea salt

## lava cakes:

8 teaspoons plus ½ cup Swerve confectioners'-style sweetener or equivalent amount of powdered erythritol or monk fruit (see page 81), divided

4 ounces unsweetened chocolate, chopped

¾ cup coconut oil, plus more for greasing

3 large eggs

3 large egg yolks

¼ cup unsweetened almond milk (or unsweetened hemp milk for nut-free)

1. To make the ice cream: Place all the ingredients in a blender and blend until very smooth. Taste and add more sweetener, if desired, and pulse once more to combine.

2. Pour into an ice cream maker and churn, following the manufacturer's instructions, until set. Store in an airtight container in the freezer for up to 1 month.

3. To make the lava cakes: Grease eight 6-ounce soufflé dishes or custard cups with coconut oil. Sprinkle the inside of each dish with 1 teaspoon of sweetener. Combine the chocolate and coconut oil in a medium saucepan over low heat and stir until smooth. Remove from the heat and set aside.

4. Using an electric mixer, beat the eggs, egg yolks, almond milk, and remaining ½ cup of sweetener in large bowl until thickened and pale yellow, about 8 minutes. Fold the warm chocolate mixture into the egg mixture. Divide the batter evenly among the prepared soufflé dishes. *Note:* At this point, you can either bake the cakes or cover them and place them in the fridge for up to 3 days. Bring to room temperature and remove the covering before baking.

5. To bake the cakes: Preheat the oven to 400°F. Place the soufflé dishes on a rimmed baking sheet. Bake the cakes until the edges are puffed and slightly cracked but the center 1 inch of each cake moves slightly when the dishes are shaken gently, about 9 minutes. (You want the centers slightly underdone.)

6. To serve, flip the soufflé dishes over onto serving dishes. Lift the dishes off the cakes; the cakes should slide out. Top each cake with a scoop of the mocha ice cream and serve immediately.

## special equipment:

Ice cream maker

| | NUTRITIONAL INFO (per serving) | | | |
|---|---|---|---|---|
| calories | fat | protein | carbs | fiber |
| 670 | 68g | 10g | 5g | 3g |
| | 91% | 6% | 3% | |

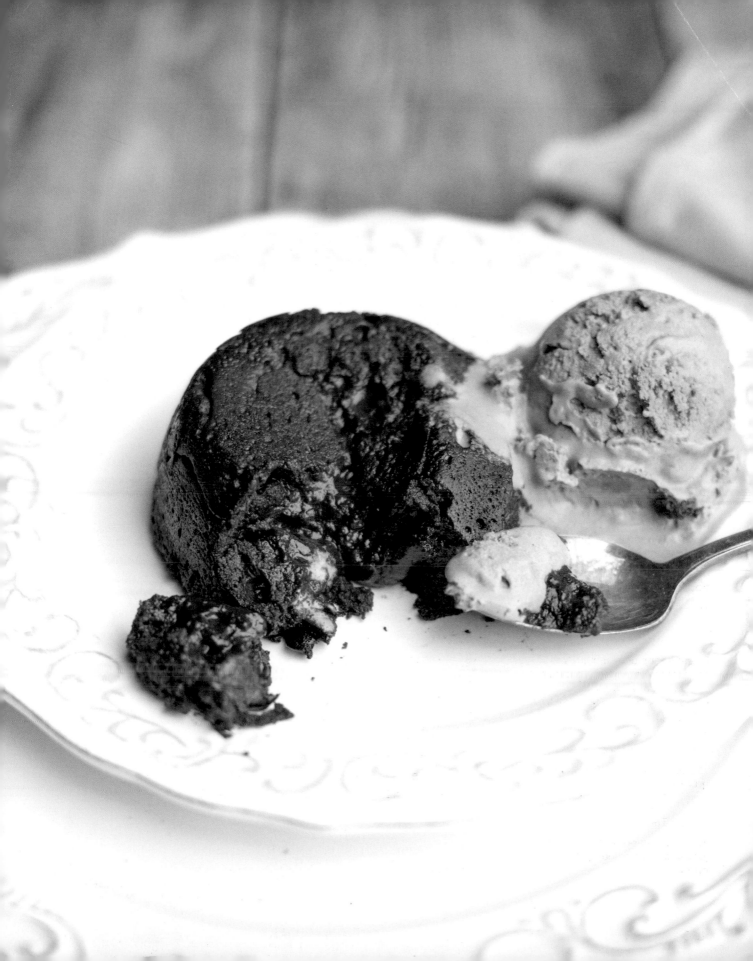

# lemon curd

prep time: 5 minutes, plus 15 minutes to chill • cook time: 15 minutes
yield: 2¾ cups (¼ cup per serving)

This lemon curd is indispensable. I serve it straight up in individual bowls for a decadent creamy treat and also use it to make my Lemon Curd Dutch Baby (page 184).

1 cup Swerve confectioners'-style sweetener or equivalent amount of liquid or powdered sweetener (see page 81)

½ cup lemon juice

4 large eggs

½ cup coconut oil

1 tablespoon grated lemon zest, for garnish (optional)

busy family tip: *Can be made up to 4 days ahead.*

1. In a medium heavy-bottomed saucepan, whisk together the sweetener, lemon juice, and eggs. Add the coconut oil and place over medium heat. Once the oil is melted, whisk constantly until the mixture thickens and thickly coats the back of a spoon, about 10 minutes. Do not allow the mixture to come to a boil.

2. Pour the mixture through a fine-mesh strainer into a medium bowl. Place the bowl in a larger bowl filled with ice water and whisk occasionally until the curd is completely cool, about 15 minutes.

3. Serve in individual bowls, garnished with lemon zest, if desired, or store in the refrigerator for up to 4 days.

NUTRITIONAL INFO (per serving)

| calories | fat | protein | carbs | fiber |
|---|---|---|---|---|
| 100 | 10g | 2g | 0.3g | 0g |
| | 90% | 8% | 2% | |

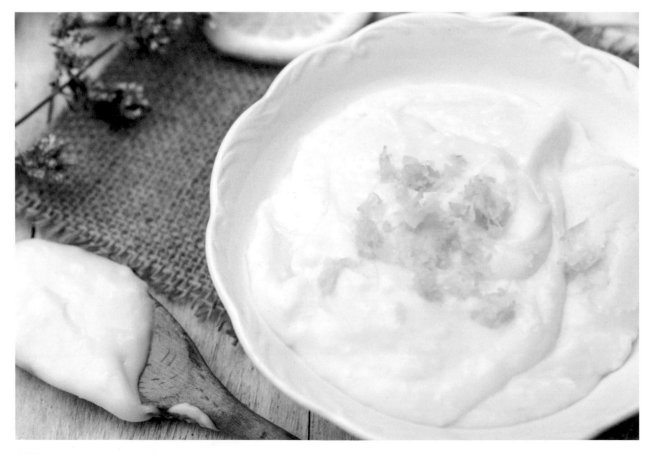

# hot fudge sauce

LMH KETO · prep time: 5 minutes • cook time: 5 minutes • yield: 1 cup (2 tablespoons per serving)

In addition to serving this sauce with ice cream, I adore it over my Chocolate Waffles (page 182).

¾ cup full-fat coconut milk

⅓ cup Swerve confectioners'-style sweetener or equivalent amount of liquid or powdered sweetener (see page 81)

2 ounces unsweetened chocolate, finely chopped

Seeds scraped from 1 vanilla bean, split lengthwise, or 1 teaspoon vanilla extract

1. Place the coconut milk, sweetener, and chopped chocolate in a double boiler or in a heat-safe bowl set over a pan of simmering water. Heat on low heat while stirring just until the chocolate melts, then remove from the heat. Add the vanilla bean seeds and stir to combine.

2. Use immediately or let cool, then cover and refrigerate until ready to serve. Store in an airtight container in the refrigerator for up to 4 days or freeze for up to 2 months. The sauce can be served chilled, or if you prefer, reheat the sauce in a double boiler or a heat-safe bowl set over a pan of simmering water while stirring until warm.

tip: *To use this sauce for drizzling over desserts, such as petits fours (page 392), thin the sauce with tablespoon or two of coconut milk to get it to a nice, pourable consistency and use warm.*

NUTRITIONAL INFO (per serving)

| calories | fat | protein | carbs | fiber |
|----------|-----|---------|-------|-------|
| 79 | 7g | 1g | 3g | 2g |
| | 80% | 5% | 15% | |

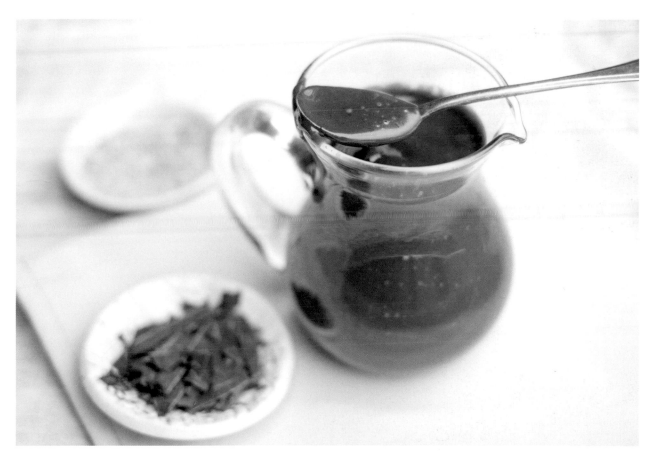

# vanilla bean crème anglaise

prep time: 5 minutes • cook time: 5 minutes • yield: 1 cup (¼ cup per serving when eaten on its own as a dessert; 2 tablespoons per serving when used with other foods)

I use this keto take on a classic dessert sauce with my Snickerdoodle Waffles (page 180) and Vanilla Bean Bread Pudding (page 396). It also tastes great on its own; it reminds me of homemade pudding.

6 large egg yolks

½ cup unsweetened, unflavored almond milk (or hemp milk for nut-free)

¼ cup Swerve confectioners'-style sweetener or equivalent amount of liquid or powdered sweetener (see page 81)

¼ cup coconut oil, melted

Seeds scraped from 1 vanilla bean, split lengthwise, or 1 teaspoon vanilla extract

1. Place the egg yolks, almond milk, and sweetener in a medium heat-safe bowl and whisk to blend. While whisking constantly, slowly drizzle in the melted coconut oil so that the eggs don't cook.

2. Set the bowl over a saucepan of simmering water. Stir the mixture constantly and vigorously until it coats the back of a spoon and an instant-read thermometer inserted into the mixture registers 140°F, about 3 minutes.

3. Remove the mixture from the heat. Using a whisk, stir in the vanilla bean seeds. Serve warm or chilled. To chill the sauce, set the bowl in a larger bowl of ice water.

4. Crème anglaise will keep in an airtight container in the refrigerator for up to 3 days. Whisk before serving. To reheat, place the sauce in a double boiler or a heat-safe bowl set over a pan of simmering water and gently reheat, stirring often; do not overheat or the eggs will curdle.

NUTRITIONAL INFO
(per ¼ cup serving)

| calories | fat | protein | carbs | fiber |
|----------|-----|---------|-------|-------|
| 202 | 21g | 4g | 1g | 0.1g |
| | 92% | 7% | 2% | |

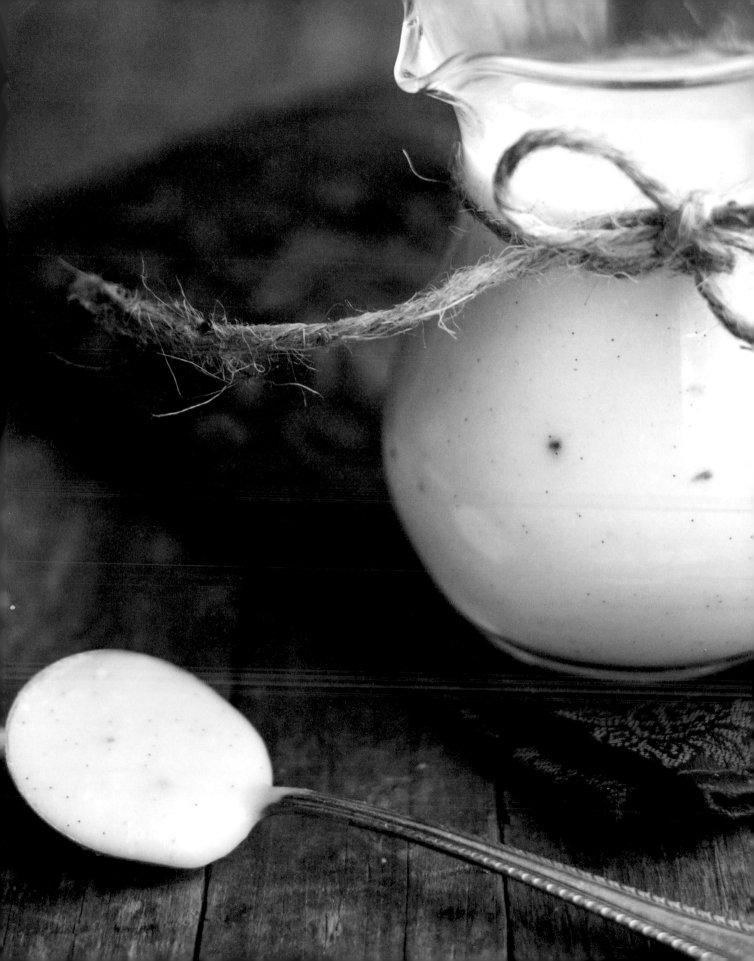

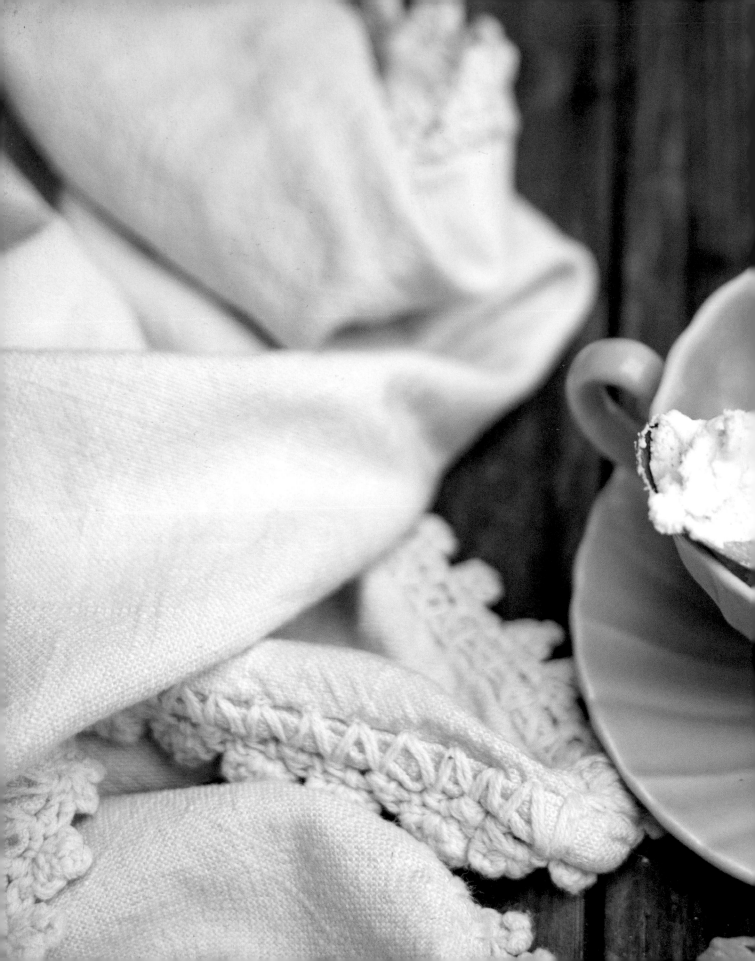

# PART 5: resources

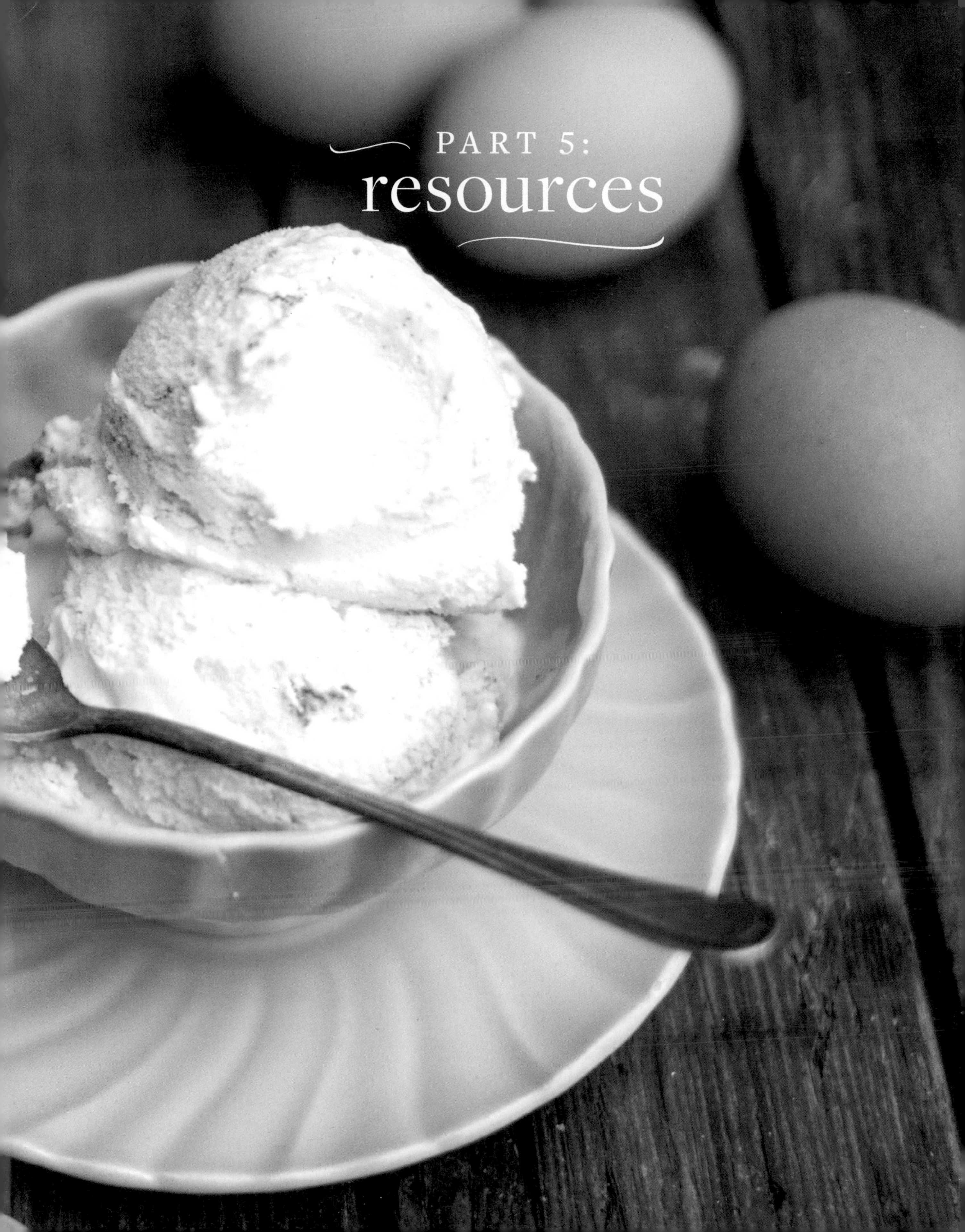

# appendix:
# taking stock of personal care products

I was enjoying a pot of tea with my friend Kristen when she told me a story about when her daughter was three years old and appeared to be drunk. It scared the living daylights out of her. After digging into the cause, she discovered that her daughter had gotten into a bottle of hand sanitizer, and it had soaked through her skin into her bloodstream!

Yep, our skin is our largest organ, and everything you put on your skin gets shuttled into your bloodstream, just as if you ate it. Pharmaceutical companies know this; that's why they use topical patches and lotions to deliver medicine. In fact, many times medications are more effective as creams than as pills because they are so readily absorbed through the skin. And so are the ingredients in *any* product you put on your skin!

Your skin also sucks in the poisons that are found in cosmetics, moisturizers, self-tanners, and products like insect repellent. The skin delivers those poisons to the bloodstream, which takes them right to your liver. The liver's job is to filter out toxins from the blood, and when toxin levels are high, the liver can become tired and congested. Your liver also governs your moods and controls how fast you lose weight, so a taxed liver can affect many aspects of your health.

Limiting the liver's exposure to pollutants enables it to heal from prior abuse. I even had a client who got out of the danger zone of high liver enzymes just by changing her makeup and skin lotions!

The chemicals in our personal care products may also be interfering with our hormones. Phthalates (found in perfume and fragrances), parabens (found in cosmetics), triclosan (found in antibacterial soaps), and oxybenzone (found in sunscreen) are all endocrine-disrupting chemicals. One study found that in teenage girls, the use of products containing lower amounts of these chemicals for just three days caused the levels in their bodies to drop significantly—by up to 45 percent! In other words, what you put on your skin truly matters.

Dihydroxyacetone, or DHA (not to be confused with docosahexaenoic acid, the beneficial DHA fatty acid found in fish oil), is a potent chemical commonly found in self-tanners. Although it's not absorbed through the skin, it does cause the upper layers of skin to be more susceptible to free radicals, cellular killers that wreak havoc by damaging DNA and altering cell membranes. Scientists now can prove that free radicals play a major role in the aging process, in addition to being associated with heart disease, stroke, cancer, arthritis, and possibly allergies, along with many other issues. To put it simply, think of your body as an apple: an apple turns brown once you slice it and expose it to air; your body basically rusts from the inside out when exposed to free radicals.

I wasn't always aware of and didn't always think about what I was putting on my skin. But just as I took baby steps to clean out my kitchen pantry, I realized that I had to take steps to clean out my bathroom cabinet and find safer alternatives for the topical products my family and I were using.

I started with shampoo and conditioner, then switched to a safer sunscreen, and over time my whole bathroom cabinet became something I was proud of, just like my kitchen pantry.

I suggest that you do the same. Think about all the products you put on your skin and gums:

- Deodorant
- Insect repellent
- Lotion
- Makeup
- Perfume
- Shampoo and conditioner
- Soap
- Toothpaste and mouthwash

Look at the brands you use and think about whether it would be a good idea to switch to other brands that use less harmful chemicals—or make your own! Some of my favorite homemade recipes appear on the following pages.

When it comes to perfume, there is a simple solution: put it on your clothes instead of your skin. I love Elizabeth Arden's Green Tea fragrance!

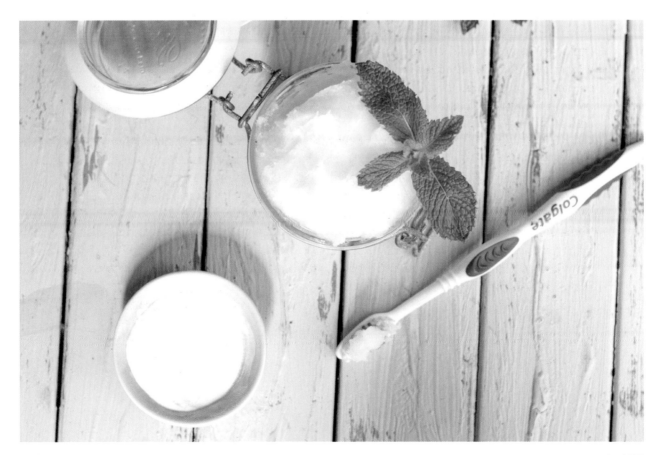

# homemade perfume

prep time: less than 5 minutes • yield: 8 ounces

12 drops clove oil

12 drops geranium oil

12 drops lavandin oil

12 drops palmarosa oil

12 drops patchouli oil

12 drops rosewood oil

12 drops sandalwood oil

1 cup water

Place the oils in a perfume spray bottle. Add the water to dilute and spray as needed!

# lip scrub

prep time: less than 5 minutes • yield: about 2¾ ounces

3 tablespoons Swerve granular-style sweetener

2 tablespoons coconut oil

2 teaspoons vitamin E oil

5 to 8 drops scented oil of choice

1. In a small bowl, mix together all the ingredients. Choose any scented oil you like!

2. Put the scrub in cute little jars. Give to friends!

# natural bug spray

prep time: less than 5 minutes • yield: 8 ounces

24 drops citronella oil

24 drops lavender oil

24 drops peppermint oil

24 drops tea tree oil

1 cup water

Place the oils in a clear dark or frosted spray bottle. Add the water to dilute and spray as needed!

note: *This recipe is easy to scale up or down. Simply use a ratio of 2 to 5 drops of each oil to 1 ounce of water.*

# bathing scrub

prep time: 5 minutes • yield: 40 ounces (about 5 cups)

A wonderful friend of mine who knows that I use only certain products on my skin gave me a thoughtful present of natural bath salts. I absolutely loved her gift, and it inspired me to make my own scrub!

4 cups large-grain sea salt

1 cup jojoba oil

2 teaspoons essential oil of choice (I like lavender)

1 teaspoon magnesium oil (optional)

1. In a large bowl, combine the salt and jojoba oil. Add the essential oil. You can use more or less essential oil depending on how strong a scent you desire. Add the magnesium oil, if desired.

2. Divide among cute jars. Share with friends!

# toothpaste

prep time: less than 5 minutes • yield: 12 ounces

1 cup coconut oil

¼ cup baking soda

⅛ to ¼ cup Swerve confectioners'-style sweetener or equivalent amount of powdered erythritol or monk fruit (see page 81), depending on desired sweetness

16 drops essential oil of choice, such as peppermint, spearmint, or cinnamon, or a combination

1. Warm the coconut oil in a small saucepan over low heat until soft and stirrable. Add the baking soda, sweetener, and essential oil and stir until well combined.

2. Place in cute jars and keep by the sink to replace store-bought toothpaste!

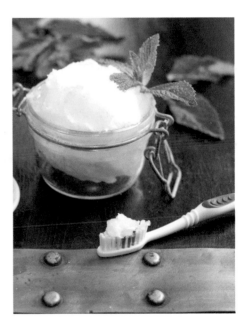

# deodorant

prep time: 5 minutes • yield: 16 ounces

½ cup coconut oil

½ cup shea butter

½ cup arrowroot powder

½ cup baking soda

10 drops lavender essential oil (optional)

1. Warm the coconut oil and shea butter in a saucepan over low heat until completely melted, about 4 minutes. Remove from the heat and add the arrowroot powder, baking soda, and lavender oil, if desired.

2. Place in a sealable jar and store in the bathroom cabinet. To apply, dip clean fingers into the jar and rub onto your underarms.

# testimonials

"I have suffered from chronic migraines with auras for the past three years. I was at the point where I had felt like I had tried everything, every pill that doctors pushed to subdue the pain, acupuncture, Botox, steroid injections, a chiropractor. I found out about your services and tried the 7-day cleanse (why not, I had tried everything else) and I was amazed. Now, I don't miss out on life because of the pain. Thank you."

—Kara

"I am now officially off my blood pressure medication!!! My BP was 160 (over something) a few years ago and I was put on medication. Today, at my first doctor appointment in quite a while, it was 112/72—and I quit my BP meds in August when I went on the keto plan, just because I was sick of taking them. Anyway, SO excited to see these numbers—especially considering my BP always goes up in the doctor's office—so it may be even lower than that! And I'm down 50 pounds! Thanks for your help!!"

—Kelly

"Today is 1 year since I started the keto-adapted lifestyle. What a journey it has been. Hiring Maria was the best money I think I ever spent. She changed the way I feel about food. I took all the processed and junk food out of my house and bought *real* food. One may think I starve myself . . . you would be wrong. I eat so well that while I eat I am always saying, 'Oh man, this is so good.' I only cook up food once or twice a week, so my meals are always ready. I use my slow cooker a lot! One year ago I had bad knee pain and needed shots every 3–4 months, and my doctor said that she might have to space the shots longer apart or someday I'd need a knee replacement. Well, that scared me. My doctor asked me about my lifestyle, so I told her a bit about my life, as many of you know I care for my brain-injured husband. She also asked how I eat and I told her the truth. I told her that I ate chocolate every day, sometimes 2–3 times a day. I craved pasta, rice, pizza, anything high in carbs and sugar. She wrote down Maria's name and told me to check out her Facebook page and just read what she does to help people like me. Well, something clicked in me when I started reading her posts, and I ordered some of her books. I started trying some of her recipes. Her homemade ranch dressing is one of my favorites. I decided to hire Maria, and we first spoke on March 7, 2015. She gave me the plan and told me the supplements I needed to heal my body. One year later I am down 85 lbs. No more pain in my knee, and I feel so happy. I have such a different feeling about life now. I feel like for the first time in my life I have control of *me*. I absolutely believe Maria saved me, and I thank god for her every day."

—Shirley

"This is what your help has done for me, a mom of 5, and business owner with employees, parents who depend on me. I reversed super high blood pressure, prediabetes, hormone imbalance (badddd), pre-arthritis, insomnia, and a slew of other things. I've lost 150 lbs in fat and massed about 20 lbs in muscle."

—Robyn

"A big thank you, Maria! For the first time in years I feel clean. By 'clean' I mean my mind, my energy, my body—the best way to describe it is 'cleansed.' My irritability is gone, and I am finding myself so grateful, grateful for my wonderful life, my terrific kids, and my amazing, supportive husband. I have always been blessed with these things, but I am just now consciously connecting to myself and my life. The funny thing is, I didn't even know that I wasn't. I am truly amazed how in a little over 2 weeks your life, health, and perspective can change. Down 13 pounds in 15 days! Thank you, Maria, for your kindness and passion to teach."

—Torri

"I was about 285 lbs at my heaviest. I first started losing weight by switching to a Paleo diet but eventually stalled at about 240. I found your site, bought your books, and switched to keto. As of this morning I weigh 181. Still have a way to go to my goal weight, but I know keto will get me there! Oh, and I no longer suffer at all from ulcerative colitis!!!"

—Sam

"I've been religiously following your advice and have lost 28 pounds. I put on 200 pounds after I had my first child (turned out pregnancy activated celiac disease for me). No matter how much I exercised and starved myself the weight kept piling on. This is the first time in 9 years I've actually felt good, and this is the first 'diet' I feel I can do for the rest of my life and am completely confident I can lose all this weight with. I have no signs of the prediabetes I was diagnosed with a year ago now. Depression and suicidal thoughts are a thing of the past. No more acid reflux (which was daily). And my periods aren't a sporadic, literal or figurative mess anymore. I can honestly say you've saved my life."

—Laura

"I have to say, when I first heard you say I should omit dairy from my meals, I panicked a little. But unbelievably, you were right! After not only removing dairy but also adding the supplements you suggested, I can now again consume lactose-free dairy without any adverse effects. I am so happy that you suggested this . . . it made a world of difference!"

—Kristen

# recipe quick reference

H $\underset{\text{KETO}}{L\overset{M}{\frown}H}$　　M $\underset{\text{KETO}}{L\overset{M}{\wedge}H}$　　L $\underset{\text{KETO}}{L\overset{M}{\curvearrowleft}H}$　　• omits this ingredient　　O option

| Recipe | PAGE | $\underset{\text{KETO}}{L\overset{M}{\frown}H}$ | DAIRY | NUT | EGG | ANIMAL PRODUCTS |
|---|---|---|---|---|---|---|
| homemade cashew milk | 106 | H | • | | • | • |
| bone broth—beef, chicken, or fish | 108 | M | • | • | • | |
| berbere spice mix | 110 | L | • | • | • | • |
| spicy and sweet hamburger spice mix | 111 | L | • | • | • | • |
| cajun seasoning | 112 | L | • | • | • | • |
| herbs de florence | 113 | L | • | • | • | • |
| ranch seasoning | 114 | L | • | • | • | • |
| dairy-free ranch dressing | 115 | H | • | • | O | |
| creamy mexican dressing | 116 | H | • | • | • | O |
| dairy-free thousand island dressing | 118 | H | • | • | O | O |
| orange-infused dressing | 119 | H | • | • | • | • |
| onion-infused dressing | 120 | H | • | • | • | • |
| fat-burning herbes de florence dressing | 121 | H | • | • | • | • |
| bacon marmalade | 122 | H | • | • | • | |
| mole sauce | 123 | M | • | | • | |
| easy blender mayo | 124 | H | • | O | | • |
| egg-free keto mayo | 125 | H | • | • | | • |
| berbere mayo | 126 | H | • | • | O | |
| basil mayonnaise | 127 | H | • | • | O | |
| garlic and herb aioli | 128 | H | • | • | O | • |
| herbes de florence red sauce | 130 | M | • | • | • | |
| worcestershire sauce | 132 | M | • | • | • | |
| hot sauce | 134 | M | • | • | • | O |
| easy dairy-free hollandaise | 136 | H | • | • | | O |
| keto lemon mostarda | 138 | H | • | • | • | • |
| guacamole | 140 | M | • | • | • | • |
| garlic confit | 142 | H | • | • | • | • |
| keto chai | 146 | M | • | O | • | • |
| breakfast chili | 148 | H | • | • | O | |
| bacon and eggs ramen | 150 | H | • | • | O | |
| florentine breakfast burgers | 152 | H | • | • | | |
| creamiest keto scrambled eggs | 154 | H | • | • | | |
| steak and eggs | 156 | H | • | • | | |
| rosti with bacon, mushrooms, and green onions | 158 | M | • | • | | |
| kimchi eggs | 160 | H | • | • | | • |
| green eggs and ham | 162 | H | • | • | | |
| bacon and mushrooms with soft-boiled eggs | 164 | H | • | • | O | |
| eggs florentine with basil hollandaise | 166 | H | • | • | | • |
| eggs in a frame | 168 | H | • | • | | O |
| keto pockets | 170 | H | O | • | | |
| ham and egg cups | 172 | H | • | • | | |
| basil deviled eggs | 174 | H | • | • | | • |
| breakfast salad | 176 | H | • | • | | |
| dairy-free yogurt | 178 | H | | | • | |
| snickerdoodle waffles | 180 | H | • | • | | |
| chocolate waffles | 182 | H | • | • | | • |
| lemon curd dutch baby | 184 | H | • | O | | |

| Recipe | PAGE | KETO (L–M–H) | DAIRY | NUT | EGG | ANIMAL PRODUCTS |
|---|---|---|---|---|---|---|
| chocolate pudding | 186 | H | • | • | | • |
| keto english muffins | 188 | H | O | | | • |
| bone broth fat bombs | 192 | M | • | • | • | |
| paleo egg rolls | 194 | H | • | • | • | |
| scotch eggs | 196 | H | • | • | | |
| bacon cannoli | 198 | H | • | • | | |
| chicken tinga wings | 200 | H | • | • | • | |
| lemon pepper wings | 202 | H | • | • | • | |
| fried prosciutto-wrapped deviled eggs | 204 | H | • | • | • | |
| chicharrón | 206 | H | • | • | • | |
| italian marinated mushrooms | 208 | H | • | • | • | • |
| chicken liver pâté | 210 | H | • | • | • | |
| pickled herring | 212 | M | • | • | • | |
| braunschweiger | 214 | H | O | • | • | |
| oscar deviled eggs | 216 | H | • | • | • | |
| herbaceous salad | 220 | H | • | • | • | • |
| asian chicken salad | 222 | H | • | O | • | |
| keto "fruit" salad | 224 | H | • | • | • | • |
| warm spring salad | 226 | H | • | • | O | |
| 7-layer salad | 228 | H | • | • | O | |
| chopped salad | 230 | H | • | • | O | |
| mixed green salad | 232 | H | • | • | | |
| panzanella salad | 234 | H | • | • | O | O |
| simple crab salad | 236 | H | • | • | O | |
| chopped salad in jars | 238 | H | • | • | O | |
| cleansing ginger soup | 240 | H | • | • | • | |
| bone marrow chili con keto | 242 | H | • | • | • | |
| chilled creamy cucumber soup | 244 | M | O | • | • | O |
| creamy mushroom soup | 246 | M | • | • | | |
| hot-and-sour soup with pork meatballs | 248 | M | • | • | | |
| bok choy and mushrooms with ginger dressing | 250 | M | • | • | • | O |
| green curry panna cotta | 252 | H | • | O | • | • |
| wraps | 254 | H | • | • | | • |
| keto bread | 256 | H | • | • | | • |
| crispy chicken skin croutons | 258 | H | • | • | • | |
| crispy pork belly croutons | 260 | H | • | • | • | |
| zoodles | 262 | L | • | • | • | • |
| chiles rellenos | 266 | H | • | • | | |
| deconstructed spicy chicken stack | 268 | H | O | • | | |
| easy egg foo young | 270 | H | • | • | | |
| doro watt chicken salad wraps | 272 | H | • | • | O | |
| slow cooker ethiopian spicy chicken stew | 274 | H | • | • | O | |
| california club wraps | 276 | H | • | • | | |
| chicken oscar | 278 | H | • | • | | |
| chicken neapolitan | 280 | M | • | • | • | |
| lemon pepper chicken | 282 | H | • | • | • | |
| tom ka gai (thai coconut chicken) | 284 | H | • | • | • | |
| keto greek avgolemono | 286 | H | • | • | • | |
| stewed chicken and sausage | 288 | H | • | • | • | |
| simple slow cooker chicken thighs | 290 | M | • | • | • | |
| smothered bacon and mushroom burgers | 294 | H | • | • | O | |
| umami burgers | 296 | H | • | • | • | |

| Recipe | PAGE | KETO | DAIRY | NUT | EGG | ANIMAL PRODUCTS |
|---|---|---|---|---|---|---|
| sloppy joes | 298 | H | • | • | O | |
| reuben meatballs | 300 | H | • | • | | |
| spicy mexican meatballs | 302 | H | • | • | | |
| herbes de florence meatballs | 304 | H | • | • | | |
| slow cooker short rib and chorizo stew | 306 | H | • | • | • | |
| slow cooker ropa vieja | 308 | H | • | • | • | |
| chili-stuffed peppers | 310 | M | • | • | • | |
| slow cooker mole short ribs | 312 | H | • | • | • | |
| texas beef sausage | 314 | H | • | • | • | |
| deconstructed BLT filet mignons | 316 | H | • | • | • | |
| steak au poivre for two | 318 | H | • | • | • | |
| steak diane | 320 | H | • | • | • | |
| hunan beef–stuffed peppers | 322 | M | • | • | • | |
| slow cooker short rib tacos | 324 | H | • | • | • | |
| deconstructed egg rolls | 328 | M | • | • | • | |
| pizza meatballs in red gravy | 330 | H | • | • | | |
| sloppy ottos | 332 | H | • | • | O | |
| reuben pork chops | 334 | H | • | • | O | |
| slow cooker hot 'n' spicy country-style ribs | 336 | M | • | • | • | |
| chive panna cotta with bacon marmalade | 338 | H | • | O | • | |
| slow cooker pastrami-style pork ribs | 340 | H | • | • | • | |
| mexican-style chorizo sausage | 342 | H | • | • | • | |
| easy smoked ham hocks | 344 | M | • | • | • | |
| porchetta | 346 | H | • | • | • | |
| chorizo sausage and mushroom casserole | 348 | H | • | • | • | |
| slow cooker asian pulled pork lettuce cups | 350 | H | • | • | • | |
| greek meatballs | 352 | H | • | • | | |
| keto BLTs with soft-boiled eggs | 354 | H | • | • | O | |
| spicy tuna stacks | 358 | H | • | • | O | |
| peel-and-eat garlic shrimp | 360 | H | • | • | O | |
| hawaiian delight | 362 | H | • | • | O | |
| spicy grilled shrimp with mojo verde | 364 | H | • | • | • | |
| seafood sausage with leek confit | 366 | H | • | • | • | |
| lemon-thyme poached halibut | 368 | H | • | • | • | |
| fried catfish with cajun keto mustard | 370 | H | • | • | • | |
| grilled trout with hollandaise | 372 | H | • | • | | |
| tom ka plaa (thai coconut fish) | 374 | H | • | • | • | |
| spaghetti al tonno | 376 | L | • | • | • | |
| zoodles in clam sauce | 378 | H | • | • | • | |
| pasta puttanesca | 379 | L | • | • | • | |
| poached salmon with creamy dill sauce | 380 | H | • | • | O | |
| keto mocha latte panna cotta | 384 | H | | O | • | |
| chai ice lollies | 386 | H | • | O | • | • |
| bone broth ice pops | 388 | M | • | • | • | |
| no-bake grasshoppers in jars | 390 | H | • | • | • | |
| no-bake vanilla bean petits fours | 392 | H | • | O | • | |
| tom ka gai savory ice cream | 394 | H | • | • | • | |
| vanilla bean bread pudding | 396 | H | • | O | | • |
| chai fat bombs | 398 | H | • | • | | • |
| lava cakes with mocha ice cream | 400 | H | • | O | | • |
| lemon curd | 402 | H | • | • | | |
| hot fudge sauce | 403 | M | • | • | • | • |
| vanilla bean crème anglaise | 404 | H | • | O | | • |

# recipe index

## sauces, dressings, and spice mixes

106
homemade cashew milk

108
bone broth—beef, chicken, or fish

110
berbere spice mix

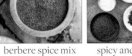
111
spicy and sweet hamburger seasoning

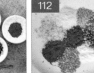
112
cajun seasoning

113
herbes de florence

114
ranch seasoning

115
dairy-free ranch dressing

116
creamy mexican dressing

118
dairy-free thousand island dressing

119
orange-infused dressing

120
onion-infused dressing

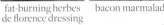
121
fat-burning herbes de florence dressing

122
bacon marmalade

123
mole sauce

124
easy blender mayo

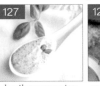
125
egg-free keto mayo

126
berbere mayo

127
basil mayonnaise

128
garlic and herb aioli

130
herbes de florence red sauce

132
worcestershire sauce

134
hot sauce

136
easy dairy-free hollandaise

138
keto lemon mostarda

140
guacamole

142
garlic confit

## break-your-fast meals

146
keto chai

148
breakfast chili

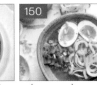
150
bacon and eggs ramen

152
florentine breakfast burgers

154
creamiest keto scrambled eggs

156
steak and eggs

158
rosti with bacon, mushrooms, and green onions

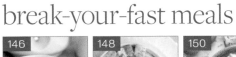
160
kimchi eggs

162
green eggs and ham

164
bacon and mushrooms with soft-boiled eggs

166
eggs florentine with basil hollandaise

168
eggs in a frame

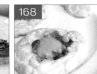
170
keto pockets

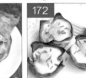

172
ham and egg cups

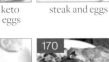

Maria Emmerich  417

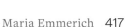
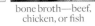
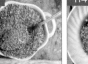

174

176

178

180

182

184

186

basil deviled eggs    breakfast salad    dairy-free yogurt    snickerdoodle waffles    chocolate waffles    lemon curd dutch baby    chocolate pudding

188

keto english muffins

# snacks and appetizers

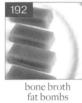
192

194

196

198

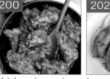
200

202

204

bone broth fat bombs    paleo egg rolls    scotch eggs    bacon cannoli    chicken tinga wings    lemon pepper wings    fried prosciutto-wrapped deviled eggs

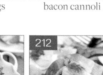
206

208

210

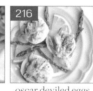
212

214

216

chicharrón    italian marinated mushrooms    chicken liver pâté    pickled herring    braunschweiger    oscar deviled eggs

# salads, soups, and sides

220

222

224

226

228

230

232

herbaceous salad    asian chicken salad    keto "fruit" salad    warm spring salad    7-layer salad    chopped salad    mixed green salad

234

236

238

240

242

244

246

panzanella salad    simple crab salad    chopped salad in jars    cleansing ginger soup    bone marrow chili con keto    chilled creamy cucumber soup    creamy mushroom soup

248
hot-and-sour soup
with pork meatballs

250
bok choy and
mushrooms with
ginger dressing

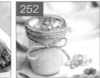
252
green curry
panna cotta

254
wraps

256
keto bread

258
crispy chicken skin
croutons

260
crispy pork belly
croutons

262
zoodles

# main dishes: chicken

266
chiles rellenos

268
deconstructed spicy
chicken stack

270
easy egg foo young

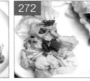
272
doro watt
chicken salad wraps

274
slow cooker
ethiopian spicy
chicken stew

276
california club
wraps

278
chicken oscar

280
chicken neapolitan

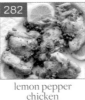
282
lemon pepper
chicken

284
tom ka gai (thai
coconut chicken)

286
keto greek
avgolemono

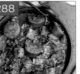
288
stewed chicken
and sausage

290
simple slow cooker
chicken thighs

# main dishes: beef

294
smothered bacon
and mushroom
burgers

296
umami burgers

298
sloppy joes

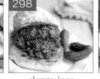
300
reuben meatballs

302
spicy mexican
meatballs

304
herbes de florence
meatballs

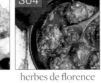

306
slow cooker short
rib and chorizo stew

308
slow cooker
ropa vieja

310
chili-stuffed
peppers

312
slow cooker
mole short ribs

314
texas beef sausage

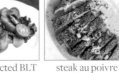

316
deconstructed BLT
filet mignons

318
steak au poivre
for two

320
steak diane

322
hunan beef–stuffed
peppers

324
slow cooker
short rib tacos

# main dishes: pork

328
deconstructed egg rolls

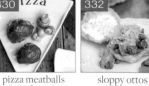
330
pizza meatballs in red gravy

332
sloppy ottos

334
reuben pork chops

336
slow cooker hot 'n' spicy country-style ribs

338
chive panna cotta with bacon marmalade

340
slow cooker pastrami-style pork ribs

342
mexican-style chorizo sausage

344
easy smoked ham hocks

346
porchetta

348
chorizo sausage and mushroom casserole

350
slow cooker asian pulled pork lettuce cups

352
greek meatballs

354
keto BLTs with soft-boiled eggs

# main dishes: fish and seafood

358
spicy tuna stacks

360
peel-and-eat garlic shrimp

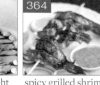
362
hawaiian delight

364
spicy grilled shrimp with mojo verde

366
seafood sausage with leek confit

368
lemon-thyme poached halibut

370
fried catfish with cajun keto mustard

372
grilled trout with hollandaise

374
tom ka plaa (thai coconut fish)

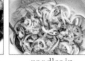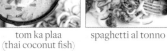
376
spaghetti al tonno

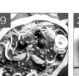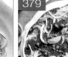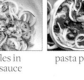
378
zoodles in clam sauce

379
pasta puttanesca

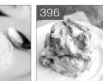
380
poached salmon with creamy dill sauce

# keto treats

384
keto mocha latte panna cotta

386
chai ice lollies

388
bone broth ice pops

390
no-bake grasshoppers in jars

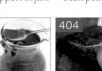
392
no-bake vanilla bean petits fours

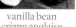
394
tom ka gai savory ice cream

396
vanilla bean bread pudding

398
chai fat bombs

400
lava cakes with mocha ice cream

402
lemon curd

403
hot fudge sauce

404
vanilla bean crème anglaise

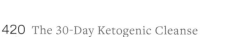

# general index

## A

A1c, increased, 17
acetoacetate, 29
acetone, 29
acid reflux, 23
acne, 23
adrenal fatigue, 57
advanced glycation end products
  (AGEs), 14, 79
afterburn effect, 39, 63
agave, 82
aging, trans fats and, 27
alcohol, 54-55, 60, 62
alcoholism, 17
allergies, 88
almond flour, 58
almond milk
  Chive Panna Cotta with Bacon
    Marmalade, 338-339
  Green Curry Panna Cotta, 252-253
  Lava Cakes with Mocha Ice Cream,
    400-401
  No-Bake Vanilla Bean Petits Fours,
    392-393
  Vanilla Bean Bread Pudding with
    Vanilla Bean Crème Anglaise,
    396-397
  Vanilla Bean Crème Anglaise,
    404-405
almond oil, 69
almonds
  about, 58
  Asian Chicken Salad, 222-223
Alzheimer's disease, 16, 17, 23
anchovies
  Pasta Puttanesca, 379
  Slow Cooker Ropa Vieja, 308-309
  Spaghetti al Tonno, 376-377
  Worcestershire Sauce, 132
antidepressants, 59
appetizers. See snacks and
  appetizers
artificial sweeteners, 82
arugula
  Breakfast Salad, 176-177
  Herbaceous Salad, 220-221
  Keto Pockets, 170-171
Asian Chicken Salad recipe, 222-223
asparagus
  Chicken Oscar, 278-279
  Oscar Deviled Eggs, 216-217
  Warm Spring Salad with Basil
    Chimichurri and Soft-Boiled Eggs,
    226-227
asthma, 23
athletes, ketosis in, 29
autism, 23
avocado oil, 69

avocados
  Breakfast Chili, 148-149
  Breakfast Salad, 176-177
  California Club Wraps, 276-277
  Chilled Creamy Cucumber Soup,
    244-245
  Chopped Salad, 230-231
  Creamy Mexican Dressing, 114
  freezing, 176
  Guacamole, 140-141
  Hawaiian Delight, 362-363
  for potassium, 31
  Spicy Tuna Stacks, 358-359
  storing, 140

## B

bacon
  Bacon and Eggs Ramen, 150-151
  Bacon and Mushrooms with
    Soft-Boiled Eggs, 164-165
  Bacon Cannoli, 198-199
  Bacon Marmalade, 122
  Bone Marrow Chili con Keto, 242-243
  Breakfast Chili, 148-149
  California Club Wraps, 276-277
  Chicken Liver Pâté, 210-211
  Chili-Stuffed Peppers, 310-311
  Chopped Salad in Jars, 238-239
  Copycat Baconnaise, 124
  Creamy Mushroom Soup, 246-247
  Deconstructed BLT Filet Mignons,
    316-317
  Eggs in a Frame, 168-169
  Keto BLTs with Soft-Boiled Eggs,
    354-355
  Keto Pockets, 170-171
  Mixed Green Salad with BLT Deviled
    Eggs and Bacon Vinaigrette,
    232-233
  Rosti with Bacon, Mushrooms, and
    Green Onions, 158-159
  7-Layer Salad, 228-229
  Slow Cooker Short Rib and Chorizo
    Stew, 306-307
  Smothered Bacon and Mushroom
    Burgers, 294-295
Bacon and Eggs Ramen recipe,
  150-151
Bacon and Mushrooms with
  Soft-Boiled Eggs recipe, 164-165
Bacon Cannoli recipe, 198-199
Bacon Marmalade recipe, 122
  Chive Panna Cotta with Bacon
    Marmalade, 338-339
  Deconstructed BLT Filet Mignons,
    316-317
bad fats, 71
Baked Scotch Eggs recipe, 196

baking products, 78
barefoot walking, 49
basil
  Basil Deviled Eggs, 174-175
  Basil Mayonnaise, 127
  Chicken Neapolitan, 280-281
  Easy Basil Hollandaise, 136
  Florentine Breakfast Burgers, 152-153
  Herbaceous Salad, 220-221
  Italian Marinated Mushrooms,
    208-209
  for potassium, 31
  Seafood Sausage with Leek Confit,
    366-367
  Warm Spring Salad with Basil
    Chimichurri and Soft-Boiled Eggs,
    226-227
Basil Chimichurri recipe, 226-227
Basil Deviled Eggs recipe, 174-175
Basil Mayonnaise recipe, 127
  Basil Deviled Eggs, 174-175
Bathing Scrub recipe, 411
beef
  about, 71, 72
  Bone Marrow Chili con Keto, 242-243
  Braunschweiger, 214-215
  Breakfast Chili, 148-149
  Chili-Stuffed Peppers, 310-311
  Deconstructed BLT Filet Mignons,
    316-317
  doneness of, 316
  Easy Egg Foo Young, 270-271
  Florentine Breakfast Burgers,
    152-153
  Herbes de Florence Meatballs,
    304-305
  Hunan Beef-Stuffed Peppers,
    322-323
  Reuben Meatballs, 300-301
  Sloppy Joes, 298-299
  Slow Cooker Mole Short Ribs,
    312-313
  Slow Cooker Ropa Vieja, 308-309
  Slow Cooker Short Rib and Chorizo
    Stew, 306-307
  Slow Cooker Short Rib Tacos,
    324-325
  Smothered Bacon and Mushroom
    Burgers, 294-295
  Spicy Mexican Meatballs, 302-303
  Steak and Eggs, 156-157
  Steak au Poivre for Two, 318-319
  Steak Diane, 320-321
  Texas Beef Sausage, 314-315
  Umami Burgers, 296-297
  using with pork, 302, 304
beef liver
  Braunschweiger, 214-215

# gratitude

I like to think of life like waves of the ocean: everyone has high points as well as low points. I have learned to accept the lows and to have gratitude for the high waves. The hardships in my life have pushed me to become the person I am today. I didn't let the hardships take me over; I struggled out of the cocoon and emerged a butterfly with strong wings. And for those struggles, I feel gratitude every day for many people in my life.

I am grateful to my love and best friend, Craig, who never complains, even though I often mess up the kitchen as soon as he cleans it. He has been a huge part of this book; he made the very detailed meal plan, added the nutritional information, and created the charts on my site, MariaMindBodyHealth.com, that supplement the material in this book.

I am grateful for my boys, Micah and Kai, who love to help me in the kitchen. Even though it takes twice as long to get dinner on the table when they help, it is totally worth it. When we had to put our adoption on hold, I was devastated, but I remember my mom telling me that my children just weren't born yet. I cry as I write this because she was totally right. These two boys were meant for me!

I am grateful for Jimmy Moore. Jimmy, when you first contacted me to do a podcast seven years ago, I was in celebrity shock. I have always admired your work and dedication. When you contacted me to write a cookbook with you, I was in awe that I was the one you chose. You have truly been a blessing, not only to me and my family, but to all dieters out there who have a trusted and respected pioneer like you.

I also need to express my gratitude to the whole Victory Belt team. I never thought I would have such amazing support and kindness from everyone at Victory Belt. Erich, your praise and fun outlook made this journey extraordinary and totally worth the hard work! I appreciate your caring phone calls just to check in on me and make sure everything was going smoothly. Holly, Erin, and Pam, you all are truly a huge part of making this book a piece of art. You all have such amazing ideas and attention to detail. I am forever grateful for all of you! Susan, I am grateful for your passion and for how magnificently you help to endorse my books! I get a smile on my face whenever I receive an email from you. Your happiness shines through!

Bill and Haley, I am honored to have your photo for the cover for this book. I've always been a big fan of your photos and cookbooks. My first Victory Belt cookbook was your *Gather* book. I was in love with your artistry from the beginning. Thank you for taking the time to make my recipes and shoot the cover.

Finally, I want to express my gratitude to you, the reader. I can't thank you enough for all your love and support throughout my journey!